5/03

Meramec Library
St. Louis Community College
11333 Big Bend Blvd.
Kirkwood, MO 63122-5799
314-984-7797

WITHDRAWN

Senior Centers

Opportunities for Successful Aging

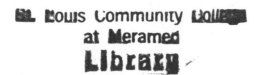
St. Louis Community College
at Meramec
Library

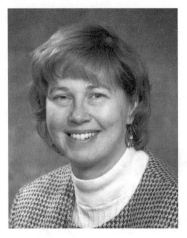

Beverly Ann Beisgen is the director of operations for development for the West Penn Allegheny Health System. She has been in health care philanthropy for 6 years. In 2001, Ms. Beisgen was awarded the professional designation of certified fund raising executive (CFRE) by the CFRE Certification Board. Prior to that, Ms. Beisgen worked in geriatrics for 19 years and was the assistant executive director of Vintage. She has her master's degree in business administration from the University of Pittsburgh and a bachelor's degree in human development/gerontology from The Pennsylvania State University.

Ms. Beisgen is the author of *Life Enhancing Activities for Mentally Impaired Elders,* published by Springer Publishing Company in 1989. She also authored the chapter "Activities to Challenge the Mind and Stimulate the Imagination" in *Activity Programming for Persons with Dementia: A Sourcebook,* published in 1995 by the Alzheimer's Association.

Ms. Beisgen has served on the board of directors of the Pennsylvania Association of Senior Centers and was a member of the Pennsylvania Department of Aging Statewide Taskforce on Senior Centers.

Ms. Beisgen is married to Henry Kacprzyk and has two children, Alex and Katie.

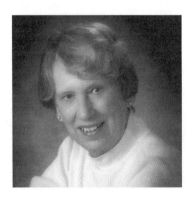

Marilyn Crouch Kraitchman has a B.S. in education. She has worked at Vintage for 15 years, where she is currently director of center services. A mother of two children and three stepchildren, she lives in Churchill, a suburb of Pittsburgh. Her hobbies are reading, traveling, and gardening.

St. Louis Community College
at Meramec
Library

Senior Centers

Opportunities for Successful Aging

Beverly A. Beisgen, MBA, CFRE

Marilyn Crouch Kraitchman

 Springer Publishing Company

Copyright © 2003 by Springer Publishing Company, Inc.

All rights reserved

No part of this publication may be reproduced, stored in a retrieval system, or transmitted in any form or by any means, electronic, mechanical, photocopying, recording, or otherwise, without the prior permission of Springer Publishing Company, Inc.

Springer Publishing Company, Inc.
536 Broadway
New York, NY 10012-3955

Acquisitions Editor: Helvi Gold
Production Editor: Janice Stangel
Cover design by Joanne E. Honigman

03 04 05 06 07 / 5 4 3 2 1

Library of Congress Cataloging-in-Publication Data

Beisgen, Beverly Ann
  Senior centers: opportunities for successful aging / Beverly A. Beisgen, Marilyn Crouch Kraitchman.
      p. cm.
   Includes bibliographical references and index.
   ISBN 0-8261-1704-X
   1. Day care centers for the aged—United States.   2. Aged—United States—Societies and clubs.   3. Aged—Services for—United States.   4. Aged—Recreation—United States.   I. Kraitchman, Marilyn Crouch.   II. Title.
   HV1455.2.U6 B45 2002
   362.6'3—dc21   2002066812
                                                                                  CIP

Printed in the United States of America by Maple-Vail.

Dedication

To Donna Holland, retired board member of Vintage, and Arlene Snyder, Vintage's first paid executive director—they led Vintage on a path to greatness with their vision and inspiration; to the Vintage staff, the unsung heroes who work so hard and with such dedication and enthusiasm; and to my family, for their support during the writing of this manuscript.

—Beverly Beisgen

To my family and to all the Vintagers.

—Marilyn Crouch Kraitchman

Contents

Foreword   *ix*

Preface   *xiii*

Acknowledgments   *xv*

PART ONE: INTRODUCTION

Chapter 1   Senior Centers and Successful Aging   3

PART TWO: DEMOGRAPHIC BACKGROUNDS

Chapter 2   A Profile of Older Adults   17

Chapter 3   Wants, Needs, and Interests of Older Adults 34

PART THREE: POSITIVE AGING EXPERIENCES

Chapter 4   Volunteerism   49

Chapter 5   Recreation   60

Chapter 6   Lifelong Learning   69

Chapter 7   Creativity   91

PART FOUR: ACTIVITIES

Chapter 8   The Arts and Aging   103

Chapter 9   Computers   139

Chapter 10   Health Promotion and Physical Fitness   153

Chapter 11   Horticulture   175

Chapter 12   Humanities   189

Chapter 13   Intergenerational Programs   198

Chapter 14   Travel   219

PART FIVE: MEETING SPECIAL NEEDS

Chapter 15   Information and Referral Programs   227

Chapter 16   Grandparenting Issues   242

Chapter 17   Developmental Disabilities   253

Chapter 18   Sensory Impairments   270

Chapter 19   Mental Health   290

Chapter 20   Caregiving   312

Chapter 21   Spirituality and Aging   335

PART SIX: CONCLUSION

Chapter 22   Creating a Culture of Philanthropy   351

Chapter 23   Looking Ahead   364

Afterword   371

Index   *373*

Foreword

I feel very privileged to have been asked to write the Foreword of a book exclusively devoted to senior centers, written by two veterans in the field. Their creativity and deeply rooted understanding of this community institution gives this book tremendous credibility and will be helpful to all who are working in the field or to those who want a better understanding of where the senior center fits in.

I can sum up the mission of senior centers in two words—aging positively. How that is accomplished varies from community to community, depending on the level of priority it is given by the community itself and the level of staff competency for which it is willing to pay. I often compare the development of senior community centers to the development of schools in this country. Just as we started with the one-room schoolhouse for our children, we started with the one-room senior center for our older adults. Both these institutions were established to provide needed services for groups as defined by chronological age.

Why were senior centers created? In a word, isolation! One social phenomena after World War II was that people were living longer and were retired from the work force with nothing to do and no place to go. In recent times, new waves of change have been added to the picture—children have become more mobile and have moved far away from their parents, and friends have moved out of the neighborhood. All these developments left a segment of the population with problems that rarely had been faced before. Many of our older adults were feeling unwanted, discarded, and were just waiting to die.

It is part of the healthy human condition to feel needed and productive and to value self-worth. The senior center was created to transition a relatively healthy, independent, older population out of their isolated state into a setting that enveloped them with security, companionship, activity, transportation, food, and advocacy. It is the one community institution that our independent elderly can identify as theirs.

In 1974, many senior centers were incorporated into the newly developing community-based aging network. Senior centers became the base service for this new network because of their easy accessibility to older people from all walks of life. Theirs are the friendly doors to the aging network.

Philosophically, it is a place people come to meet and greet rather than a place you go if you need help. The social service supports are accessible and after a level of trust is built between the center and a member, it is much easier for older persons to accept the help they need, when they need it, through their senior center. Problems are not generally the reason that people identify as why they come to a center.

Today, senior centers range in their development from the bingo, cards, and lunch brigade to complex programs that incorporate primary health care, computer labs, fitness centers, sophisticated arts programs, celebrations that commemorate both happy and sad moments, trips, Senior Environment Corps, and an array of volunteer opportunities. In fact, I define the senior center's possibilities as almost infinite. I see every interest group as a support group built on the strengths of people rather than on their weaknesses. The senior center becomes the important link to new friendships and to positive feelings about the purpose of living life as an older person. These are important keys to healthy living. With so many negative stereotypes of older people, feeling positive about oneself and one's capabilities is often harder to accomplish. For so many, accessing low-cost senior-center group services has been the answer, but it is no longer recognized by many for its value. It is the cheapest preventive medicine that can be bought for our older population, yet there is very little support for it. This is a very shortsighted view if a penny saved is a penny earned. Senior centers keep people out of hospitals and maintain their independence with appropriate low-cost supports.

In closing, I would like to suggest that one of the most effective ways a senior center would serve its community better is if all stakeholders would walk through a center and think about what it would have to be like for them to feel comfortable there. What would it have to look like? Where would it have to be located, and what should be offered?

What kind of staff would they want to have on site? Who would they want to be there? My staff and members of my board have used this process every time we take on a major project and it has enhanced the quality of what we produce enormously.

Rennie Cohen
Executive Director
Center in the Park
Philadelphia, PA

Preface

This book describes how to create a successful community center, recreational program, or environment for older adults based on our more than 20 years' experience working with older adults at Vintage Senior Community Center. The real-life vignettes featured in the book bring the text to life, providing the reader with a rare opportunity to see how older adults benefit from senior centers and how, in turn, the senior center benefits from their participation. The book provides a case for supporting senior centers and serves as a comprehensive guide to innovative programs and resources for older adults.

The ideas and insights developed through our experiences are relevant to professionals in the field of aging, including social workers, recreation therapists, nurses, gerontologists, educators, administrators, students, and interns. The suggestions for activities are applicable in a wide range of settings, including senior community centers, assisted-living facilities, adult day-living centers, residential facilities, and recreational programs.

Vintage, and the Vintagers, are the inspiration for this book. Identified as a need in the community because of the large aging population, Vintage was established in 1973 by local churches and the Junior League as Pittsburgh's first senior center. A dietitian and dedicated group of volunteers prepared sandwiches for lunch and offered socialization and recreation in the rented hall of the East End Christian Church. It was an immediate success. Later, when the Area Agency on Aging was established, Vintage received funding to operate as a senior center and community focal point, providing information and referral and congregate meals. Some of the early participants are still active today.

By 1976, the need for health services was apparent and a relationship that continues today was established with The Western Pennsylvania Hospital. A nurse practitioner was placed at Vintage to provide health screenings, health promotion, and educational programs. A counselor at the center worked closely with the nurse practitioner and the center's staff to address Vintager needs.

When Vintage outgrew its space in the church, it purchased a mansion in 1978 and relocated there following extensive renovations. A resale shop and adult day-care programs were added as well as an ever expanding curriculum of educational programs. Satellite senior center programs at a local high-rise and the YWCA were added but Vintage continued to focus on providing a comprehensive range of services at its main site.

When the center once again outgrew its space in 1994, the closed supermarket next door was purchased, renovated, and connected to the existing building. Following a successful $3 million capital campaign to build the new center and renovate the mansion, Vintage totaled 35,000 square feet. The office of the chief of geriatrics at West Penn Hospital was relocated to Vintage. Participants worked closely with the architect to design the space to suit their needs, including space for an art gallery, health center, a handicapped accessible stage, ceramic studio, card and game room, billiards room, adult day center, and classrooms with natural lighting for art classes. A café and atrium were added as an alternative to the congregate meal program.

Even the most carefully made plans require revising and by 1998, the craft shop was closed to accommodate the ever increasing demand for computer classes. Two years later, the center added a country store to sell staples, take-out foods, and gifts, as well as a beautiful new sitting room and space for programs to serve older adults with mental illness.

Vintage serves more than 2,500 older adults a year—an inner-city population that is primarily low-income, has an average age of 77, is 75% female, 60% Black, and 40% White. Vintage is well known nationally for its innovative programs and facilities.

Acknowledgments

We would like to thank Phyllis Abt, Michelle Bruno, Marilyn Fischer, Lois Folino, Earl McCabe, Heather Parker, and Cheryl Schell for their help in preparing this manuscript.

A special thank you is extended to the following people whose stories are featured in this book: Annette Balsamico, Albert Blumer, Mario Camerota, Mary Cerchiara, Millie Coles, George Cottam, Charles Davis, Paula Davis, Albert Goldsmith, Michael Graziano, Sidney Hills, Donna Holland, Dorothy Hollingsworth, Myrtle Hutchins, Ellouise Keen, Jerry Kraitchman, Edward Jones, Jay and Vicy Lewis, Margretta Lutz, Earl McCabe, Jr., Alban Mockenhaupt, Louise Murphy, "Smokey Joe" Preston, Jayne Rhodes, Felix Robinson, Jr., Ruth Rupp, Cheryl Schell, Shirley Steele, Harry White, and Bea Williams.

PART ONE

Introduction

CHAPTER ONE

Senior Centers and Successful Aging

AL

Every senior center needs an Al. I say this because Al has been a link with the men who play billiards and the rest of the center. Ninety-five percent of the men who play pool are involved in nothing else in the center. It was Al, along with staff, who started holding some events in the poolroom. He said the guys would never come upstairs for a holiday party or a wellness lecture. With his help, we learned that we needed to take the holiday luncheon to them, as well as a health lecture on prostate cancer.

Al came to Vintage about 20 years ago, recently retired from the retail business. To this day he has an eye for retailing. He will tell any staff person how to make the center's country store more attractive or how to better advertise an event. Vintage has been a social outlet for Al. He frequently arrives early enough for coffee with some of his friends in the Arbor Café and occasionally hangs around until after lunch. Although age has slowed him down, he still retains a great spirit and a true love for Vintage.

A number of years ago he and his wife attended our holiday parties. Boy, could they dance! They made a very attractive couple. Unfortunately, his wife began experiencing problems with dementia and Al turned to Vintage for help. Along with the physicians at The Western Pennsylvania Hospital, we were able to treat her illness and place her in our adult day care. When she passed away, Vintage was able to assist and support Al.

Not long ago I received a call from Al's sister-in-law. She lives out of town and had tried several times to reach him by phone. She became worried and thought perhaps we knew his whereabouts. After asking a couple of his friends in the café, I learned he had moved to another apartment in his building and his phone had been temporally disconnected. I was able to reach his sister-in-law and assure her that Al was tired from the move, but otherwise fine.

This story is a good example of how we have been able to provide many services to Al over the years, and how Al has given back to Vintage. He helped us provide needed services to the men in the poolroom. He is sensitive to their needs and though not a gossip has alerted us to possible problems in that area. Al has also been very generous financially to Vintage. His gifts have made it possible for Vintage to purchase items we could not have afforded otherwise. Most recently he paid for every Vintage member to have a name tag attached to a lanyard. This encouraged participants to become members and it also helped to learn the names of everyone. I have a feeling this was part of the "retail" in Al.

Al is a standard fixture at Vintage. It is good to know we can count on seeing him at Vintage every day.

BEA AND CHUCK

There is a great song verse in the musical 70 Girls 70 *that goes like this.*

Do we? Do we? That's what you want to know, isn't it?
Do we? Do we? That's what disturbs you so, isn't it?
You sit there wondering what are those two all about.
Do we? That's for us to know and you to find out.

Ask Bea and Chuck and they'll tell you love is alive and well at senior centers. They were both widowed when they met at Vintage. Actually Chuck saw Bea before they even met. A friend had invited Chuck to come to Vintage and when he walked past the trip office, a lovely lady caught his eye. That very day they were introduced as both were leaving the center after the line-dancing class. It didn't take Chuck long to make his first move. Family obligations required him to make a trip to New York, and while out of town he phoned Bea and asked her out for an upcoming New Year's Eve party. She agreed and their relationship soon blossomed.

When they met, Bea was already very active at Vintage, including serving as president of House Council, the advisory board. It wasn't long before Chuck was equally busy, volunteering his time and talents at the center. Currently they are both members of the Vintage Voices, a choral group directed by the music therapist, who perform both at Vintage and in the community. They continue to serve on House Council, but perhaps their major joint effort has been the summer picnic, which can easily draw well over 200 participants. Together they organize the food and games for everyone and motivate people to come out and have a good time. In addition to their formal commitments, they are both willing to assist whenever asked. As members of House Council they feel comfortable discussing possible problems with the staff, either as a couple or alone. Their contributions to Vintage have been immeasurable.

Recently I asked Bea and Chuck what Vintage meant to them. Bea spoke first saying, "Vintage was the place to lift me over my troubles when I lost my husband. Getting involved in activities and meeting new friends helped a lot." Chuck listened closely, nodding his head in agreement, and then he added, "Well after all, we met here!"

The National Institute of Senior Centers (NISC) of the National Council on the Aging (NCOA) describes a senior center as

a community focal point on aging where older adults come together for services and activities that reflect their experiences and skills, respond to their diverse needs and interests, enhance their dignity, support their independence and encourage involvement with the community. As part of a comprehensive community strategy to meet the needs of older adults, senior centers offer services and activities within the center and link participants with resources offered by other agencies. Center programs consist of a variety of individual and group services and activities. The center also serves as a resource for the entire community for information on aging, support for family caregivers, training professionals and lay leaders and students; and for development of innovative approaches to addressing aging issues.

NISC estimates that 10 million older adults are served each year by senior centers. The oldest senior center in the country is the William Hodson Senior Center in New York City, started in 1943.

According to the National Institute on Aging, there is no census of the number and types of senior centers in the United States. There are an estimated 12,000 to 16,000 senior centers, many funded entirely by local organizations and governments and others supported with funds raised by national charitable, voluntary, and religious organizations. More than 8,000 centers receive some funds that originate from the Older Americans Act and are allocated through state and area agencies on aging. In 1997, these centers provided services to almost 7 million people aged 60 and older.

The Older Americans Act, signed into law in 1965, has provided a wide range of community-based services, including congregate and home-delivered meals, adult day services, transportation, information and referral, advocacy assistance, telephone reassurance, and legal and employment services. Many of these services are based in senior centers, a setting that is familiar and accessible to older persons, their families, and the community. Consistent with the targeting requirements of the Older Americans Act, considerable emphasis has been placed on services to persons with the greatest social and economic need, including members of racial and ethnic minority groups. Among the Older Americans Act Title III service recipients, 21.8% were members of racial and ethnic minority groups. Nearly half of the minority clients were African American, more than one third were of Hispanic origin, 6% were American Indian or Alaskan Native, and approximately 10% were Asian American or Pacific Islander. Within this minority group cohort, nearly 60% were poor, with a poverty rate more than 2 1/2 times higher than the minority elderly population overall. Programs operating through the Older Americans Act provide vital support for those older persons who are at significant risk of losing their ability to remain independent in their own homes and communities.

The Older Americans Act requires area agencies on aging to designate focal points for comprehensive and coordinated service delivery to older persons. The majority of organizations designated as focal points are senior centers, and a majority of senior centers are focal points.

According to the Administration on Aging, a typical senior center/focal point may offer

- meal and nutrition programs
- information and assistance
- health, fitness, and wellness programs
- recreational opportunities
- transportation services
- arts programs
- volunteer opportunities
- educational opportunities
- employment assistance
- intergenerational programs
- social and community action opportunities
- other special services

However, senior centers vary considerably in terms of programs, services, facilities, staffing, and resources. Most senior centers are multipurpose, providing a range of activities and services and working with a large number of organizations to meet the needs of older adults in their community. In general, senior center participants draw from a fairly limited geographical area and a center's participants reflect the population of that area. As highly visible community focal points, they are part of, as well as a gateway to, the aging network and home, community, and social supports that enable older adults to maintain their health and independence.

❷ In 1998, the National Institute of Senior Centers of the National Council on the Aging launched a national effort to accredit senior centers. Accreditation of a senior center is a certification by official peer review of compliance with the national standards of senior center operation as adopted by the National Institute of Senior Centers of the National Council on the Aging. Accreditation positively portrays the senior center as a viable, fundable, and qualified provider of services within the community. The *Senior Center Self-Assessment and National Accreditation Manual* can be used as an internal evaluation instrument to define areas that need improvement, expansion, and new direction or it can serve as a part of the accreditation process.

Longevity and earlier exit from the work force has led to a growing number of persons who are spending extended years in retirement. Senior centers help bridge the gap that older adults experience between work and retirement, and they are poised to help retirees reach their goal of a vital and successful aging. The National Survey of Health and Supportive Services in the Aging Network conducted by the National Council on the Aging in 2001 has contributed to the growing body of evidence that community-based organizations, including senior centers, are empowering and assisting thousands of older people to achieve vital aging. The programs in the study appeared to be serving those older adults with the greatest needs—low income, over age 75, minorities, and rural residents.

❷ By 2010, the baby-boom generation will constitute more than two thirds of the population over 50 years of age.❷ Senior centers will also experience changing populations, including increasing numbers of immigrant and non-English speaking and minority older persons. Senior centers will be called upon to offer new ways to improve the health status of seniors, reduce health disparities, increase economic security, decrease caregiver stress, and increase the independence of older persons. As they have in the past, senior centers will have to adjust and refine their programs and services with new and improved methods and systems for addressing the needs of their ever changing constituency.

SUCCESSFUL AGING

Retirement deprives older people of a major source of social interaction and mental stimulation. For much of adult life, employment provides the opportunity to perform productive activities and participate in meaningful relationships. In retirement, older people must discover alternative sources of stimulation. Older adults who continue to work prefer a healthier balance between work and leisure. At the same time, older people today experience longer life and less illness, resulting in the emergence of a mentally fit, nondisabled older population with the potential for a prolonged active life. This is causing a shift in focus from medically prolonging life to ensuring that a prolonged life is worth living.

Although some elders lead productive lives in retirement, many do not. Erik Erikson's research led him to the conclusion that each successive stage of life involves assuming new, more mature challenges. During the eighth stage, old age, individuals evaluate their life and accomplishments. The key psychological achievement is wisdom, fueled by generativity, or the desire to give back. Erikson feels that this stage of life provides individuals with the opportunity to contribute back to society what they have learned. The older adult and society both benefit when this goal is achieved; failure can result in despair and a sense of meaninglessness.

In the book *Successful Aging*, John Rowe, MD, and Robert Kahn, PhD, describe successful aging as the ability to maintain three key behaviors or characteristics:

- low risk of disease and disease-related disability
- high mental and physical function
- active engagement with life (maintaining relationships and performing activities that are productive)

They defined productive behavior as any activity, paid or unpaid, that generates goods or services of economic value. Key features that promote productivity and predict strong mental function in old age are health and overall ability to function; regular physical activity; friendship and a strong social support system; and personal characteristics, including a better education and belief in one's ability to handle what life has to offer.

Another key research finding for promoting successful aging is the need to stay connected with other people. The John D. and Catherine

T. MacArthur Foundation assembled a group of scientists from different disciplines to form a research network to develop a new concept for gerontology that emphasizes the positive aspects of aging. The MacArthur Foundation study on aging has shown that the more older people participate in social relationships, the better their overall health. In fact, being part of a social network of friends and family is one of the most dependable predictors of health and longevity. Yet even as research has shown for years the value of promoting and developing social support programs, they are often overlooked.

A variety of social contacts and support were found to promote successful aging, including telephone contact, visits with family and friends, participation in religious groups, and attendance at meetings of organizations. Active participation and making a meaningful contribution have a greater impact on health than mere attendance.

Emotional support, including expressions of affection, love, esteem, and respect, is extremely important for successful aging. The life-giving effect of close social relations holds throughout the life course. In coping with stressful life events, people who have more support do better than those with less or none at all.

Another element in successful aging is a positive mental attitude. Leonard Giambra, PhD, research psychologist at the National Institute on Aging's Gerontology Center in Baltimore, found that it is the positive habits accumulated over a lifetime, including a positive mental outlook, that will help ensure successful aging.

Research has found that older people are just as happy and may be happier than younger people. In a 10-year, ongoing study of 1,800 older and younger adults, M. Powell Lawton, PhD, found that the prevalence of positive emotional states such as happiness, elation, contentment, and interest does not decrease with aging. Subjects who were 65 years and older were less anxious than the younger subjects. Older subjects managed the aging process by learning to avoid situations and people they found disturbing or draining.

A Stanford University study by Laura Carstensen, PhD, on people aged 70 and older found that those who age happily have formed emotional goals that bring satisfaction. Successful agers are those who focus on what is really important and meaningful to them.

Another component of successful aging appears to be continually challenging oneself. Creativity continues into old age and can contribute significantly to successful aging.

Older people with higher mental function are more likely to retain physical function. A major benefit of pursuing a physical exercise program is for its influence on memory. Physically active people are more likely to maintain sharp mental acuity. Active mental stimulation and keeping up relationships with friends and relatives helps to promote physical ability. Frequent emotional support is also associated with improved physical function in old age.

Researchers are proving that humans in their later years have far more physical and mental strength than imagined. They are showing that memory can be enhanced by personal strategies such as regular mental exercise. A team of Princeton University psychologists found that adults continue to grow new brain cells throughout life and that late-generated cells may allow older people to bolster their learning and memory capabilities or even prevent declines.

The mental decline most people experience is due to the atrophy of connections between nerve cells in the brain. Routine behaviors requiring little brainpower contribute to such atrophy. Daily life, especially in retirement, can be predictable and free from surprises. Older people need to experience the unexpected, participate in something that challenges and engages the mind, and use all of their senses daily.

Studies are finding that older people's expertise can compensate for cognitive losses, as expertise remains intact with age and in some cases increases. In addition, mental stimulation can enable the brain to maintain and even increase its capacity. Even if mental activity is lost through inactivity, it can be reclaimed through retraining.

Aging bodies need good food and exercise to flourish—and so does the brain. The brain needs positive training, education, and experience throughout the life span. According to science writer Ronald Kotulak, scientists now realize that the brain's plasticity means that new learning and relearning can take place at any age, thus older adults can still do much to keep mentally fit. Mental training in old age can boost intellectual power, help maintain mental functions such as problem solving, and reverse memory decline. The old adage "Use it or lose it" is proving to be true.

The Seattle Longitudinal Study of the intellectual abilities of aging people involved more than 5,000 people. The study found that intellectual decline varies widely, mainly depending on how much stimulation the brain receives. Seven factors were identified regarding elders who maintain their mental acuteness: a high standard of living marked by above-average education and income; lack of chronic diseases; active engagement in reading, travel, cultural events, educational clubs, and professional associations; willingness to change; having a smart spouse;

an ability to grasp new ideas quickly; and satisfaction with accomplishments.

Marilyn Albert, a Harvard University neurologist and director of gerontology research at Massachusetts General Hospital, studied more than 1,000 people ages 70 to 80. She found that both physical and mental factors seem to determine which elders hold on to their intellects. Key elements revealed in the study were education, which appears to increase the number and strength of synaptic connections; strenuous activity, which improves blood flow to the brain; lung function, which ensures that the blood is adequately oxygenated; and the feeling that what people do makes a difference in their lives.

Many of the factors that contribute to successful aging can be found at the senior center, which provides opportunities to

- participate in disease prevention and health promotion activities
- maintain and develop social relationships and a strong social support system
- perform productive activities
- experience satisfaction from accomplishments
- develop emotional supports
- actively engage in meaningful activities
- participate in travel, cultural and educational programs, and mentally stimulating activities
- develop and maintain a positive mental attitude
- focus on what is really important and meaningful
- learn new skills and information
- be challenged
- be creative

BIBLIOGRAPHY

Erikson, E. (1997). *The life cycle completed.* New York: Norton.

Kotulak, R. (1997). *Inside the brain: Revolutionary discoveries of how the mind works.* Kansas City, MO: Andrews McMeel.

Krout, J. (1989). *Senior centers in America: A brief overview.* Fredonia: State University of New York, College at Fredonia.

Margoshes, P. (1995). For many, old age is the prime of life. *APA Monitor, 26*(5), 36–37.

National Council on the Aging. (2001). *National Institute of Senior Centers.* Washington, DC: Author.

National Council on the Aging. (2001). *A National Survey of Health and Supportive Services in the Aging Network.* Washington, DC: Author. [On-line]. Available: www.ncoa.org/research/cbo.html

Rowe, J. W., & Kahn, R. L. (1998). *Successful aging.* New York: Dell.

Thompson, A. (2000). *Inside the brain: New research prescribes mental exercise.* American Society on Aging. [On-line]. Available: www.asaging.org/at/at-204/thompson.htm

U.S. Department of Health and Human Services, Administration on Aging. (2001). *Factsheets: Senior centers.* Washington, DC: Author. [On-line]. Available: www.aoa.gov/factsheets/seniorcenters.html

U.S. Department of Health and Human Services, Administration on Aging. (2001). *Minority participation in older Americans act programs—profile of older Americans 2000.* Washington, DC: Author.

U.S. Department of Health and Human Services, Administration on Aging. (2001). *Notes: Senior centers.* Washington, DC: Author. [On-line]. Available: www.aoa.gov/NAIC/Notes/seniorcenters.html

Volz, J. (2000, January). Successful Aging: The Second 50. *APA Monitor, 31,* 1. [On-line]. Available: www.apa.org/monitor/jan00/

RESOURCES

Administration on Aging (AoA)
U.S. Department of Health and Human Services
Washington, DC 20201
202-619-0724
http://www.aoa.gov
The Older Americans Act of 1965 established the Administration on Aging, an agency of the U.S. Department of Health and Human Services.

National Council on the Aging, Inc. (NCOA)
National Institute of Senior Centers
409 Third Street SW, Suite 200
Washington, DC
202-479-6688
http://www.ncoa.org/
The National Council on the Aging works to promote the dignity, self-determination and well-being of older persons through a wide variety of services and programs. The National Institute of Senior Centers is a network of professionals who represent the senior center field.

National Association of Area Agencies on Aging (N4A)
1112-16th Street NW, Suite 100
Washington, DC 20036
202-296-8130 (nationwide AAA listings)
800-677-1116 (national Eldercare locator)
http://www.n4a.org/
The National Association of Area Agencies on Aging is the umbrella
organization for the 655 area agencies on aging (AAAs) and more than
230 Title VI Native American aging programs in the U.S. N4A advocates
on behalf of the local aging agencies to ensure that needed resources
and support services are available to older Americans.

Vintage
401 N. Highland Avenue
Pittsburgh, PA 15206
412-361-5003
http://www.vintageseniorservices.org
Vintage is a private, nonprofit human service agency founded in 1973
to meet the needs of elderly residents in Allegheny County. Programs
include the Vintage senior center, adult day services and wellness
programs.

PART TWO

Demographic Backgrounds

CHAPTER TWO

A Profile of Older Adults

HELEN

I was leaving the agency one afternoon when I saw Helen cutting through the parking lot. "It must be Tuesday," I thought, and it certainly must be after 2:00, because one could almost set one's watch by Helen's comings and goings over the past 20 years. We can always count on Helen to come to Vintage on Tuesdays and Fridays, first for lunch and then for the Vintage Drama Group.

As I watched Helen on this particular fall day, I noticed her flowered polyester dress hanging 3 inches below her green all-weather coat, left open as the summer breeze made its final bow. During the summer, the coat is replaced by a lightweight sweater and a wide-brim straw hat to shield her eyes from the sun. She always wears a smile. During all four seasons her footwear remains the same, a sturdy pair of sneakers. In her hand she carries a blue plastic bag from a local grocery store. Actually, there are probably two or three bags, one inside the other to ensure that her belongings will remain safe should one of the bags break. The contents would reveal a script from the group's latest play, Vintage newsletters, and, tucked in napkins or small plastic bags, part of her or her neighbor's lunch saved from the noon meal at the center.

The congregate meal program is provided by the Allegheny County Area Agency on Aging. It has always been the policy of the county that with the exception of bread, milk, and fruit, all food must be consumed in the dining room. This "policy" is not understood by Helen or her friends, as a lifetime of thrift brought on by a depression and a world war have taught them to waste nothing. Chicken was on the menu this particular day, so my guess is that at least one chicken leg and some mixed vegetables are packed away someplace in Helen's bag.

The drama group has always been important to Helen and indeed this seems a paradox: Until she gets on stage, Helen is often shy and quiet.

Another volunteer writes, directs, and is often the lead actor in the play—an amateur performance, but one that serves Helen well. The drama group has provided more than just an outlet for Helen's creativity; its members have become her second family.

Helen was widowed 2 years ago and is the mother of two adult children. Occasionally, the three of them are seen walking home after a party at Vintage, each with a handful of helium-filled balloons that had been used as decorations.

Helen celebrated her mother's 100th birthday at the center with the staff and her friends from the drama group. Helen is typical of the original members of Vintage; her needs are easily met by the center. Helen is happy to enjoy a lunch with her friends and take part in a drama performance. She is always ready with a friendly hello, appreciates what Vintage has done for her, and is more than willing to volunteer.

JAYNE

It's shortly after 9:00 a.m. as Jayne pulls her late-model car into the Vintage parking lot. She's dressed in an attractive running outfit and her hair is well coiffed as she hurriedly enters the building to assume her volunteer job in the Arbor Café.

Recently retired from a local bank, Jayne was first recruited to act as a mentor in the computer studio. Twice a week over a period of 2 years, Jayne has helped other seniors navigate everything from word-processing to the Internet. She is not interested in teaching the class, but is more than willing to assist on a one-to-one basis. Jayne was also agreeable to volunteering in the Arbor Café one morning a week or more, if needed. She sells items ranging from bagels to juice. Many Vintage members come to this eatery for breakfast, while others enjoy a second cup of coffee with friends. Making change and simultaneously toasting a bagel is no problem for Jayne as it is for some of our older participants. Jayne has simply transferred her skills from her professional life, whether it is computer knowledge or customer relations, to Vintage, and we are happy to be the recipient of such talent. Participants also recognized her abilities and she was nominated and elected to the advisory board where she has become involved on several committees.

Jayne has met new friends at Vintage. In addition to her volunteer duties, she enjoys the weekly bowling outings as well as trips to local museums and restaurants. Asked recently what brought her to Vintage, she responded, "I wanted to help others." Asked why she stays, she replied,

"I love it here. I like the people and the staff, and I find the volunteering that I do to be very rewarding."

ANNETTE

The name "godmother" fits Annette perfectly. She rules her domain with ease. For as long as any of us can remember, Annette has led the Friday super bingo, the Pittsburgh history class, the Columbus Day celebration, the Italian holiday display, plus numerous smaller projects. A lifelong resident of East Liberty, she has a tremendous sense of pride in her Pittsburgh community. Once a vital shopping and theater district, now the area is almost beyond recognition. That is unless you ask Annette. How many participants have an entire wall in a classroom for a permanent display? The answer would be one: Annette. The wall is covered with photographs and copies of pictures depicting East Liberty as she remembers it. Any guest to her domain receives a ten-minute history lesson. With any encouragement, a file drawer reveals numerous scrapbooks and a detailed lesson. Annette has not accomplished this feat alone. Depending on the project, she recruits the "soldiers" necessary to get the job done. Tony assisted with all the photography; Olympia and Felix helped during the Columbus Day celebration by making hundreds of pasta shells; numerous family members and friends have made thousands of cookies for various events over the years. Annette is the first to admit that she is the general when it comes to her soldiers, and like any good soldiers, they all follow orders as expected. Over the years she has lost some of her more faithful helpers, but she carries on, recruiting new people to her cause.

Vintage has seen a handful of volunteers like Annette over the years. Because of their desire to get tasks accomplished, they will often wield a lot of power, and sometimes that power will extend beyond the project. Participants like Annette are the type of leader every agency needs. She is dedicated to her church, her family, her community, and to Vintage. I have often asked Annette to pull together a group of participants for a guest speaker or a small program. I can always be sure that at the appointed date and at the appointed time, the job will have been done perfectly by Annette and, of course, her soldiers.

SMOKEY JOE

Getting to know the people who come to Vintage and learning the lifetime of experiences they bring with them is probably the best part of our job. This was especially true with Joe.

Occasionally Joe would show up in the billiards room for a couple games of pool or perhaps join his friends at the annual men's group picnic, but the one time we knew for sure that we would see Joe was in February for Black History Month.

Early in the history of Vintage, the African American Committee was formed to highlight and celebrate the history of our Black members. Joe immediately volunteered to co-chair this committee. He was very proud of his heritage. The group was active in several programs from the Martin Luther King celebration to the June garden party. Joe faithfully attended all the meetings, sometimes as the only man there.

In February, Joe's attendance increased as preparations for the Black-History event got underway. For years, Vintage has had speakers, performers, and Joe's display of Black-history memorabilia, including a wonderful collection of books, posters, pictures, and smaller items gathered over a lifetime. The display was always worthwhile, but it was Joe's presentation and presence that made it so meaningful. Even as his health began to fail, Joe was at his table dressed in a handsome suit, ready to share with others his pride in his heritage. Before and after the formal program, Joe was only too happy to tell you detailed stories about Black celebrities, from Jesse Owens to Marian Anderson. Martin Luther King, Jr. was a favorite of Joe's, and he could tell you little-known facts about this famous American.

In the mid-1990s, Vintage hosted a program on the Negro Baseball Leagues. Several of the men attended, including Joe. The speaker focused on the Homestead Grays and the Pittsburgh Crawfords, both local teams. At the conclusion of the program, Joe revealed that as a young man he had played for the Negro Leagues and was known as Smokey Joe. He spoke quietly of the discrimination he felt as a man and as a baseball player, as he was denied entrance into restrooms and hotels. To hear him tell of his life during this period is something that many of us will never forget. Smokey Joe lost his battle with heart disease this past year, but for all of us who knew this quiet, dignified man, we felt we knew a piece of history, and we certainly had a better understanding of why Reverend King was his hero.

It is important to understand characteristics that make up the older adult population. Only by understanding who they are can senior centers serve them effectively.

In 2000, the size of the older population (persons aged 65 and older) was 34.9 million, representing 12.7% of the population in the United States. There were 4.2 million Americans aged 85 years and older, representing about 1.5% of the population. Another 24 million persons were aged 55 to 64. The 65-plus population is projected to double over the next three decades to nearly 70 million, or 20% of the population; the population of those 55 to 64 will grow to 37 million.

There were 20.4 million older women and 14.5 million older men, a ratio of 141 women for every 100 men. The gender ratio increases with age to a high of 237 women for every 100 men among persons 85 and over. Women represent 58% of the population aged 65 and older, and 70% of the population aged 85 and older.

Since 1900, the percentage of Americans who are 65-plus has more than tripled. In addition, the older population itself is getting older. In 1999, the age group of 65 to 74 (18.2 million) was 8 times larger than in 1900, but the 75 to 84 group (12.1 million) was 16 times larger and the 85 and older group (4.3 million) 34 times larger.

The older population will continue to grow significantly in the future. This growth slowed somewhat during the 1990s because of the relatively small number of babies born during the Great Depression of the 1930s. But the older population will burgeon between the years 2010 and 2030 when the baby-boom generation reaches age 65. This growth will affect every aspect of our society and has important implications for the services provided by aging organizations, including senior centers.

The population aged 85 and older is currently the fastest growing segment of the older population. By 2050, this age group is projected to increase to almost 5% of the U.S. population. The size of this group has important implications for the future as they tend to be in poorer health and require more services than the younger-old. The number of centenarians is projected to grow quickly as well, from about 68,000 people aged 100 or older in 2000 to over 1 million by 2050.

Half of all adults 65 years and older live in the suburbs, 27% live in central cities, and 23% live in nonmetropolitan areas. According to the National Academy of Aging, those aging in place in suburban and rural environments will face problems living in areas where housing is designed for single-family living and the distance to services, amenities, and family may be relatively significant. As this population grows frail, they may experience growing problems with social isolation and inadequate access to necessary supports and services.

In 1999, 4 million Americans who were 65 years of age and older were in the labor force, were working, or were actively seeking work.

RACIAL AND ETHNIC POPULATION

Racially, today's older people are the most homogenous of all Americans: 89% are White, 8.3% are Black, 5.2% are Hispanic, 2.3% are of

Asian origin, and .5% are American Indian, Eskimo, and Aleut. In 2000, more than 3 million U.S. residents aged 65 and older were foreign-born. As the older population grows larger, it will also grow more diverse, reflecting the demographic changes in the U.S. population as a whole over the past century. Over the next 50 years, programs and services for the older population will require greater flexibility to meet the demands of a diverse and changing population.

Minority populations are projected to represent 25% of the older population in 2030, up from 16% in 1999. Between 1999 and 2030, the White population of 65 and over is projected to increase by 81% compared with 219% for older minorities, including Hispanics (328%), Black (131%), American Indians, Eskimos, and Aleuts (147%), and Asians and Pacific Islanders (285%). Although the older population will increase among all racial and ethnic groups, the Hispanic older population is projected to grow the fastest, from about 2 million in 2000 to more than 7 million by 2030.

MARITAL STATUS

Marital status can strongly affect a person's emotional and economic well-being by influencing living arrangements and availability of caregivers among older Americans with an illness or disability. Among people aged 65 and older, more than 55% were married and living with a spouse in 2000.

Because women as a group outlive men, men aged 65 to 84 are more likely to be married (75% in 1998) compared to older women (45%). Almost half of all older women in 1999 were widows, outnumbering widowers four to one. Among people aged 85 or older, about 53% of men are married, compared with only 12% of women. Older women are more likely to be widowed than are older men due to a combination of factors, including gender differences in life expectancy, the tendency of women to marry men who are slightly older, and higher remarriage rates for older widowed men than for widowed women.

About 8% of all older persons are divorced or separated. Their numbers (2.2 million) have increased significantly since 1990, when approximately 1.5 million of the older population were divorced or separated.

LIVING ARRANGEMENTS

Most people aged 65 and older live with family members; about two out of three live with spouses or other family members (80% of men and 58% of women). However, the proportion living in a family setting decreases with age so that only 45% of those 85 and older live in family setting.

In 1998 about 31% of all noninstitutionalized older persons lived alone. Older women are more likely to live alone than are older men. Older women were as likely to live with a spouse as they were to live alone, about 41% each. Eighty percent of older men lived with their spouses or other relatives, 3% lived with nonrelatives, and 17% lived alone.

Living alone correlates with advanced age. Older White and Black women are also more likely to live alone compared with older Hispanic, Asian, and Pacific Islander women.

INCOME

Adequate income and assets are of critical importance to virtually all dimensions of well-being in old age. Poverty is associated with poor nutrition, health status and self-care, and diminished access to health care and social service.

The median income of older persons in 1999 was $22,812, compared to a median of $40,816 for all households. In 1995 the median net worth for householders 65 and over was $92,399 compared to $40,200 for all householders. Thirty four percent of older persons reported incomes of less than $10,000; only 23% reported incomes of $25,000 or more.

Retirement income is influenced by employment and earnings history—Social Security benefits, pensions, employer-provided health benefits, and the employee's ability to save. According to the Social Security Administration, the major sources of income for older persons in 1998 were Social Security (reported by 90% of older persons), income from assets (62%), public and private pensions (44%), and earnings (21%).

According to a 1998 AARP study, the income trajectories of baby boomers indicate improved economic circumstances relative to age cohorts born 20 years earlier. Mean family income of baby boomer women is more than 50% higher than that of women born in the 1920s and 1930s. However, this improvement in family income largely reflects increased labor force participation by married women and declining family sizes, rather than improvement in wages. It has not been determined if boomer retirement income will be adequate relative to their preretirement income.

POVERTY

The poverty rate in 1999 for people 65 and over was 9.7%, or about 3.2 million individuals (11.8% of women and 6.9% of men were poor). Another 2 million, or 6.1% of older persons were classified as near-poor (income between the poverty level and 125% of this level). Among the older population, poverty rates were higher among women, the nonmarried, and minorities compared with non-Hispanic White persons. Divorced Black women aged 65 to 74 have one of the highest poverty rates for any subgroup of older Americans.

Older persons living alone or with nonrelatives were much more likely to be poor (20.2%) than were older persons living with families (5.2%). The highest poverty rates (58.8%) were experienced by older Hispanic women who lived alone.

Only 8.3% of elderly Whites were poor in 1999, compared to 22.7% of elderly Blacks and 20.4% of elderly Hispanics. Higher than average poverty rates for older persons correlated with living in central cities, rural areas, and the South. The poverty rate is also higher at older ages. Poverty rates are lower for baby-boomer households than for earlier generations.

There is a large disparity in net worth between Black and White households headed by older Americans. The median net worth among older Black households was estimated to be about $13,000, compared with $181,000 among older White households. Older members of various ethnic and racial groups will be at particular risk because of the vulnerability of old age and a life course of relative poverty and discrimination. A disproportionate number are likely to enter advanced age with few assets and limited ability to provide for their needs. Minorities are more likely to be employed in lower-wage jobs not covered by pensions and are more likely not to own their homes. The need for sensitivity in service provision to ethnically and racially diverse subgroups of older persons will be greatly magnified in the future. Diversity poses unique challenges to senior centers and other aging service providers.

EDUCATION

Educational attainment influences socioeconomic status and thus can play a role in well-being at older ages. Higher levels of education are usually associated with higher incomes, higher standards of living, and above-average health status. In 1999, 75,000 people aged 65 and older were enrolled in college.

The educational level of the older population is increasing. Between 1950 and 1999, the percentage who had completed high school rose from 18% to 68%. About 15% of the older population in 1999 had a bachelor's degree or higher. Income differences between college graduates versus those who did not finish high school were substantially greater among boomers than earlier generations, indicating a larger educational premium for boomers than for earlier generations.

Despite the overall increase in educational attainment among older Americans, there are still substantial educational differences among racial and ethnic groups. In 1999, about 73% of Whites, 68% of Asians and Pacific Islanders, 45% of Blacks, and 32% of Hispanics completed high school.

HEALTH AND DISABILITY

Seventy-two percent of older adults who responded to a 1996 National Health Interview Survey reported their health as good, very good, or excellent. Women and men reported comparable levels of health status. However, positive health evaluations decline with age. Also, among older men and women in every age group, minority older persons were less likely to report good health than their White counterparts. Asking people to rate their own health provides an indicator of health and well-being. Good to excellent self-reported health correlates with lower risk of mortality.

Functioning in later years may be diminished if illness, chronic disease, or injury limits physical and mental abilities and has important implications for the well-being of the older population. Limitations on activities because of chronic conditions increase with age. Among those 65 to 74 years old, 30% reported a limitation caused by a chronic condition. In contrast, over half of those 75 years and over reported they were limited by chronic conditions.

More than half of the older population (52.5%) reported having at least one disability. One third had at least one severe disability. The percentages with disabilities increase sharply with age, and disability takes a much heavier toll on the very old. Almost three fourths of those 80 and older report at least one disability. The percentage of that age group having difficulty with their activities of daily living (bathing, dressing, eating, preparing meals, shopping, managing money, and taking medication) is double that of the 65 and older population in total.

Most older persons have at least one chronic condition and many have multiple conditions. The most frequently occurring conditions are arthritis, hypertension, hearing impairments, heart disease, cataracts, orthopedic impairments, sinusitis, and diabetes. Five of the six leading causes of death among older Americans are chronic diseases. The prevalence of chronic conditions also varies by race and ethnicity in the older population. Non-Hispanic Black persons were also more likely to report having diabetes, stroke, and hypertension than either non-Hispanic White persons or Hispanic persons.

LIFE EXPECTANCY

Americans are living longer than ever. In 1900, life expectancy at birth was about 49 years. By 1960, it had increased to 70 years, and in 2000, life expectancy at birth was 77 years. The major part of this increase occurred because of reduced death rates for children and young adults.

Life expectancies at ages 65 and 85 have also increased. People who survive to age 65 can expect to live an average of nearly 18 more years, more than 5 years longer than persons who were 65 in 1900. The life expectancy of persons who survive to age 85 today is about 7 years for women and 6 years for men. Life expectancy does vary by race, but the difference decreases with age. In 1997, life expectancy at birth was 6 years higher for White persons than for Black persons. At age 65, White persons can expect to live an average of 2 years longer than Black persons do.

The leading cause of death among persons age 65 or older is heart disease, followed by cancer and stroke. Death rates were higher for older men than for older women at every age except the very oldest, persons aged 95 or older, for whom men's and women's rates were nearly equal.

According to the Federal Interagency Forum on Aging, certain causes of death vary according to sex and race and ethnic origin. For example, diabetes was the third leading cause of death among older American Indian and Alaska Natives, fourth among older Hispanics, and sixth among older Whites and older Asian and Pacific Islander men.

Educational attainment is also associated with higher life expectancy. The life expectancy of high school graduates at age 65 is approximately

1 year longer than the life expectancy at that age for persons who did not graduate from high school.

SEXUAL ORIENTATION

Experts estimate that between 1.75 million and 3.5 million Americans aged 60 and over are lesbian, gay male, bisexual, or transgender. Their numbers should increase as the older population grows in the next 30 years. Existing research suggests that older lesbian, gay, bisexual, and transgender adults' concerns about aging are often the same that other older people typically report.

Older lesbian, gay, bisexual, and transgender persons may face discrimination based on their age and sexual orientation. Consequently, they may not feel comfortable either in organizations serving older people or in lesbian, gay male, bisexual, and transgender community organizations, and thus may not receive services from these groups. Years of experience dealing with discrimination based on their sexual orientation does appear to help them cope with age discrimination. Research also suggests that this resilience may depend on the older person's integration into the older lesbian, gay male, bisexual, and transgender communities, which varies widely. Older lesbian, gay male, bisexual, and transgender people differ in the extent to which they have revealed their sexual orientation to family, friends, and health care and social service providers. Moreover, there are generational differences that are based largely on society's changing attitudes toward diverse sexual orientations.

Most studies indicate that older lesbian, gay male, bisexual, and transgender people report high levels of satisfaction with their social support networks. Some have less support from families than other older people, possibly as a result of the tensions families experience when they reveal their sexual orientation. Many rely primarily on partners and close friends for social support. Older persons who are gay or lesbian are more likely to live alone than are older people overall.

Older lesbian, gay male, bisexual, and transgender persons express concerns about access to high-quality health care. Some are reluctant to reveal their sexual orientation to health care providers because of fears of discrimination or concerns about confidentiality. Some research indicates that lesbians are more likely than heterosexual women to smoke, be overweight, or abuse alcohol, and lower lifetime rates of pregnancy may also affect long-term health. The major health concern associated with gay men continues to be HIV/AIDS. The number of older people of all sexual orientations with HIV/AIDS may increase in the future, in part because people with the disease are living longer as a result of improved treatment.

GENERATIONAL DIFFERENCES

People born around the same time, a cohort, will share many values and attitudes about life, which were acquired because they share a series of common life experiences formed in youth and young adulthood. Each cohort exhibits preferences particular to the influences that shaped their formative years. These differences affect the interests, needs and behaviors of the participants of senior centers and consequently are important to understand.

In the early years of senior centers, the GI generation dominated and influenced the activities and services provided. By the early 1990s, with a growing influx of the younger elderly and a decline in the numbers and vitality of the older participants, centers were scrambling for ideas to maintain and increase participation while serving the needs of both groups. Understanding the generational differences helped senior centers design programs and market to their target audiences. Preparing for the participation of baby boomers will require the same kind of understanding.

William Strauss and Neil Howe provide an in-depth look at these differences in *Generations, The History of American's Future, 1584–2069*. A few of their observations are described below.

THE GI GENERATION

Strauss and Howe defined the GI generation as those born between 1901 and 1924. The GI's history included the Great Depression and World War II. Their members include seven U.S. presidents, Walt Disney, Charles Lindbergh, John Wayne, Billy Graham, Joe Dimaggio, and Walter Cronkite.

Strauss and Howe described the GI generation as civic-minded, a generation of achievers, organizers, and problem solvers, with a powerful work ethic and a sense of duty. They achieved the largest single generation jump in education—their average length of schooling increased from the 9th grade level to 12th. As senior citizens, and throughout their life, the federal government directed its attention to their benefit, creating the first White House Conference on Aging, the first federal age-discrimination law, and the National Institute on Aging. They have a high degree of confidence in government and other traditional authority figures such as unions, doctors, church leaders, and politicians. They have been active volunteers at senior centers, spending entire days and weeks volunteering in the kitchens, classrooms, and wherever needed.

THE SILENT GENERATION

Strauss and Howe described the *silent generation* as a product of a birthrate trough, with fewer members than either the GIs who preceded them or the baby boomers who followed. Born between 1925 and 1945, their history included the Korean War and the cold war. Their achievements include civil rights, sexual liberation, and mainstreaming for those who are handicapped. Their members include Martin Luther King, Jr., James Dean, Ralph Nader, Gloria Steinem, Elvis Presley, Bob Dylan, Abbie Hoffman, and no U.S. Presidents.

The silent generation experienced a lifetime of steadily rising affluence. They married earlier than any previous generation in American history but they also experienced the largest age-bracket jump in the divorce rate. An amazing 94% of the 1931–1935 female cohort became mothers, the most fertile of the twentieth century.

The silents produced many of the nation's prominent feminists and major figures in the Civil Rights movement. Silent professionals also accounted for the surge in the helping professions and public-interest advocacy groups. Their nostalgia for youth has fueled a booming market in dietary aides, health and fitness activities, plastic surgery, hair replacements, and relaxation therapies. They enjoy social activities that bring them in contact with youth and adventure. They want to be actively engaged and will use their time, money, and talents to help others.

THE BABY BOOM GENERATION

The *baby boom generation*, born between 1943 and 1960, are described by Strauss and Howe as idealists. Because of their massive size, whatever age bracket boomers have occupied has been the cultural and spiritual focal point for American society. They already have two U.S. Presidents as members, as well as Al Gore, Jr., Bill Gates, Janis Joplin, David Letterman, Spike Lee, and Oprah Winfrey. They grew up in the age of TV, watching as the Vietnam War, Woodstock, and Watergate unfolded. Interestingly, only 1 in 16 male boomers ever saw combat in Vietnam, as they effectively avoided military service during that era.

As they moved into adulthood, boomers moved out of the mainline and established churches in New Age and evangelical sects, resulting in the most active era of church formation in the twentieth century. The baby boomers have also experienced many worsening trends— increased rates of accidental death, crime, drunk driving, suicide, and illegitimate births. The rates of premarital sex and adultery increased substantially for women but not for men.

Boomers narrowed the sex-role distinctions—men became more nurturing fathers and women took on roles previously reserved for men. Boomer family incomes would be below what the silents earned at the same age were it not for working women and dual income households. Married couples and single women are doing better but single men are not. However, when asked to compare themselves with their fathers at the same phase of life, they overwhelmingly consider their careers better, their personal freedoms greater, and their lives more meaningful.

CULTURAL DIVERSITY

With the current and projected demographic changes in the U.S. population, senior centers have both an opportunity and a challenge to serve the needs of an older group that is diverse racially, ethnically, culturally, linguistically, and in sexual orientation. The Administration on Aging developed the following principles to serve as a guide for the development of policies, strategies, practices, and procedures to support the delivery of culturally and linguistically competent services.

Cultural competency means knowing and understanding the people you serve, appreciating the importance of culture, and understanding the sociopolitical influences that help to shape the participants' attitudes, beliefs, and values. Cultural awareness efforts should be part of a system-wide program within the senior center and are a vital component of how services are both delivered and received. It is important to promote mutual respect and to recognize that acculturation occurs differently and at different rates for everyone.

It is important to build skills that enhance communication. Senior-center staff must be open, honest, respectful, nonjudgmental, and, most of all, willing to listen and learn. Letting people know that staff are interested in what participants have to say is vital to building trust. Communication strategies must capture the attention of the intended audience. This means not only using the language and dialect of the people being served, but also using appropriate audio and visual materials. Multilingual brochures and other written material do not help those persons who cannot read regardless of the language they are written in.

The environment should provide a culturally and linguistically friendly interior design with pictures, posters, and artwork to make the senior center more welcoming and attractive to participants. Providing services in a comfortable setting enhances program participation for all.

A "community" can refer to the people who live within a geographic boundary, as well as a group of people who have similar beliefs, a similar culture, or shared identity and experiences. Senior centers must know the community, its people, and its resources in order to identify useful strategies for service delivery. Involve the community at the planning and development stage because involved participants are invested participants.

Cultural and linguistic competence must be infused throughout the senior center and throughout everything the staff does. Policies, planning, structures, and procedures must provide support and resources for culturally competent services. This includes the following:

- mission statements that articulate principles, rationale and values for culturally and linguistically competent service delivery
- consumer and community participation in the planning, delivery, and evaluation of services
- policies and procedures for the recruitment, hiring, and retention of board, staff, and volunteers that will achieve a goal of a diverse and culturally competent work force and leadership
- training and staff development
- outreach, translation, and interpretation services

Staff development is essential to cultural and linguistic competence. It is also important to provide informal opportunities such as brown-bag lunches for staff to explore their attitudes, beliefs, and values. Specialized training for staff who are involved in the interpretation process is often overlooked. There is an assumption that if you are bilingual you can interpret. Training bilingual staff in interpreter skills enhances their ability to communicate effectively in both directions. Five elements have been identified that contribute to an organization's cultural competence:

1. valuing diversity
2. having the capacity to conduct a cultural self-assessment
3. being conscious of the dynamics inherent when cultures interact by taking into consideration how and where services are provided
4. institutionalizing cultural knowledge so that everyone in the organization is culturally competent, from the receptionist, to the director, to the custodian
5. adapting service delivery so that programs and services are delivered in a way that reflect the culture and traditions of the people being served

BIBLIOGRAPHY

Crystal, S., & Johnson, R. W. (1998). *The changing retirement prospects of Americans: Impact of labor market shifts in economic outcomes—executive summary*. Washington, DC: American Association of Retired Persons, Public Policy Institute. [On-line]. Available: www.research.aarp.org

Federal Interagency Forum on Aging-Related Statistics. (2001). *Aging Stats*. Hyattsville, MD: Author. [On-line]. Available: www.agingstats.gov

National Academy of Aging, the Maxwell School of Citizenship and Public Affairs, Syracuse University. (1994). *Old age in the twenty-first century: A report to the assistant secretary for aging, U.S. Department of Health and Human Services, regarding his responsibility in planning for the aging of the baby boom*. Syracuse, NY: Author.

National Council on the Aging. (2000). *Facts about older Americans*. Washington, DC: Author. [On-line]. Available: www.ncoa.org/news/mra_2000/factsheet.html

Strauss, W., & Howe, N. (1991). *Generations, the history of American's future, 1584–2069*. New York: William Morrow.

U.S. Census Bureau. (2001). Country's Older Population Profiled by the U.S. Census Bureau. *U.S. Department of Commerce News*. [On-line]. Available: www.census.gov/press-release.www/2001/cb01-96.html

U.S. Department of Health and Human Services, Administration on Aging. (2001). *Facts and figures: Statistics on minority aging in the U.S.* Washington, DC: Author. [On-line]. Available: www.agingstats.gov

U.S. Department of Health and Human Services, Administration on Aging. (2001). *Lesbian, gay, bisexual, and transgender older persons*. [On-line]. Washington, DC: Author. Available: www.aoa.dhhs.gov/may2001/factsheets/LGBT.html

U.S. Department of Health and Human Services, Administration on Aging. (2001). *A profile of older Americans: 2000.* Washington DC: Author. [On-line]. Available: www.aoa.dhhs.gov

U.S. Department of Health and Human Services, Administration on Aging. (2001). *Fact for Features from the Census Bureau.* Washington, DC: Author. [On-line]. Available: www.aoa.gov/aoa/STATS/2001pop/factsforfeatures2001.html

U.S. Department of Health and Human Services, Administration on Aging. (2001). *Achieving cultural competence: A guidebook for providers of services to older Americans and their families.* [On-line]. Available: www.aoa.gov/minorityaccess/guidbook2001/

RESOURCES

U.S. Census Bureau
Washington, DC 20233
301-457-4608
http://www.census.gov
The Census Bureau collects and provides timely, relevant, and quality data about the people and economy of the United States.

Stanford Geriatric Education Center
703 Welch Road, Suite H-1
Palo Alto, CA 94304-1708
650-723-7063
http://www.stanford.edu/dept/medfm/gec/page1.html
The Stanford Geriatric Education Center provides a variety of ethnogeriatric programs and curriculum resource materials to educate health care professionals on the cultural issues associated with aging and health. The Stanford Geriatric Education Center promotes cultural sensitivity and cultural competence to improve the quality of health care delivered to the rapidly growing population of ethnic minority elders in the United States.

CHAPTER THREE

Wants, Needs, and Interests of Older Adults

VICY AND JAY

With Vintage nearing its 30th anniversary, we should not be surprised to find a second generation of participants involved in programs and using the many services Vintage offers. Jay's mother came to Vintage during the 1970s and early 1980s. A proud woman, she did not want to admit her age, and she instructed her son not to come to Vintage because she did not want anyone to know she had a son old enough to become a member.

In 1993, Vicy's daughter was terminally ill, and she and Jay found their way to Vintage as an escape from their troubles. Jay had retired from U.S. Steel and Vicy, at age 51, had given up her job to care for her daughter. Friends who attended Vintage encouraged Vicy to get away for a few hours, and knowing how much both she and Jay enjoyed dancing, invited them to come for the line-dancing class. This turned out to be a wonderful outlet for both of them.

My first remembrance of Vicy is when she shared with me her concern for her daughter. She told me how devastating this was for her and how grateful she was to be able to come to a place like Vintage. The staff encouraged Vicy to do what she felt comfortable doing and acted as a sounding board when she just needed to talk. She started to do needlework, which was especially helpful as she could continue to work on the projects at home. She wanted to volunteer, but couldn't commit to any particular time, so she was given the lunch tickets, which she faithfully numbered at home.

Following her daughter's death, she and Jay became more involved in the center. They took computer classes, assisted in a variety of volunteer efforts, and were instrumental in bringing the duplicate-bridge class to Vintage. Additionally, they have acted as spokespersons for the agency, allowing others to know what Vintage has meant to them. Jay has also served as president of House Council (the advisory board) for 2 years.

On two occasions The Western Pennsylvania Hospital/Vintage Community Care for Seniors has been available to detect and assist with health care issues. Jay was diagnosed with diabetes during a routine screening at Vintage, and Vicy was hospitalized when the wellness coordinator detected a very rapid heartbeat.

Vicy and Jay will both say that Vintage has been their salvation. Vicy added that at first she thought Vintage was just for "old people," but now she will tell you there are things for everyone. If anything, she feels younger as her involvement at Vintage has grown. She often says you come to Vintage and "lose yourself in activities and forget any troubles you may have."

If Vicy and Jay are part of the second generation to find Vintage, can the third generation be far behind?

Who makes up the senior market and what do they want? Demographic, generational, gerontographic, and other descriptive information help identify who and where they are and what motivates them. Variables such as age, education, economic status, and ethnicity are important indicators in understanding the older market. The first step that senior centers need to take is to define who their customers are now, and who they want to reach. Everyone is different and everyone attends a senior center for different reasons.

Market research has found that, in general, an aging population is interested in home products, health care, wellness and youth-enhancing products, recreational and leisure services, financial services and products, and educational services. With more education, better health, and greater financial well-being than in the past, older adults are more active, independent, and able to enjoy their retirement years. This trend will continue.

However, older consumers are highly heterogeneous. Different generations have different attitudes and consumer behaviors. They differ in their family and marital status, ethnicity, geography, education, and social class as well as age, and all of these factors affect their consumption patterns. The 50-plus mature market is the most affluent age segment, controlling more than 50% of total discretionary income in the U.S. The over-65 population consists of several very different marketplaces—the relatively healthy, affluent group of younger seniors (65–74), and the rapidly growing, less prosperous over-age 75 group that includes the middle-seniors (75–84) and the old-old (85+). Each age group is concerned about what matters to them at each stage of their life. For example, the young-old are more interested in travel and leisure services than the old-old.

The United States has begun to experience one of the greatest demographic and cultural shifts of focus in history. The traditional demographic balance is reversing at an accelerated rate. In 1970, the youth culture was dominant and children under 18 far outnumbered adults 50 years and older (70 million versus 50 million). By 2030, it is estimated there will be 83 million children under 18 and 127 million adults 50 years and older. David Foot in *Boom, Bust and Echo 2000* predicts this shift will create an economic and social revolution. The cause of this phenomenon will be the maturing of the baby boomers, combined with a dramatic increase in their longevity. The boomers have dominated American culture through every stage of their life as the issues that concerned them became the outstanding social, political, and marketplace themes of the time. Their massive numbers have amplified and intensified the importance of whatever experiences they've had at each stage of their lives. Their mature years will be no exception. Boomers have always done it differently than before, transforming relationships, the workplace, and the fashion, dining, health-care, and technology industries.

In contrast to earlier generations who defined success from the outside-in through their title, status, wealth, and power, boomers are redefining success from the inside-out, through personal fulfillment and an emphasis on self-esteem, quality of personal relationships, and personal freedom.

Ken Dychtwald, in *Age Power: How the 21st Century Will Be Ruled by the New Old*, predicts that as the boomers pass through their middle years into maturity, five key factors will reshape supply and demand:

1. concern about chronic disease and the desire to postpone physical aging
2. increasing amounts of discretionary dollars
3. entry into new adult stages including empty-nesting, caregiving, grandparenting, retirement, and widowhood
4. a shift from acquiring material possessions to participating in enjoyable and satisfying experiences
5. the continued absence of disposable time due to complex lifestyles

He predicts the aging-boomer leisure market will create these needs:

- elders with a desire to help solve social problems or community issues
- lifelong learning programs at colleges and community centers, and on cable TV and the Internet
- adventure-travel services
- apprenticeships with masters to learn new skills or crafts
- stores and Web sites featuring products and technologies for retirees
- sabbaticals and informal work-leave programs for renewal and refreshment

David Foot suggests looking at where the front-end boomers are today to forecast the changes of the future as the rest of the massive boomer population catches up. He also examined the traditional leisure interests of the 50-plus population to predict future growth areas.

Both serious and recreational gamblers tend to be in their 50s or 60s as they also tend to have the discretionary income to afford this pastime. Upscale travel, ecotourism, and other forms of educational travel are another growth area. Elders want to see interesting sites while learning new things from qualified experts. Travel is a booming senior market because older adults have the time and income to travel and they are healthy enough to do so.

A great deal of importance is placed on personal health, including the amount and kinds of food eaten, and adequate recreation, relaxation, and physical exercise. However, as they get older and become less inclined to engage in strenuous activities, their recreation and leisure habits will change. David Foot suggests that through the impact of these changes will be dramatic, they are also predictable. The data on the impact of aging on leisure pursuits is remarkably stable over time. Two factors determine the growth of leisure activities: the size of the population and the rate of participation. The rate of participation changes dramatically as the population ages. Studies confirm that even though all age groups are more active, a declining level of activity accompanies the aging process. Projections show that resting, reading, hobbies, and attendance at museums, theaters, and places of worship will become the most popular leisure activities in the years to come. Birdwatching, golfing, gardening, and walking are all activities that people do more of as they age. Birdwatching combines gentle exercise, travel, and the intellectual challenge of finding and identifying birds. Golf is one sport in which participation increases with age and golfers actually play more as they get older because they have more time to play. Golf is a wonderful sport for retired people because it offers companionship and exercise. Adult education and gardening are also seen as growth industries.

According to a special report from *Modern Maturity* magazine and the Roper Organization, "Mature America in the 1990s," adults 50 years and older identified how they want to spend their leisure time:

- with their families (70%)
- relaxing (66%)
- with companions (55%)
- helping other people (50%)
- learning new things (44%)
- keeping informed (40%)
- exercise, creativity (29%)
- amusement (28%)
- culture (26%)
- challenge (25%)

Leisure hours are a time for personal interests and hobbies. The top 10 hobbies identified by the report are

- reading (41%)
- cooking (32%)
- gardening (31%)
- music (25%)
- travel (20%)
- needlework (18%)
- pets (18%)
- fishing (18%)
- crafts (15%)
- sewing (14%)

The report found that dining out and socializing with friends are the most popular entertainment activities. Travel ranks among the top leisure activities. Grandchildren are an important part of mature Americans' lives. Eighty percent are interested in environmental issues and are concerned for future generations, especially protecting human health.

They are taking proactive steps to remain healthy and are concerned about healthful eating and feeling attractive. They want to look their best by eating right, exercising, dressing well, and observing a regular grooming routine (regular skin care, professional hairstyling, and wearing cosmetics and fragrances). They are balanced media users, enjoying TV, radio, newspapers, and magazines; they are above-average newspaper readers. They are generous and give back to their communities, in both time and money.

To access these markets, businesses may need to go out of their way to test new products, services, and ways of servicing these customers.

GERONTOGRAPHICS

Gerontographics is another way to understand the mature market. The older people get, the more dissimilar they become with respect to their needs, lifestyles, and consumption habits. Gerontographics is a market-segmentation approach based on the premise that older consumers' market choices are related to their needs and lifestyles, which are influenced by changing life conditions. Of course, life-changing events can and do occur at varying ages. They can be physiological, such as the onset of a chronic illness, or social and psychological, such as the loss of a spouse. George Moschis uses gerontographics to gain insight into human behavior in later life and describes four distinct consumer segments with different ways of responding to marketing efforts. Older people who experience similar circumstances in late life are likely to exhibit similar patterns of consumer behavior. Older adults can move from one stage to another.

The gerontographics life-stage model classifies older adults, 55-plus, into the following four groups based on the amount and type of aging they have experienced:

1. *Healthy indulgers* (18%) have experienced the fewest life-changing events. They are the group most likely to behave like younger consumers, except that they are financially better off. One of their main interests is enjoying life.

2. *Healthy hermits* (36%) are likely to have experienced life events that have affected their self-concept and self-worth, such as the death of a spouse. They react by becoming psychologically and socially withdrawn.

3. *Ailing outgoers* (29%) maintain positive self-esteem and self-concept despite life events such as health problems. Unlike hermits, outgoers accept their "old-age" status and acknowledge their limitations, but are still interested in getting the most out of life.

4. *Frail recluses* (17%) are likely to have accepted their old-age status and have adjusted their lifestyles to reflect physical declines and changes in social roles.

Some changes occur slowly, such as providing long-term care for a spouse with a dementing illness. Other changes are abrupt, such as a sudden death of a spouse. The consumer behavior of older people depends on the experiences they have had and the way they adapt to them.

For example, ailing outgoers and frail recluses are the more important mature markets for health-care products and services. When it comes to money, healthy indulgers value both convenience and personal service; they can afford to take more expensive trips by air and cruise ship, although they won't complain about special group rates and senior discounts. They enjoy the convenience that packaged travel services provide. Over time, many ailing outgoers will become frail recluses. In the process, they will become less concerned with where the nearest shopping center is and more concerned about the nearest hospital. Because mature Americans can and do move from one life-stage segment to another in a somewhat predictable fashion as they experience and react to life changes, it is possible to identify those who are at risk for moving into a given life stage. Senior centers and other aging service providers can then be proactive about targeting people even before they enter the next life stage. Those centers and providers that track the progress of mature consumers will stay ahead of the competition.

WHAT THE OLDER CONSUMER WANTS

The Oasis Institute conducted research to learn what is most important to people as they become part of the 65-plus senior market. They found that seniors don't want to be stereotyped and they dislike being lumped into one group.

In general, older consumers want

- information that will help them maintain their health and independence;
- to know all about products and services; they need to know why they should buy them, so if necessary, give them a sample, a taste, a trial period or a coupon;
- security and safety as key factors in their decision making;
- financial security;
- to feel appreciated;
- to be regarded as individuals, without age being a major factor;
- to not be thought of as old; in fact, they tend to feel 10 to 20 years younger than their actual age;
- a response to their concerns, not their age;
- to be comfortable;
- to play an active role as a consumer;
- products and services that enhance their personal enjoyment of life;
- to know about new things;
- romance in their lives;
- to feel attractive, fashionable, and desirable;
- quality and service, but they are interested in discounts;
- convenience and access;
- experiences rather than things.

MARKET STRATEGIES

Compete on the basis of quality and service because the older consumer is interested in quality and service. As the average age of the population increases, quality and service will assume an even greater importance.

There are three ways to look at marketing to the senior market:

1. Choose a market segment and focus on it.
2. Find a way to differentiate the same product so that it can be marketed to different segments of the senior market.
3. Change, improve, or alter a product to expand its demographic reach.

Relying on word of mouth and using the same promotions will attract more of the same participants a center already has, therefore, it is important to identify who you have and who you want. To reach different age cohorts, aim products, service, or facilities to appeal to two or more markets. To reach new markets, new methods must be used, such as employer publications, direct mail, Web sites, e-mails, posters at places such as toy stores, and ads in the sports, business, and lifestyle sections of newspapers. Print advertising earns the most respect from older consumers, and they find the advertising they read in magazines and newspapers to be useful and informative.

A market research study sponsored by the Pennsylvania Department of Aging found that 91% of those between 55 and 60 years of age preferred activities off-site—a senior center without walls. Senior centers are a sponsor and a center of activities, not just a physical space. Alternative settings permit and encourage market segmentation.

In promotional materials, it is important to focus on the benefits to the participant, and promote the product (retirees having fun and learning), not the center. Appeal to the older consumer by solving their problems, answering their wants and needs, and providing personal satisfaction and gain. Older consumers are risk-adverse and they need lots of information before they buy. Depict them handling problems, rather than anguishing over them. Be specific in showing how the center can help by documenting any claims; case histories are effective.

In promotional materials, use positive images of aging. Portray older adults as healthy, vigorous, alert, and leading active lives. It is ability, not age, that matters. Older people want to see themselves represented in advertising as intelligent, attractive, and useful. Communicate the feeling of achievement. Show the age they feel, 10 to 20 years younger than the target audience. Use upbeat testimonials and the key motivators for older people: independence, self-sufficiency, social and spiritual connectedness, altruism, personal growth, and revitalization.

Picture older consumers laughing and with friends and family, having fun with different generations of people. Use photographs and films showing older people engaged in useful work and helping others. Present mature people who are happy with their newfound free time, pleased with their options, and relishing life. Mature people take pleasure in their food; show them enjoying it with friends and family. Depict them expanding their horizons, learning new skills, and growing, giving as well as getting. Mature people like to mingle with everybody. When promoting goods and services, mix voices, colors, and backgrounds.

Senior centers can also target lifestyle affinities by addressing lifestyle needs and interests—empty-nesting, caregiving, retirement, grandparenting, and widowhood. Another strategy is to expand programs and services in order to expand markets. Senior centers can provide

- services for caregivers
- novelty food services such as a café with specialty coffees, desserts, and healthful foods, or a juice bar as an alternative to the congregate meal
- restaurant outings with commentary by the chef
- wine appreciation
- the foods and flavors of other cultures (Thai, Indian, Vietnamese, etc.)
- employment and volunteer services
- computers and Internet access
- experiential travel opportunities
- apprentice opportunities with master craftspersons and artists
- evening and weekend activities
- a 50s party with plenty of rock and roll
- investment and money management programs
- activities and services for grandchildren
- preretirement planning

Use focus groups of younger, nonparticipating elders to find out what message the physical location, appearance, amenities, and services send. Create opportunities for participants to share suggestions, complaints, opinions and comments (and one hopes) praise.

IDEAS FOR ATTRACTING THE YOUNGER OLDER ADULT

The National Institute on Senior Centers asked its delegates for solutions to attract and retain members from younger age groups. Their ideas include

- computer classes
- investment clubs
- reading or discussion groups; programs that bring in local authors
- speakers on alternative health care and medicines (natural-healing information, pressure point therapy, and biofeedback)
- competition via juried fine art and photo shows
- fitness
- wellness
- languages

- dine-around
- trips and tours
- massage therapy
- caregiver workshops
- special events
- healthful-food programs
- focus on fine arts instead of crafts
- self-empowerment and improvement classes
- senior leadership training
- humanities
- dart, baseball, and basketball tournaments
- tai chi
- yoga
- community service opportunities
- senior leadership
- intergenerational programs
- programs for the newly divorced and support for how to succeed on their own

The delegates suggested redesigning volunteer programs to recruit younger groups, including providing leadership opportunities, challenges, involving participant leadership in mission and goal development for change, and recruiting and training volunteers to plan and implement entire projects. Participant leadership must be vibrant.

Evening programs and preretirement seminars are important to those older adults who are still working. To attract a younger audience, the center may need a "spring cleaning," including furnishings, programs, staff, volunteer services, publications, and a more appealing menu.

BIBLIOGRAPHY

Dyhtwald, K. (1999). *Age power: How the 21st century will be ruled by the new old.* New York: Tarcher/Putnam.

Foot, D. K., & Stoffman, D. (1998). *Boom, bust and echo 2000. Profiting from demographic shift in the new millennium.* Toronto: Macfarlane, Walter and Ross.

Fudemberg, G. (2000). *The importance of the senior market.* (2000). Chicago: GRF Marketing. [On-line]. Available: www.seniorsessions.com/Insightsarticle.htm

Mature Marketing and Research. (2001). [On-line]. Available: www.maturemarketing.com

Modern Maturity. (1992). *Mature America in the 1990s. A Special Report from Modern Maturity Magazine and the Roper Organization.* Washington, DC: Author.

Moschis, G. P. (1996). Life stages of the mature market. *American Demographics, 18,* 9. [On-line]. Available: www.demographics.com.

Newton, G. (1995). *Marketing to Recruit the New Senior Market.* State College, PA: Presentation at the Pennsylvania Association of Senior Centers State Conference.

The Office of Senior Interests. (1997). *Breaking the Ice: A Guide to Marketing to Maturity.* The State of Western Australia: Author. [On-line]. Available: www.osi.wa.gov/au/pubs/index.htm

Senior Centers. (2001). *NISC Nuggets.* [On-line]. Available: www.ncoa.org/nisc/nisc_news/nuggets_mar2001.html

RESOURCES

American Geriatrics Society
The Empire State Building
350 Fifth Avenue, Suite 801
New York, NY 10118
212-308-1414
http://www.americangeriatrics.org/
The American Geriatrics Society is a professional organization of health-care providers dedicated to improving the health and well being of older adults.

American Society on Aging
833 Market Street, Suite 511
San Francisco, CA 94103-1824
415-974-9600
http://www.asaging.org/
The American Society on Aging is a membership organization dedicated to providing up-to-date information, research, training, and resources to professionals concerned with all aspects of aging.

Gerontological Society of America
1030 15th Street NW, Suite 250
Washington, DC 20005
202-842-1275
http://www.geron.org/
The Gerontological Society of America promotes interdisciplinary research in aging by expanding the quantity of and improving the quality of gerontological research.

PART THREE

Positive Aging Experiences

CHAPTER FOUR

Volunteerism

EDDIE

"When I help others I feel I am fulfilling God's will." This is the reason Eddie gave me recently for being a home-delivered-meal volunteer. For 10 years, every Tuesday without fail, you will find Eddie in the home-delivered-meal area, first packing and then transporting the food to between 15 and 20 homebound clients. If people happen to stop in during the packing process they'll find a very friendly group, but also a group intent on getting the food ready and on the road. The homebound anxiously await and look forward to the meal and the visitor each day. They need the food to sustain the physical body as well as the friendly hello and a few words to sustain the spirit. For some, it is the only contact they have each day with the outside world.

The one day Eddie would rather not drive for home-delivered meals is Wednesday. This is the day the photography group meets. He has been as much a part of this group as he has been delivering meals. In addition to taking pictures, they also have a darkroom where they can develop black-and-white photos. Eddie, along with the other men, are very proud of the yearbook they worked on for the 25th anniversary of Vintage. In the traditional yearbook style they took numerous pictures not only of individuals, but also of events and classes.

As all the volunteers will tell you, they genuinely care about the people they visit and the homebound person responds in kind. Eddie is one of the few drivers who is also the visitor, preferring to do both jobs. This is extra work, as one must find a parking place on a busy city street, collect the food, travel over snow-covered sidewalks in the winter, and often climb flights of steps to deliver the meal. Eddie does all of this every week, and often twice a week if a substitute is needed.

Many people think working on home-delivered meals is a real chore, going out in all kinds of weather and keeping this commitment, which *can and often does extend to years. Ask Eddie and he will tell you just the opposite. Every morning he wakes up, thanks God for another day, and once again sets off to help someone less fortunate than himself.*

Older adults make important social contributions through voluntary commitments. They represent a large reservoir of knowledge, skills, cultural continuity, wisdom, and civic responsibility. The volunteer efforts of older people amount to the equivalent of more than 1 million full-time employees. Upwards of 50% of retired seniors gave more than 4 hours of their time each week to volunteer. Even among seniors who work full or part-time, 54% reported volunteering. When other factors such as uncompensated child-care are added in, it is clear that the voluntary activities of older persons add significantly to our economic and social well-being.

Volunteer action is a tradition in the United States and all older people have time and talents to share. Every culture has developed ways in which people help people, and organizations have a never-ending need for the time and talents of volunteers. With many Americans retiring earlier and baby boomers in their 50s forming a large part of the maturing population, older people represent a growing force of potential volunteers. Many older people have the time to volunteer and are free from the distraction of raising a family. Through volunteer service, older people can enrich their own lives and enhance the quality of life in their communities.

The federal government encourages volunteerism in older citizens. Many federal programs provide volunteer opportunities. Older Americans Act programs, including senior centers, largely depend upon the efforts of half a million volunteers to deliver services. These volunteers work through the state and territorial units on aging, area agencies on aging and more than 20,000 local organizations. Volunteer activities include assisting at group meal sites, delivering meals to the homebound, telephone reassurance, counseling older persons, serving as nursing home ombudsmen, and assisting in senior centers, adult day-service centers, and other group programs.

The senior center can expand opportunities for older people to contribute to society. There are many barriers to broader participation in volunteer activities that could be overcome through efforts to recognize and address them. Barriers include difficulty obtaining information about volunteer opportunities, unrealistic expectations and perceptions about the role of volunteers, lack of skills or the training needed to be effective as a volunteer, and impediments such as transportation and out-of-pocket expenses. Volunteer experience can be enhanced by offering nontraditional avenues for seniors to express their talents and contribute to the well-being of society.

Lack of time is the number one reason people do not get involved as a volunteer. Another reason is also time-related—the unwillingness to make a year-round commitment. Though these barriers diminish with age and retirement, organizations need to offer short-term volunteer experiences for people whose lifestyles will not accommodate a year-round or long-term commitment.

VOLUNTEER STATISTICS

The demographic profile of volunteers is changing. Full-time homemakers no longer constitute the majority of volunteers. Volunteer opportunities draw older adults, students, full-time professionals, and people with disabilities. According to a survey conducted by the Independent Sector, "Giving and Volunteering in the United States," 56% of the adult population does volunteer work, more than 100 million people in 1998. A higher percentage of women volunteer (62%) compared to men (49%). The percentage of people reporting volunteer work increased in all demographic groups since the 1995 survey, including those who are unemployed and part-time workers.

Forty-seven percent of African Americans and 46% of Hispanics volunteered, while 43% of people aged 75 and over reported volunteering. As the level of education and household income increased, so did the rate of volunteering. College graduates were more than 50% likelier to volunteer than were those respondents with only a high-school education.

Changing demographics require volunteer managers to revise management practices and offer new types of volunteer tasks to accommodate the needs of an increasingly diverse pool of volunteers. Organizations must be in tune with the attitudes and values of people today to attract the volunteers they need.

For example, a new area of volunteer activity is computer technology. Cyber-volunteers create or maintain Web sites, perform on-line research, provide technical assistance, and help with on-line marketing and activism for organizations they volunteer with. Though fewer than 10% of survey respondents reported wanting to volunteer on-line as an alternative to traditional volunteer activities, those who do so cited convenience and schedule flexibility as the reasons. The Internet is an important medium to educate the public about the work of senior centers and to stimulate giving and volunteering. A cyber-volunteer can help the senior center develop and maintain their on-line presence.

The National Center for Charitable Statistics develops the national average hourly value of volunteer time, which is derived from the annual report of economic indicators. The 1999 U.S. average value of volunteer time was $14.83. This represents a range of tasks that might be valued at minimum wage as well as services from doctors, lawyers, and other professionals that are valued at a higher rate.

Family volunteering is part of family life for more than a third of American households. The most common partnership is husband and wife. Once established, family volunteering tends to become a tradition. Early life experiences bear some relationship to the likelihood of volunteering in adult years. The rate of volunteering is higher among people with specific volunteer experience during their youth.

Formal volunteering involves regular work for an organization. Informal volunteering involves helping others or organizations on an ad hoc basis, such as baby-sitting or making cookies for a bake sale. According to the Independent Sector, the most popular areas of volunteer activity include

- direct service activity such as serving food (24%)
- fund-raising (16%)
- informal volunteer (15%)
- religion (14%)
- giving advice or counseling (11%)
- youth (11%)
- organizing an event (10%)
- visiting people or offering companionship (9%)

For 41% of volunteers, volunteer service is a sporadic, one-time activity. Thirty-nine percent of volunteers prefer to volunteer at a regularly scheduled time. The remaining 9% reported volunteering only around special holidays such as Christmas or Hanukkah.

Volunteering is at the heart of philanthropy. One clear trend emerged from the Independent Sector survey: volunteers give more than nonvolunteers. As the percentage of volunteers increased, giving rose. Being asked personally to give money and time continued to be the most effective way to recruit donors and volunteers.

Volunteers reported three ways they learned about their volunteer activities: (a) they were asked by someone; (b) through participation in an organization; or (c) through a family member or relative. An incredible 90% of individuals reported volunteering when asked, but only 22% did so when not asked. The majority of older volunteers found volunteer opportunities through their places of worship. More than 50% of senior volunteers reported that they volunteered because they wanted to give back to society some of the benefits they received individually.

Volunteering provides a variety of personal benefits and satisfaction, in addition to the benefits received by nonprofit organizations such as senior centers. Older volunteers are motivated by their desire for purpose, affiliation, growth, and meaning. The most important reasons people cited for volunteering were

- feeling compassion for those in need (86%)
- having an interest in the activity or work (72%)
- gaining a new perspective on things (70%)
- the importance of the activity to people whom the volunteer respects (63%)

Other reasons people volunteer are to share their good fortune, to show gratitude for what they have received, because they now have the time to do what they want to do, and to fulfill court-ordered community service requirements.

Ninety-seven percent of older volunteers were motivated to do so because they believe in the particular cause. Other motivating factors are the opportunity to use skills and experience, being personally affected by the organization or service, fulfilling religious obligations, exploring one's own strengths, wanting to learn more about a specific cause or area, and volunteering with a friend or friends. For some, learning new skills for career advancement or exploring job options is an important motivation. For others, skills and experiences gained through volunteer service fulfill a need for relationships, personal growth and development, achievement, or affiliation.

THE BENEFITS OF VOLUNTEERING

Volunteers experience personal fulfillment and satisfaction. Through volunteerism, older people can put a lifetime of skills and experience to good use. In a study commissioned by Volunteer Canada, Manulife Financial and Health Canada, the links between volunteering and health were examined. People who gave their time to a volunteer activity, especially if it involved helping others, were happier and healthier in their later years. The personal benefits of volunteering should be used as a way to recruit volunteers.

One of the major benefits of volunteering is a sense of personal satisfaction from helping others. Volunteering can positively affect an individual's outlook on life and help provide a new perspective on their problems. The social benefits can be tremendous. Volunteers meet new people, work together as part of a team, gain new experiences and create new memories. Volunteering helps to keep the body and mind active. Other benefits to volunteering include

- increased self-esteem and confidence
- feeling needed
- improved interpersonal skills
- the opportunity to share knowledge and expertise with others
- learning new skills
- pursue new interests
- empowerment
- creativity
- renewed vigor and enthusiasm for life
- having fun
- obtaining career-related experience and transferable skills
- exercising leadership and problem-solving skills
- enhancing personal development
- fulfilling the need to achieve
- being involved in the community
- having an impact on the lives of those in need
- being a good citizen
- supporting a good cause

VOLUNTEER MANAGEMENT

The field of volunteer management shows increased movement toward professionalization as practitioners establish standards for practice. Managing volunteers effectively is a problem for many not-for-profit organizations, including senior centers. More could be accomplished if senior centers could better recruit, train, manage, and recognize the work of volunteers. Senior centers often lack the resources to effectively use and retain volunteers. A 1998 United Parcel Service (UPS) study on volunteer management found that the American public sees the inefficient management of volunteer time as a basic obstacle to increased volunteerism. People are more likely to volunteer when they feel an organization is well-managed and will make good use of their time and talents. Time is the most limiting factor in volunteering, and volunteers expect the time they donate to be well managed. Many potential and active volunteers are discouraged from volunteering because of the inefficient use of their time.

The most common reason people gave for stopping volunteering for an organization was they had more important demands on their time (65%). However, two out of five volunteers have stopped volunteering for an organization at some time because of one or more poor volunteer management practices—the organization did not make good use of their time or their talents, skills, and expertise; volunteers' tasks were not clearly defined; or they were not thanked or recognized for their efforts.

The UPS study found that although half of those surveyed were content with their current level of volunteering, 38% would like to do more. Those who have never volunteered are the least likely to be interested in becoming more involved. The best way for organizations to receive more hours of volunteer service is to be careful managers of the time already being volunteered. Organizations that are able to recruit and make effective use of volunteer resources are positioned to make the greatest contributions to those in need.

Volunteers want an opportunity that is of personal interest to them and will allow them to put their skills and experience to good use. To ensure that volunteers are matched to an appropriate activity, senior centers should have prospects complete an application. Through the application and a personal interview, a volunteer's skills, interests, and experience can be determined. A reference check is another important element to the screening process.

Volunteers want to know about the position, including how much time is involved, a description of the position, the skills and abilities required, what opportunities they will have to learn new skills, what kind of training or orientation they can expect, what kind of feedback they will receive, who they will be working with and supervised by, and if references will be checked or if a background report is required.

Comprehensive orientation and volunteer-training programs show that the organization values volunteers enough to make an investment in them. Orientation and training ensures that the volunteer under-stands the organization and the expectations of the position. It also ensures that volunteers have the information and the preparation needed to undertake their responsibilities. Learning is a crucial factor in a volunteer's satisfaction with his or her experience, and satisfied participants are more likely to remain committed to the organization. Volunteers frequently report learning by experience, interaction, or observation. Informal and incidental learning that occurs in the process of activity is a significant part of the volunteer experience. Personal empowerment obtained through learning is a motivation for volunteer-ing, and acknowledging its value adds to organizational effectiveness.

Studies comparing volunteer management and adult education sug-gest that an organizational climate that recognizes the motivation of volunteers to both serve and learn is an essential element in the success of the volunteer program. Volunteer managers need to focus on how their organizational culture supports learning. Learning through the volunteer experience can be enhanced by

- including mentoring, peer support, and information needs to facili-tate learning;
- educating volunteer managers about self-directed learning, pro-gram development, and assessment of adult learners;
- providing greater recognition and support for informal learning by increasing the individual's capacity for critical reflection, enabling them to recognize and document their volunteer activities as learn-ing experiences.

The volunteer program should enhance and extend the work of the organization's paid staff but should never replace it. Volunteer manag-ers should develop a philosophy of volunteerism and create and pro-mote a climate of volunteerism that recognizes the rights of volunteers. Volunteers have the right

- to be assigned a volunteer position that is worthwhile and challenging
- to be able to use existing skills and develop new ones
- to have the information and training needed to carry out the assignment
- to receive supervision, encouragement, and feedback
- to expect that their time will not be wasted by lack of planning or coordination

- to be reimbursed for out-of-pocket expenses
- to be given appropriate recognition

SUGGESTED ACTIVITIES

- Volunteer job descriptions for every volunteer position.
- Application and interview process to determine the volunteer's interests and skills.
- Orientation and training program to orient volunteers to the organizational history, structure, services, climate, staff and volunteers, and the expectations of the volunteer position.
- Educational programs for volunteers to develop leadership, guest relation, and team building skills.
- Recognition and appreciation activities and events to thank volunteers for their contributions. Volunteers should be thanked often— following each assignment—through personal notes, in newsletters and other organization publications, and through formal recognition events.
- Evaluation program to provide and obtain feedback from volunteers.
- Special events: The Points of Light Foundation and the Volunteer Center National Network sponsor national Seasons of Service Opportunities to promote volunteerism. Seasons of Service Opportunities include Martin Luther King Day, www.mlkday.org; Join Hands Day (youth and adults volunteering together), www.joinhandsday.org; and Make a Difference Day (a national day to help others), www.makeadifferenceday.com.

BIBLIOGRAPHY

The Benefits of Volunteering. (2001). [On-line]. Available: www.mysask.com/community/moosejaw/lifestyle/selfimprovement/volunteer.shtml

The Benefits to Volunteering. (2001). [On-line]. Available: www.nextsteps.org/net/career/81yecp3b.htm

Independent Sector. (1999). *Giving and volunteering in the United States. National survey.* Washington, DC: Author.

Kerka, S. (1998). *Volunteering and adult learning. (No. 202).* Washington, DC: ERIC Clearinghouse on Adult, Career and Vocational Education, Office of Educational Research and Improvement, U.S. Department of Education.

National Academy on Aging, Maxwell School of Citizenship and Public Affairs, Syracuse University. (1994). *Old age in the 21st century: A report to the assistant secretary for aging, U.S. Department of Health and Human Services.* Syracuse, NY: Author.
Points of Life Foundation. (2001). *International Year of the Volunteer 2001 U.S.* Washington, DC: Author.
United Parcel Service. (1998). *Managing Volunteers. A Report from United Parcel Service.*
U.S. Department of Health and Human Services, Administration on Aging, ElderAction. (1997). *Volunteer opportunities for older Americans.* Washington, DC: Author.
Volunteer Canada. (2000). *Volunteering . . . A Booming Trend.* Ottawa, Canada: Author.

RESOURCES

Association for Research on Nonprofit Organizations and Voluntary Action (ARNOVA)
Indiana University Center on Philanthropy
550 West North Street, Suite 301
Indianapolis, IN 46202-3162
317-684-2120
http://www.arnova.org
The Association for Research on Nonprofit Organizations and Voluntary Action is an international, interdisciplinary network of scholars and leaders fostering the creation, application and research on voluntary action and non-profit organizations.

Association for Volunteer Administration (AVA)
PO Box 32092
3108 N. Parham Road, Suite 200-B
Richmond, VA 23294
804-346-2266
www.avaintl.org.
AVA is an international professional organization for individuals working in the field of volunteer management.

Helping.org
AOL Time Warner Foundation
22000 AOL Way
Dulles, VA 20166
http://www.helping.org
Helping.org is an online resource designed to help people find volunteer and giving opportunities in their own communities and beyond.

Independent Sector
1200 18th Street, NW, 2nd floor
Washington, DC 20036
202-467-6100
www.independentsector.org
The Independent Sector is a national membership organization that encourages giving and volunteering through public education, research and advocacy.

International Association for Volunteer Effort (IAVE)
1400 I Street NW, Suite 800
Washington, DC 20005
202-729-8250
www.iave.org.
International Association for Volunteer Effort promotes, supports and celebrates volunteering.

National Center for Nonprofit Boards (NCNB)
1828 L Street, NW Suite 900
Washington, DC 20036
800-883-6262
www.ncnb.org
The National Center for Nonprofit Boards is dedicated to increasing the effectiveness of nonprofit organizations by strengthening their boards of directors.

The Points of Light Foundation
1400 I Street, NW, Suite 800
Washington, DC 20005
202-729-8000
www.pointsoflight.org.
The Points of Light Foundation works to involve more people in community service through volunteer initiatives, volunteer services and products, and membership programs. The Volunteer Center National Network is a local/regional organization serving the community through promoting volunteerism, training and assisting non-profit organizations, and recruiting and recognizing volunteers. 1-800-VOLUNTEER.

CHAPTER FIVE

Recreation

EARL

There are a lot of reasons why one might attend a senior center, but redemption and the environment are usually not the ones mentioned. This was, however, the case with Earl. A retired mechanical and chemical engineer, he had heard about a project Vintage was doing with a national organization, EASI (Environmental Alliance for Senior Involvement), where several counties in Pennsylvania are involved in the monitoring of surface stream water. Various volunteer teams monitor the streams monthly to test for nitrates, sulfates, pH, specific conductance, phosphates, and dissolved oxygen. In addition they make a physical assessment of the stream and its surroundings. Monitoring each stream at the same site for several years, they provide a baseline for the health of the stream.

In his professional life, Earl had worked with uranium and, in those days industry and government did not realize the danger of discharging such substances into a stream or creek near the plant. It was with this background that he came to Vintage in the late 1990s. When I first met this tall, thin Irishman with white hair and blue eyes, I knew immediately he felt committed to the project. He told me that 2 years prior to learning about the EASI project, he had picked up a book at a college bookstore and had studied extensively the tests and techniques for quality water monitoring.

Shortly after joining the group, Earl volunteered to be the team leader for not just one but two teams. They would monitor a total of four sites on tributaries leading into a very polluted stream located within the boundaries of a city park. There were many challenges that came with monitoring this particular stream, the least of which was the inability to calculate the flow (how fast the water was moving). This presented no problem to the engineer in Earl, as he quickly took advantage of an existing weir, using a bucket and a stopwatch.

60

There are presently close to 60 volunteers monitoring the streams in Allegheny and surrounding counties. Earl's enthusiasm for this project has been evident as he has become a trainer for chemical testing, training other volunteers to monitor even more streams. Earl recognizes that the future of a healthy environment lies not in the hands of senior adults, but in the hands of young people. As a result, he and other volunteers will be working with schools in the coming months to show how pollution in one area can move through the aquifer and create problems in other areas.

When he talks about why he finds this program so important he will say: "To get a more comprehensive survey of the health of the state's waterways, the people must lend a hand. The job is too big. Many streams would go unmonitored because the state doesn't have the manpower to do the work."

Earl and the other volunteers are an example of how a senior center can be a conduit for volunteers to extend services to the larger community.

"EASY"

Her real name is Eloise, but 79 years ago her mother nicknamed her Easy because she was such a good baby. For the past 16 years she has been coming to Vintage, we've all known her as "Easy."

Like many senior centers, Vintage has created numerous questionnaires over the years in an attempt to find out why people come to Vintage and how they came to hear about us. Easy's story is both unique and amusing. Sixteen years ago, she had just retired from The Western Pennsylvania Hospital, and like many new retirees she wondered what she would do with all her free time. During a routine visit to West Penn Hospital for an x-ray, Easy began talking to another patient, Anne. Anne remarked that everyone seemed to know her and Easy explained that she had just retired from the hospital. As they continued their conversation, Anne told Easy about Vintage and all its great activities including her favorite card game, 500. Easy perked up when cards where mentioned and before they were taken away to get their x-rays, Easy had promised Anne she would go to Vintage the following Monday to join the 500 club. It wasn't long before she was playing cards at Vintage almost every day.

I remember when Vintage took a bus trip to Canada and the "card players" as we often called them, joined us. Before the bus pulled away from the curb, they were all set up and the card games were already underway. They played cards morning, noon, and night and when we arrived home, they all declared it had been a great trip. I often wonder if they saw much beyond the deck of cards. The card players were such an active group that when we moved into our new building, a room was set aside for their exclusive use.

Like many of the card players, Easy became and remains to this day a vital part of the volunteer force. She has assisted with blood pressure screenings in the wellness office, has worked in the kitchen, helped with home-delivered meals, served on the Advisory Board and, currently, works at the registration desk.

Her mother was right: "Easy" is easygoing, has a friendly hello for everyone, loves a good time, and continues to enjoy a good game of cards.

Activities are an essential part of life, and men and women benefit from physical and social activity at older ages. Those who continue to interact with others tend to be healthier, physically and mentally, than those who become socially isolated. Active recreation is vital to the promotion and maintenance of general health and wellness. It can reduce the risk of certain chronic diseases, relieve symptoms of depression, help to maintain independent living, and enhance overall quality of life.

A growing body of research in gerontology recognizes the importance of social engagement and productive activity as essential features of healthy aging. Participants in a variety of social, expressive, artistic, and nature-based activities demonstrated decreased loneliness and increased affiliation with others; increased verbal interaction; improved morale and life satisfaction; enhanced perceptions of personal control and competence; increased relaxation and ability to effectively manage stress; and reduced levels of depression. Social and productive activities lower the risk of death and are a complement to physical fitness activities. Senior centers that offer a broad range of activities and opportunities for social interaction can help to increase the quality and length of life of participants. Social interactions can provide emotional and practical support that enable older persons to remain in the community and reduce the likelihood that they will need formal health care services.

The relationship between recreation, disease prevention, and health promotion is substantiated by findings that recognize that light to moderate activity, typical of many recreational activities, can help prevent and manage many chronic diseases, including cardiovascular disease and high blood pressure. Research has shown that even among adults who are frail and very old, mobility and functioning can be improved through physical activity. Recreation also positively impacts mental health by reducing anxiety and stress and increasing self-esteem.

Activity can positively affect physical and emotional health, and inactivity is one of the major underlying causes of premature death. According to the National Center for Health Statistics, inactivity accounts for as many as 23% of all deaths from major chronic diseases. *Older Americans 2000: Key Indicators of Well-Being* reports that 34% of persons aged 65 or older had a sedentary lifestyle. Women were more likely than men to have a sedentary lifestyle. The percentage reporting social activities declines with age. By age 75, about one in three men and one in two women engage in no physical activity. The percentage reporting volunteer work in the past year also declines with age, from 20% among persons ages 70 to 74 to 7% among persons aged 85 or older.

The majority of persons aged 70 or older reported engaging in some form of social activity in the past 2 weeks. Interactions with family were the most common type of interaction reported. The most common types of exercise among older Americans were light to moderate activities such as walking, gardening, and stretching.

The benefits of active living include meeting new people, sleeping better, feeling more relaxed, and having more fun. In addition, regular physical activity can result in

- continued ability to remain independent
- better physical and mental health
- improved quality of life
- more energy
- improved self-esteem
- reduced stress
- healthier muscles, bones, and joints
- weight maintenance
- fewer aches and pains; less joint swelling and pain associated with arthritis
- better posture and balance
- fewer falls and fractured bones
- reduced risk for heart disease, high-blood pressure, adult-onset diabetes, stroke, osteoporosis, colon cancer, and premature death
- reduced symptoms of anxiety and depression and improvements in mood and feelings of well-being

In retirement, the individual has more time to fill. Meaningful leisure activities are vital to prevent boredom and isolation and provide a bridge between pre- and postretirement. Continuity in satisfying leisure activities helps to prevent and minimize the negative effects of physical and psychological aging. Senior centers provide lifelong learning programs and new opportunities for older persons in education, recreation, and the arts by encouraging learning and self-expression. Recreation preserves and maintains self-esteem, motivation, mobility, social interaction, and mental agility. Older adults who remain active are more likely to be satisfied with their lives than those who are inactive.

Cards and games, popular senior-center activities, are fun and cost-effective ways to facilitate and maintain cognitive, perceptual, and motor skills as well as a means to support social relationships. The card groups and chess and billiards players at Vintage have developed a camaraderie that extends well beyond the center's walls.

Many people have a competitive spirit and they enjoy events and activities that challenge them. Some of the most successful special events at Vintage have enabled participants to compete with one another and with other senior centers—the Bake-off, the Vintage 5K Masters Race and Walk, bowling and pool tournaments, spelling championship, talent shows, and juried art shows.

Retirees are looking for diverse experiences in their leisure time and experiential trips rather than spending their time relaxing, with obvious implications for providers of recreational activities, including senior centers. Like Elderhostel, senior centers need to provide high quality educational adventures that include field trips, engaging discussions, and expert instructors.

OUTDOOR RECREATION

Outdoor recreation is a component of physical fitness that can lead to a better quality of life physically, mentally, and socially. There is an increased recognition of the role that the immediate natural environment can play in relation to the well-being of older adults, through both aesthetic appeal and the presence of green space. Studies found that older adults considered nature to be very important, with resources such as nearby flower gardens, places to relax, places to watch wildlife, and nature trails being the most important outdoor settings. Parks are a valuable resource for a certain segment of the older adult population

A study of Cleveland metropolitan-area park-users who were 50 years of age and older found walking or hiking and relaxation as two commonplace activities in which older adults participated during their park visits. Results also indicate that older adults' use of parks drops off with age, particularly among individuals 75 years of age and older. People in this age bracket comprised only 2% of all park visitors. Visitation drops off with age for females more than it does for males, as fear of crime and a lack of companionship are two critical factors that limit older women's use of public parks. Women were significantly more likely than men to visit a park in the company of children; men were more likely to engage in self-directed activities, such as running or jogging.

Lifestyle trends influence how people recreate and how they use their leisure time. Adventure activities, including camping, hiking, scuba diving, white-water rafting, biking, and rock climbing have seen significant increases in the level of participation by women. Urban residents are more likely to participate in activities utilizing specialized facilities, such as city parks and recreational facilities, whereas rural residents are more likely to participate in activities associated with wilderness areas.

The aging of the baby boom generation is one of the most significant trends affecting outdoor recreation. Baby boomers are major participants in outdoor recreation and will have even more leisure time as they reach retirement. Although participation in outdoor activities declines and becomes more selective as one grows older, activities such as walking, birdwatching, and observing nature will continue to be popular.

Preserving the environment offers an opportunity that combines outdoor recreation with public service. The Environmental Alliance for Senior Involvement (EASI) is a national nonprofit coalition of senior, environmental, and volunteer organizations. EASI's mission is to encourage and develop opportunities for older Americans to apply their experiences and wisdom to the environmental challenges facing their communities. EASI's organizational tool is the Senior Environmental Corps, a model program being implemented in more than 35 states and 30 countries.

The Pennsylvania Senior Environment Corps was established in 1997 with the support of the Departments of Aging and Environmental Protection. More than 400 volunteers maintain a volunteer water-quality-monitoring program at 400 sites along Pennsylvania waterways. Training and evaluation are essential components of the program, ensuring that the monitoring experience is fun and productive for all involved. Volunteers also work with youth to inspire environmental stewardship, carry out public relations campaigns, and develop and implement restoration projects along waterways. Senior centers coordinate sites throughout the state. Vintage coordinates 36 volunteers at 16 sites in Allegheny County. In addition to their monitoring activities, the volunteers produce a bimonthly newsletter and engage in educational activities to inform the community about the monitoring program and why it is important. They are planning to work with youth as well, as their involvement is a key to the project's future success.

Senior centers need to consider including outdoor recreation opportunities for senior center participants. Departments of parks and recreation and other providers of outdoor recreation and senior centers can work together to expand the available options for older adults to participate in outdoor recreation, including the following:

1. Provide recreation programs with health and wellness objectives and that demonstrate or reinforce recreation, health, and wellness relationships.

2. Form partnerships and networks with providers of outdoor recreation to provide outdoor recreation opportunities for older adults.

3. Form partnerships and networks with institutions of higher learning, governments, private foundations, businesses, and health care organizations to exchange information and support research on the relationship of recreation, health, and wellness.

4. Promote the importance and increase public awareness of the value of recreation and the relationship of recreation, health, and wellness.

5. Provide opportunities for seniors to be involved in efforts to address environmental challenges in the community.

SUGGESTED ACTIVITIES

- Competitive activities such as cooking contests, sporting events, and juried art shows
- Championship games and tournaments at and between centers
- Holiday and historical celebrations
- High-quality educational adventures led by qualified experts
- Educational programs and activities involving wildlife, ecology, nature, and the environment

- Birdwatching, fishing, and wildlife-watching trips
- Water activities—rafting, float trips, kayaking, canoeing
- Hiking and biking programs

BIBLIOGRAPHY

Active Living Coalition for Older Adults. (2000). *Benefits of active living.* [On-line]. Available: www.alcoa.ca/e/whatis/exampl.htm

Federal Interagency Forum on Aging-Related Statistics. (2000). *Older Americans 2000: Key indicators of well-being.* Hyattsville, MD: Author.

Glass, T., deLeon, C., Marottoli, R., & Berkman, J. (1999). Population based study of social and productive activities as predictors of survival among elderly Americans. *British Medical Journal, 319,* 478–483.

National Recreation and Parks Association. (2000). *Policy on recreation and health.* [On-line]. Available: www.nrpa.org/branches/ntrs/rec&health.htm

National Center for Chronic Disease Prevention and Health Promotion. (2000). *Physical activity and health. A report of the surgeon general* Atlanta, GA: Author. [On-line]. Available: www.cdc.gov/nccdphp/sgr/olderad.htm

Pennsylvania Senior Environment Corps. (1999). *Environmental alliance for senior involvement. 1998–1999 annual report.* Harrisburg, PA: Author.

Pressley, R. (1997). *Therapeutic Recreation in an Elderly Persons Care Setting.* Health Studies at the Centre for Nurse Education, Hilary House, Prospect Hill Douglas, Manchester Metropolitan University.

Raymore, L., & Scott, D. (1998). The characteristics and activities of older adult visitors to a metropolitan park district. *Journal of Park and Recreation Administration, 16*(4), 1–21.

RESOURCES

Environmental Alliance for Senior Involvement
P.O. Box 250
Catlett, VA 20119-0250
540-788-3274
http://www.easi.org/
The mission of the Environmental Alliance for Senior Involvement is to build, promote, and utilize the environmental ethic, expertise, and commitment of older persons to expand citizen involvement in protecting and caring for our environment for present and future generations.

National Recreation and Parks Association
22377 Belmont Ridge Road
Ashburn, VA 20148
703-858-0784
http://www.nrpa.org.
The National Recreation and Parks Association's mission is to advance parks, recreation and environmental conservation efforts that enhance the quality of life for all people.

CHAPTER SIX

Lifelong Learning

ALBERT

As Albert prepares for his latest role in STAR, an intergenerational reading program, the huge hat he will be wearing as the villain in the story will surely get the attention of the students in the classroom if nothing else does. Albert loves the melodramatic. He also believes in the importance of education. "Former" teacher does not really apply when it comes to Albert. He is teaching something to someone everyday.

He is also taking advantage of increasing his knowledge whenever possible. All you need is to look at the stacks of papers in his car just waiting to be read, to know that Albert never throws anything away that may contain valuable information.

He came to Vintage in 1985. He has taught or been involved in more classes than then he or any of us can begin to remember. Most of his classes have to do with the humanities, the arts, or literature. Creative writing is a class he started over a dozen years ago, and the class still meets every Monday. His students respect him so much that they refer to him as "Professor." The group has published two literary books of poetry under his guidance. Albert is also very active in the drama group as well as being director of the Community Singers. He is the founder of the adult literacy group, which meets twice weekly at Vintage. Albert has been elected to and served four terms on the advisory board.

Albert is a fixture in the community as well. Many of the staff have seen him at the symphony or at the opening of an art show at a local gallery. It is not his being there that is unique or different, but that he is so well known in the community. I have often wondered how he has time for Vintage.

Some years ago he had open-heart surgery. Following his recovery he was back at Vintage and teaching all of his classes. I now know there are days when he isn't feeling well, but he will carry on without complaining. For him, the importance of his attending the adult literacy class far outweighs how he is feeling on any given day.

Much can be written of Albert and the many contributions he has made to Vintage, but when you stop and think for a moment about this man who is nearing 90, you realize something else about him. He always displays a sincere kindness for the underprivileged or those with some type of disability. Albert goes out of his way to befriend the person who seems to need it most. He has indeed left a legacy with Vintage. When someone asks, "Have you see Albert today?" that person can only be speaking about one Albert.

Education is an investment in the well-being of older adults because engagement in learning enhances quality of life, lessens dependency, and increases self-confidence and motivation. The capacity to learn is lifelong and older adults maintain a continuing desire to learn. Research indicates that individuals can retain 98% of mental capacity into their 80s as long as there is no physical deterioration. Reaction time and speed of learning may be slower for older adults but the ability to learn is not impaired by age. Positive, nurturing, and stimulating environments can foster continued development into old age. Stereotypes older people have about themselves ("I'm too old to learn") can be overcome by exposure to people who are active learners. Senior centers create the conditions under which lifelong learning can be nurtured and achieved.

INTERESTS OF OLDER ADULT LEARNERS

The needs and interests of the older adult learner provide a direction for planning educational programs. In the report from *Modern Maturity* magazine and the Roper Organization, *Mature America in the 1990s,* older adults identified the subjects they want to know more about:

- developments in health and medicine (44%)
- current events (39%)
- history (29%)
- music (24%)
- politics (23%)
- business world (20%)
- best-sellers (20%)
- art (16%)

In 2000, the American Association of Retired Persons (AARP) commissioned Harris Interactive Inc. to conduct a survey of adults 50 years and older, to explore how and why people over 50 learn about new things. More than 60% use newspapers, magazines, books, and journals when they want to learn, and these methods are used in greater proportions than all other learning methods. More than half of the older adults interviewed search the Internet to learn about something they want or need to know. Ninety percent said they learn best by watching, listening, and thinking, and by putting their hands on something and manipulating it or figuring it out. More than 90% agree they want to learn in order to keep up with what is going on in the world, for spiritual or personal growth, or to learn something new.

Older adults are most interested in learning about the subjects that would enrich the quality of their lives, build upon current skills, or enable them to take better care of themselves. In the AARP study, six topics generated the greatest interest: learning more about a favorite hobby or pastime (62%); learning more about advanced skills (52%); getting more enjoyment or pleasure out of life (51%); having a healthful diet and nutrition (49%); measuring personal health status (48%); and managing stress (46%).

Older adults prefer to learn in loosely structured groups, in workshop settings or by teaching themselves. Individual settings are preferred for learning about topics that are of direct personal benefit, including health-related subjects. More than half said they experienced at least one event that had a major impact on their life in the past year. Of those experiencing a major event, health-related and caregiving events had the greatest reported impact on their everyday lives. Older learners are eager to put what they learn into practice and want to have at least some control over the learning process. AARP study participants indicated they are willing to invest modest sums of money to learn, up to about $100.

Other reasons older adults enroll in classes include to meet interesting people, to be able to contribute to society, to improve one's social life, and to become more cultured.

Urban elders have different educational values than their rural counterparts. Both groups rate learning more things of interest first, but rural elders rate learning a practical skill, gaining an education, and contributing to society as more important while urban elders valued meeting new people, becoming more cultured, and gaining an education.

To help identify what older adults find meaningful, it is also useful to look at the needs of the older adult learner. Howard McCluskey contends that educational interests are needs driven for the older adult learner. These needs include the following:

- Coping needs—to deal with the changes and losses of age
- Expressive needs—arts, crafts, and music
- Altruistic needs—to contribute to others and the community
- Influence needs—the need to feel they are a master of their own fates
- Transcendence needs—the need to grow and develop

PRINCIPLES OF ADULT LEARNING AND EDUCATION

Andragogy is the art and science of helping adults learn. Understanding the principles of adult learning is essential for planning and implementing educational programs. In most circumstances, adults are not captive learners, and if the learning situation does not suit their needs and interests they will simply stop coming. In learner-centered instruction, learners are mutual partners in the learning endeavor. The use of learner-centered instruction addresses the needs and interests of learners and is an effective way to teach adults.

There appears to be no limit to the development of the human mind. Eduard Lindeman, who wrote *The Meaning of Adult Education* in 1926, identified several concepts that have been supported by later research and are the foundation of modern adult learning theory:

1. Adults are motivated to learn as they experience needs and interests that learning will satisfy.
2. Adult orientation to learning is life-centered.
3. Experience is the richest resource for adult learning.
4. Adults have a deep need to be self-directing.
5. Individual differences among people increase with age.

Effective instructors understand how adults learn best. Adults have special needs and requirements as learners. According to Malcolm Knowles, considered by many to be the father of adult education in the United States, a critical characteristic of adult learners is that they see themselves as capable of self-direction and they work best with teachers who see themselves as facilitators of learning. He identified the following characteristics of adult learners:

1. Adults are autonomous and self-directed. They learn best when they are actually involved in the learning process, are free to direct themselves, and take responsibility for their own learning. Teachers should treat adult students as peers—accepted and respected as intelligent experienced adults whose opinions are listened to, honored, appreciated. Students should work with their instructors to design individual learning programs that address their needs and wants. Teachers must get participants' perspectives about what topics to cover and let them work on projects that reflect their interests. Participants should be allowed to assume responsibility for presentations and group leadership. Educators must act as facilitators, guiding participants to their own knowledge rather than supplying them with facts. Teachers must show participants how the class will help them reach their goals. In some situations, learners may need direction because they do not have the requisite skills and knowledge to be self-directed or they may need support because they lack confidence or need help progressing from being a dependent to a self-directing learner.

2. Adults have a rich reservoir of experience that can serve as a resource for learning. They have accumulated a foundation of life experiences and knowledge that may include work-related activities, family responsibilities, and previous education. Educators need to connect learning to this knowledge and experience base and focus on the strengths learners bring to the classroom, not just gaps in their knowledge. Instructors should draw out participants' experience and knowledge relevant to the topic, relate theories and concepts to the participants, and provide opportunities for dialogue within the group. It is important to individualize learning, provide a wide range of subject options, and plan what, how, and when learning will occur. Peer helping, group discussion, field experience, and experiential techniques are important to adult learning.

3. Adults are goal-oriented. Upon enrolling in a course, they usually know what goal they want to attain. Adults appreciate an educational program that is organized and has clearly defined elements. Instructors must show participants how the class will help them attain their goals. This can be accomplished by using examples and anecdotes that show how other people have used the material.

4. Adults are relevancy-oriented. They must see a reason for learning something and the content must be meaningfully presented. Learning has to be applicable to their work or other responsibilities to be of value to them. Instructors must identify objectives for adult participants before the course begins. Theories and concepts must be related to a setting familiar to participants. Because adults' readiness to learn is frequently affected by their need to know or do something, they tend to have a life-, task-, or problem-centered orientation to learning as opposed to a subject-matter orientation.

5. Adults are practical, focusing on the aspects of a lesson most useful to them. They may not be interested in knowledge for its own sake. Instructors must tell participants explicitly how the lesson will be useful to them, specifying what procedures will be used to facilitate content acquisition.

Even though learners may need direction and support, they can still be involved in designing and directing their learning in meaningful ways. Information about the amount and type of direction that learners require can be obtained through a needs assessment. Adult learner involvement in assessing their needs and learning objectives initiates a partnership with the instructor or program director. Input from adult learners should be obtained before designing a course for them and they should evaluate the extent to which the objectives have been met.

Support for adult learners is provided through a learning environment that meets both their physical and psychological needs. Learning is enhanced when all energies can be devoted to the leaning situation. Senior centers must create an effective adult learning environment in which adults feel safe and challenged and intellectual freedom, experimentation, and creativity are encouraged. Students need to be involved actively in learning, as opposed to passively listening to lectures.

Older adult learners must be able to work at their own pace. Research indicates that older people need more time to receive and store incoming information. Response time can be improved with the right conditions. Any anxieties that learners might have about appearing foolish or exposing themselves to failure should be eased, but they should not feel so safe that they do not ask questions or are not challenged in other ways. Optimal pacing means challenging people just beyond their present level of ability. If challenged too far beyond that, people give up. An ideal adult-learning climate has a nonthreatening, nonjudgmental atmosphere in which adults are permitted and expected to share the responsibility for their learning.

Health-related problems and a decline in overall health status can also impact learning ability, including such problems as fatigue, reduced mobility, and declines in hearing or visual acuity. Hearing and vision loss decreases informational input that can affect perceived ability to learn and interact with others. There are ways of accommodating such limitations and it is important that the classroom environment compensate for visual or auditory impairments by combining audio and visual presentations of new material, good lighting, amplification, and elimination of distractions. Such problems can create barriers to learning or instructional success.

There is a need for a multicultural perspective on adult education, and curriculum development has to be sensitive to cultural and religious factors. Current theories of adult learning have been criticized for their lack of cultural understanding and the role that race, economics, and gender play in learning. Andragogy and self-directed learning focus heavily on the individual and do not recognize the value of groups, a concept preferred by some racial and ethnic groups. It is important to give voice to all people and groups about how and where they learn and their learning values.

Many older adults—especially women, the less affluent, members of minority communities, persons with disabilities, and the educationally disadvantaged—have not experienced support or equality in the learning environment. Engaging all learners as partners in the learning process requires that instructors consider their own attitudes toward, and knowledge about, the people they teach. Their expectations, behavior, and language may say something about the way they perceive the learners. Instructors must act on the belief that change and development are possible for all people and that their role is to assist the process in all learners. In order to be effective, senior center staff or volunteers who have little training in teaching older adults should participate in professional development activities related to adult learning theory and application. Senior centers need to collaborate with employers, educational institutions, and other organizations in order to develop and improve educational opportunities for older adults.

MULTIPLE INTELLIGENCES AND LEARNING STYLES

Using a variety of delivery methods and incorporating multiple intelligences facilitates learning and adds to the enjoyment of the educational program. The theory of multiple intelligences was developed by Dr. Howard Gardner, professor of education at Harvard University. Dr. Gardner proposes eight different intelligences to account for a broader range of human potential in children and adults. He identified the following distinct types of intelligence:

• *Linguistic*—Linguistic intelligence is the capacity to use language to express what's on your mind and to understand other people. A poet, writer, orator, speaker, lawyer, or person for whom language is important specializes in linguistic intelligence. People with this kind of intelligence enjoy oral communication, writing, reading, storytelling, or crossword puzzles. This learner is good at remembering names, places, and dates. Given an opportunity to hear, see, and say words associated with the desired outcome, they will learn practically anything of interest to them.

• *Logical-mathematical*—People with logical intelligence are interested in patterns, sequences, and relationships, arithmetic problems, reasoning, and strategy games. This learner likes to figure things out by asking questions, exploring, and experimenting and is usually good at math, logic, and problem solving. They learn best when provided with opportunities to classify, categorize, and work with abstractions and their relationship to one another. People with highly developed logical-mathematical intelligence understand the underlying principles of a causal system, the way a scientist or a logician does; or they can manipulate numbers, quantities, and operations the way a mathematician does.

• *Spatial*—Spatial intelligence refers to the ability to represent the spatial world internally in the mind; it can be used in the arts or in the sciences. These adults use mental imagery and pictorial presentations to learn. They enjoy drawing, designing, and looking at pictures, slides, videos, and films. They are likely to be proficient at imagining, sensing changes, doing puzzles, and reading charts and maps. Painters, sculptors, or architects are spatially intelligent in the arts, and certain sciences like anatomy or topology emphasize spatial intelligence.

• *Intrapersonal*—Intrapersonal learners are very aware of their own feelings and are self-motivated. They need time for reflection. This person really does better alone, pursuing self-defined interests. New information is absorbed best when projects are individual, self-paced, and singular-oriented. Intrapersonal intelligence refers to having an understanding of yourself, of knowing who you are, what you can do, what you want to do, how you react to things, which things to avoid, and which things to gravitate toward.

- *Interpersonal*—Interpersonal intelligence is understanding other people. Anybody who deals with other people (teachers, clinicians, salespersons, or politicians) has to be skilled in the interpersonal sphere. These are people who are joiners, always with a group of people and talking with friends, leaders among their peers, good at communicating, and who seem to understand others' feelings and motives. They like to learn through group interaction and support. They are skilled at organizing, mediating, communicating, and generally understanding people and how to work well with them. Impart new information to this person by giving opportunities to compare and contrast, interview others, share ideas, and cooperate to accomplish any given task.
- *Bodily-kinesthetic*—Bodily-kinesthetic intelligence is the capacity to use the whole body or parts of the body—hands, fingers, arms—to solve a problem, make something, or put on a production. These adults process knowledge through physical experience, bodily sensations and movement, learning by doing, and using the body to express ideas. They are often athletic, dancers, actors, or producers of a variety of crafts, such as sewing or woodworking. Learning here has to have a kinetic component; interacting with space in some way to process and remember the new information through the body. The most evident examples are people in athletics or the performing arts, particularly dance or acting.
- *Musical*—Musical intelligence is the capacity to think in music, to be able to hear patterns, recognize them, remember them, and perhaps manipulate them. Musical learners are always singing, humming, or tapping to themselves and are usually listening to music. They are aware of sounds others may miss and are good listeners. Musical learners get new information via melodies, musical notation, or rhythm.
- *Naturalistic*—Naturalistic intelligence has to do with observing, understanding, and organizing patterns in the natural environment, the ability to discriminate among living things (plants, animals), and a sensitivity to features of the natural world (clouds, rock configurations). This ability was clearly of value in our evolutionary past as hunters, gatherers, and farmers. This could be anyone from a molecular biologist, botanist, or chef to a traditional medicine man using

herbal remedies. Naturalistic learners would enjoy activities like drawing or photographing natural objects; nature hikes; gardening; caring for pets; visiting zoos, botanical gardens and museums of natural history; and bird watching.

A ninth intelligence, existential ability, is currently under consideration.

By the time people reach adulthood, they have settled into a learning style that works well for them. Individuals process, absorb, and remember new information in different ways. When material is presented in a way that complements a learner's preferred style, that individual will learn more readily and have a better chance of retaining what is learned.

Our culture focuses the most attention on linguistic and logical-mathematical intelligence. Equal attention must be given to individuals who show gifts in other intelligences, such as artists, musicians, naturalists, designers, and dancers. This has implications for adult learning and development as many adults find themselves in jobs that do not make optimal use of their most highly developed intelligences. Retirees have the opportunity to develop the potential they left behind in their youth (such as love for art or drama) through programs in self-development at the senior center.

It is not necessary to teach or learn something in all eight ways, just to see what the possibilities are and then decide which pathways seem to be the most effective for teaching or learning. The theory of multiple intelligences expands the horizon of available teaching and learning tools beyond the conventional linguistic and logical methods. Instructors should use a variety of teaching strategies and auditory, visual, tactile and participatory teaching methods. Learning results from stimulation of the senses. In some people, one sense is used more than others to learn or recall information. Instructors should present materials that stimulate as many senses as possible in order to increase their chances of teaching success.

Adults have barriers against participating in learning. Some of these barriers include lack of time, money, confidence, or interest; lack of information about opportunities to learn, scheduling problems, red tape, and problems with transportation. The best way to motivate adult learners is simply to enhance their reasons for enrolling and decrease the barriers.

Attrition is the number one problem in adult education. Studies have found the first few weeks, and especially the first class, are crucial to retaining student interest. One cause of early withdrawal is a gap between learner expectations and reality. Adult learners may get frustrated early by lack of progress or if they are not given enough information before enrollment to know what to expect from the class. Social integration helps to motivate students to persist and positively affects retention.

HELPING OLDER ADULTS LEARN

Four elements of learning must be addressed to ensure that participants learn.

1. *Motivation.* People learn best when they are highly motivated to learn. Adults are motivated more by intrinsic factors such as a desire for increased self-esteem, creative expression, or a better quality of life than by extrinsic factors such as grades. At least six factors serve as sources of motivation for adult learning:

- Social relationships: They want to make new friends or meet a need for associations.
- External expectations: They need to comply with the instructions, expectations or recommendations of someone with formal authority, such as a job requirement.
- Social welfare: They want to improve their ability to serve mankind and prepare for and participate in community service.
- Personal advancement: They want to achieve higher status in a job, advance professionally, and stay abreast of competitors.
- Escape or stimulation: They want to relieve boredom and provide a break in the daily routine.
- Cognitive interest: They want to learn for the sake of learning, or to satisfy an inquiring mind.

2. *Reinforcement.* Reinforcement is a very necessary part of the teaching and learning process; through it, instructors encourage correct modes of behavior and performance. Adults need immediate feedback concerning their progress and want to know how they are doing all along the way. They are not content to continue plugging away at course material without knowing whether they are on the right track. Both kinds of feedback are useful: recognition for work well done and guidance when improvement is needed. Regular feed-

back mechanisms must be in place for students to tell teachers what works best for them and what they want and need to learn.

3. *Retention.* Students must retain information from classes in order to benefit from the learning. If they do not learn the material well initially, they will not retain it. The instructor's job is not finished until the learner has been helped to retain the information. In order for participants to retain the information taught, they must see a meaning or purpose for that information. The must also understand and be able to interpret and apply the information.

4. *Transference.* The transfer of learning is the ability to use the information taught in the course in a new setting. Older adults want to be able to practice new skills immediately.

SUPPORTING THE OLDER ADULT LEARNER

Adult learners need as much, or even more, than their younger counterparts in the way of quality academic and student support. Without positive human connection, adult students are likely to become disaffected, no matter how technically excellent the program may be. It is important to build community among learners and support the older learner in learning activities by designing appropriate learning conditions:

• Provide personal attention, assistance and support to enhance the students ability to become self-directed.
• Design educational experiences with learning outcomes in mind.
• Use self-discovery techniques such as self-study kits, learning guides and study groups.
• Incorporate group work. Well-designed group work can contribute to the development of a collaborative, participative learning environment in which the instructor is perceived as a partner. Small group activities foster the development of positive peer relationships among learners, which frequently have a much greater influence on learning than teacher-learner relationships. The social environment created by small groups of peers also motivates adult learners to persist.
• Employ a teaching-learning process that includes a high degree of interaction among learners and between learners and teachers.

- Use multiple methods of instruction, including technology.
- Instructors need to be highly organized as this will help learners organize their learning efforts. Cueing devices such as headings, summaries, and visual images will enhance learning.
- Encourage learners to become involved in all aspects of the learning process.
- Encourage the older person to become more self-directed in selecting goals, learning approaches, and resources.
- Utilize instructional leadership from within the group of learners.
- Help learners relate new knowledge to their own experiences. Use concrete examples tied to past experiences.
- Recognize experience and work-based learning that already has been obtained.
- Identify participants' life and educational goals.
- Be flexible; break the traditional classroom routine. Deviating from the conventional practices associated with classrooms can help create an effective adult-learning environment. A potluck or snacks during a class break can create opportunities for interaction and break down barriers between instructors and learners. For classes that meet more than a few times, varying the meeting place can help add interest.
- Use humor, which can free creative capacities by providing novelty and helping learners break out of ruts. Humor can assist in building relationships among learners.
- Speed is a factor that works against the older student, so fast-paced drills and competitive exercises and activities may not be successful with the older learner.
- Minimize time pressures and allow learners to work at their own pace. Provide adequate time for response to questions.
- Move from easy to difficult material to promote success. Avoid sudden or drastic changes in content.
- Provide opportunities to succeed at something in every class meeting, including the first.
- Provide small amounts of information at a time. Summarize frequently to increase retention and recall.
- Plan frequent breaks.
- Individual differences among people increase with age. Take into account differences in style, time, types, and pace of learning.
- Use practice, repetition, case studies, problem-solving groups, and participatory activities to enhance learning.

- Positive reinforcement enhances learning.
- Differing needs, interests, and abilities will exist and change over time among older learners so instructors must be flexible; life stages and life changes will impact learning needs.
- Overcome barriers of time and place to ensure access to learning opportunities.

OLDER WOMEN LEARNERS

Older women have more expressive needs, more self-directed preferences, and are more heavily involved in learning than men and differ from older men as learners. They are more likely to study personal or self-fulfillment-type topics and are more likely to use reading and travel as educational resources.

Suggestions for enhancing older women's ways of learning include the following:

- Encourage older women to form autonomous learning and support groups.
- Provide older women, including older minority women, with opportunities to assume leadership roles.
- Enable and support older women as they develop their leadership skills and become more empowered.
- Develop mechanisms for more social interaction and networking among older women in leadership roles.
- Create places within senior centers where older women as learners can gather, obtain learning resources, and support each other.
- Develop individualized resources, create self-study materials, and establish appropriate learning settings to encourage self-directed learning.

LITERACY

Twenty four percent of older Americans have an eighth-grade education or less. A majority of persons aged 60 and older have limited skills in reading, using information from texts such as newspaper articles, filling out forms, following directions, and using schedules. Functional literacy skills are important to older adults, particularly for those older adults who are in the workplace. Many older workers would like to continue working but are handicapped by a lack of training opportunities to meet the demands of America's changing job market. This is particularly true of older minorities and those with limited English-speaking skills.

As information and technology increasingly shape our society, the skills we need to function successfully have gone beyond reading. The Workforce Investment Act of 1998 defines literacy as "an individual's ability to read, write, speak in English, compute and solve problems at levels of proficiency necessary to function on the job, in the family of the individual and in society." When *literacy* was simply a synonym for *reading skill*, it was typically measured in grade-level equivalents. In other words, an adult's literacy skill was described as equivalent to reading at a level keyed to the kindergarten–12th grade system.

To determine the literacy skills of American adults, the 1992 National Adult Literacy Survey (NALS) used test items that resembled everyday life tasks involving prose and quantitative skills. The NALS classified the results into five levels that are now commonly used to describe adults literacy skills. Almost all adults in level 1 can read a little but not well enough to fill out an application, read a food label, or read a simple story to a child. Adults in level 2 usually can perform more complex tasks such as comparing, contrasting, or integrating pieces of information but usually not higher-level reading and problem-solving skills. Adults in levels 3 through 5 usually can perform the same types of more complex tasks on increasingly lengthy and dense texts and documents.

Very few adults in the U.S. are truly illiterate. Rather, there are many adults with low literacy skills who lack the foundation they need to find and keep decent jobs, support their children's education, and participate actively in civic life. According to the National Adult Literacy Survey (NALS), between 21% and 23% of the adult population, or approximately 44 million people scored at level 1. Another 25% to 28% of the adult population, or between 45 and 50 million people, scored at level 2. Literacy experts believe that adults with skills at levels 1 and 2 lack a sufficient foundation of basic skills to function successfully in our society.

Many factors help to explain the relatively large number of adults in level 1. Twenty-five percent of adults in level 1 were immigrants who may have just been learning to speak English. More than 60% didn't complete high school; more than 30% were over 65; more than 25% had physical or mental conditions that kept them from fully participating in work, school, housework, or other activities; and almost 20% had vision problems that affected their ability to read print.

Older Americans with literacy needs should have access to services that can help them gain the basic skills necessary for success in the workplace, family, and community. As a non-threatening location, senior centers can partner with literacy organizations on projects to make literacy programs more relevant and more widely available to older adults.

THE OLDER LANGUAGE LEARNER

Research shows that older adults can successfully learn foreign languages. There is no decline in the ability to learn as people get older, and except for minor considerations such as hearing and vision loss, the age of the adult learner is not a major factor in language acquisition. The context in which adults learn is the major influence on their ability to acquire the new language. The difficulties older adults often experience in the language classroom can be overcome through adjustments in the learning environment, attention to affective factors, and use of effective teaching methods.

English classes offer older immigrants the opportunity to decrease their isolation and facilitate their access to services and community activities. Studies of aged second-language learners have established that the right physical and learning environment can compensate for physiological and sociocultural variables such as perceptual acuity, psychomotor coordination, and language-memory that are likely to affect their performance and progress. Recommendations include highly contextualized language relevant to the learners' experiences, concrete tasks, multisensorial methods, recycling of content at increasingly difficult levels, and optimal physical conditions. Learner anxiety can be reduced by creating supportive relationships within the class, slowing the pace of instruction, putting the emphasis on receptive rather than productive skills, downplaying the role and formality of assessments, and providing a comfortable learning environment.

The greatest obstacle to older-adult language-learning is the doubt—in the minds of both learner and teacher—that older adults can learn a new language. Most people assume that "the younger the better" applies in language learning. However, many studies have shown that this is not true. Studies comparing the rate of second-language acquisition in children and adults have shown that although children may have an advantage in achieving nativelike fluency in the long run, adults actually learn languages more quickly than children in the early stages. Studies indicate that attaining a working ability to communicate in a new language may actually be easier and more rapid for the adult than for the child.

Factors such as motivation and self-confidence are very important in language learning. Many older learners fear failure more than their younger counterparts, maybe because they accept the stereotype of the older person as a poor language-learner or because of previous unsuccessful attempts to learn a foreign language. When such learners are faced with a stressful, fast-paced learning situation, fear of failure only increases. The older person may also exhibit greater hesitancy in learning. Thus, teachers must be able to reduce anxiety and build self-confidence in the learner.

Small classes of around 10 students in a quiet and pleasant environment that is close to learners and their community are recommended for English-language classes. Nonthreatening learning conditions, access to information technologies, and appropriate teaching methodology provide the conditions needed for learning. Students of all ages and backgrounds learn English fast and well in classes where they feel safe, where lessons are focused on current language needs, where students are asked for input on what helps them most to learn, where they are actively involved in interesting and fun exercises, and where there's lots of laughter and congeniality. In classes where students are made to feel inadequate and threatened, little is learned.

Class activities that include frequent oral repetition, extensive pronunciation correction, or an expectation of error-free speech will inhibit the older learner's active participation. On the other hand, providing opportunities for learners to work together, focusing on understanding rather than producing language, and reducing the focus on correcting errors can build learners' self-confidence and promote language learning.

Older adults studying a foreign language are usually learning it for a specific purpose. They are not willing to tolerate boring or irrelevant content or lessons that stress the learning of grammar rules out of context. Adult learners need materials designed to present structures and vocabulary that will be of immediate use to them, in a context that reflects the situations and functions they will encounter when using the new language. Materials and activities must incorporate real-life experiences to succeed with older learners.

An approach that stresses the development of the receptive skills (particularly listening) before the productive skills may have much to offer the older learner. According to research, effective adult-language-training programs are those that use materials that provide an interesting and comprehensible message, delay speaking practice and emphasize the development of listening comprehension, tolerate speech errors in the classroom, and include aspects of culture and nonverbal language use in the instructional program. This creates a classroom atmosphere that supports the learner and builds confidence.

LIFELONG LEARNING AND LIFELONG WORKING

Increased longevity has transformed the traditional life pattern of school, work, raise a family, retire. A more cyclic life plan is taking shape as people change careers and intersperse them with creative breaks and retraining. With the speed of technological innovation, worker's skills become obsolete much faster. Today's workers are also more likely to change jobs many times in their careers. Full-time work may be interspersed with periods of flexible working arrangements such as part-time, seasonal, occasional, and project work. This has created the need for adult basic education, literacy, English as a second language, training and retraining programs for older adults, personal enrichment through the arts, and volunteer training, all of which reduce unnecessary dependency on the part of older persons. As the need to continuously upgrade skills becomes a requirement, senior-center educational programs can help meet this need.

In the future, a declining birthrate may result in a shortage of skilled and knowledgeable employees. Increasing demands for work force productivity, a projected shortage of skilled and experienced workers, and older adults who are healthier and living longer are powerful forces that will shape employment in the future. Retirement as a permanent separation from the workplace is being replaced with the idea of bridge employment. *Bridging* is a form of partial retirement in which an older worker alternates periods of disengagement from the workplace with periods of temporary, part-time, occasional, or self-employed work at a job other than a career job. Work provides income, status, personal achievement, structure to the day, and opportunities for interpersonal relationships. Bridging allows older workers to "practice" retirement, to fill labor market shortages, or to try a variety of other occupational positions.

The American Association of Retired Persons conducted a working life survey of workers aged 50-plus who had returned to the workplace after an initial period of retirement. The three most frequently cited reasons for returning to work were financial need, liking to work, and keeping busy. "Liking to work" included feeling successful, enjoying the excitement of the workplace, and making a contribution. "Keeping busy" included working with a spouse, staying healthy, or fulfilling a social need. In a 2000 study by Stein, Rocco, and Goldenetz, older workers mentioned not planning wisely, the need to contribute, appreciation from others, and the desire to create something as reasons for not retiring from the workplace.

Employers need to change the attitudes and expectations of managers and younger employees toward an increasing number of older workers and to reengineer the work environment to account for physiological changes due to aging. Education and job redesign are the means by which older workers can enter, reenter, and advance in the workplace, which can be a dynamic place for older workers rather than a one-way path leading to retirement. These work-choice patterns will challenge employers to provide a workplace that embraces older workers as capable, productive, and knowledgeable lifelong workers. Older workers will need organizational and social supports and career guidance to make the transition to part-time work, returning from periods of retirement, or leaving the work force. Senior centers can take advantage of the opportunity to work with educational institutions and employers to counsel, train, retrain, and prepare older workers for life and career transition.

SUGGESTED ACTIVITIES

Classes in the areas of

- adult literacy
- English as a second language
- foreign languages
- conversational foreign language for travel
- workplace development skills
- sign language
- personal development, including such topics as Feng Shui (the ancient Chinese art of harmoniously arranging living and working

spaces to enhance well-being), qi energy (the body's life force), and visual journaling
• social activism
• mentoring

BIBLIOGRAPHY

American Association of Retired Persons. (2000). *AARP survey on lifelong learning—Executive summary*. [On-line]. Available: www.research.aarp.org/general/lifelong_1.html

American Association of Retired Persons. (1992). *Mature America in the 1990s. A special report from Modern Maturity Magazine and the Roper Organization*. Washington, DC: Author.

Armstrong, T. (1993). *7 Kinds of smart: Identifying and developing your many intelligences*. New York: Plume.

Billington, D. D. (2000). Seven characteristics of highly effective adult learning programs. *New Horizons for Learning*. [On-line]. Available: www.newhorizons.org

Campbell, B. (2000). *The naturalistic intelligence*. [On-line]. Available: www.newhorizons.org/article_eightintel.html

Council for Adult and Experiential Learning. (2000). *Serving adult learners in higher education. Principles of effectiveness. Executive summary*. Chicago: Author.

Daniel, D. E., & Templin, R. (1977). The value orientation of old adults toward education. *Educational Gerontology, 2*(1), 39.

Dickinson, D. (1991). *Positive trends in learning: Meeting the needs of a rapidly changing world*. Commissioned and printed by IBM.

Dychtwald, K. (1990). *Age wave*. New York: Bantam Books.

Dyhtwald, K. (1999). *Age power. How the 21st century will be ruled by the new old*. New York: Tarcher/Putnam.

Gardner, H. (1993). *Multiple intelligences: The theory in practice*. New York: Basic Books.

Hiemstra, R. (1993, April 1). *Older women's ways of learning: Tapping the full potential*. Paper presented at the conference entitled The Enduring Spirit: Woman as They Age. Omaha: University of Nebraska at Omaha.

Imel, S. (1994). Guidelines for working with adult learners. *ERIC Digest No. 154*. [On-line]. Available at ericacve.org

Kerka, S. (1995). Adult learner retention revisited. *ERIC Digest No. 166*. [On-line]. Available at ericacve.org

McClusky, H. (1974). Education for aging. *Learning for aging*. Washington, DC: Adult Education Association.

National Council on the Aging. *NCOA's 1999–2000 Public Policy Agenda*. Washington, DC: Author. [On-line]. Available at www.ncoa.org

The National Institute for Literacy. (2001). *Frequently asked questions*. Washington, DC: Author. [On-line]. Available at www.nifl.gov/nifl/faqs.html#literacy

Rowland, M. L. (2000). African Americans and self-help education: The missing link in adult education. *ERIC Digest No. 222*. [On-line]. Available at ericacve.org

Schleppergell, M. (1987). The older language learner. *ERIC:ED287313.* [On-line]. Available at ericacve.org

Stein, D., Rocco, T. S., & Goldenetz, K. A. (2000). Age and the university workplace. A case study of remaining, retiring, or returning older workers. *Human Resource Development Quarterly, 11*(1), 61–80.

Stein, D. (2000). The new meaning of retirement. *ERIC Digest No. 215.* [On-line]. Available at ericacve.org

Winters, E. *Seven styles of learning. The part they play when developing interactivity.* [On-line]. Available at www.bena.com/ewinters/styles.html

Yenerall, J. (1996). *The educational values and interests of older students: Consensus and variation.* Pittsburgh, PA: Duquesne University.

RESOURCES

Council for Adult and Experiential Learning
55 East Monroe, Suite 1930
Chicago, IL 0603
312-499-2600
http://www.cael.org
The Council for Adult and Experiential Learning is a national, non-profit organization and leader in pioneering strategies to advance life-long learning.

Educational Resources Information Center (ERIC)
Clearinghouse on Adult, Career, and Vocational Education
Center on Education and Training for Employment, College of Education
The Ohio State University
1900 Kenny Road
Columbus, OH 43210-1090
614-292-7069 or 800-LET-ERIC
http://ericacve.org
ERIC, a national education information network, is part of the National Library of Education, U.S. Department of Education. The goal of ERIC is to identify, select, process, and disseminate information in education.

Harvard Project Zero
Graduate School of Education
124 Mount Auburn Street, Fifth Floor
Cambridge, MA 02138
617-496-7097

http://pzweb.harvard.edu/
Project Zero's mission is to understand and enhance learning, thinking, and creativity in the arts, as well as humanistic and scientific disciplines, at the individual and institutional levels.

National Institute for Literacy
1775 I Street NW, Suite 730
Washington, DC 20006-2401
Phone: 202-233-2025
http://www.nifl.gov/
The National Institute for Literacy is an independent federal organization leading the national effort toward a fully literate nation in the 21st century.

CHAPTER SEVEN

Creativity

DOROTHY

Sometimes the nicest things happen to the nicest people and that surely is true with Dorothy. I first met her when she stopped in at Vintage at the YW, a satellite site at the YWCA in downtown Pittsburgh. She and her husband were interested in taking a trip with us. I remember that she reminded me of the actress Jessica Tandy. Dorothy had a slight build and her white hair was pulled back. She was somewhat reserved, but always very friendly. I learned later that she had graduated from college with a degree in chemistry. She had worked during World War II, but following the war had married and remained at home to raise their children.

In the early 1990s Vintage founded the Pennsylvania Spelling Championship for Older Adults. We had heard about this happening in other states and decided to try it in Pennsylvania. The participants needed to compete first at the local level (a senior center), followed by the countywide competition, and finally the state competition. Dorothy easily won the local and county competition and moved on to the state competition that was held at Vintage. There were 13 other spellers and they were all very good. The competition lasted well over 2 hours and finally we were down to two spellers, Dorothy and another woman. You could have heard a pin drop as the two contestants went back and forth. Finally, Dorothy won by spelling a misspelled word correctly and a second word correctly. Everyone declared the event a success, and we all went off to celebrate on the Gateway Clipper, a riverboat in our city. I suppose one might say this was a very special happening in Dorothy's life, but it didn't end that evening. A freelance writer for the Wall Street Journal *read about the competition in our local paper and she interviewed Dorothy. Shortly thereafter the article appeared on the front page of the* Journal. *The producers of the David Letterman show read the* Journal, *and within a couple of days they were on the phone asking Dorothy to come to New York to be on the show. Much conversation followed and Dorothy was somewhat uncertain but also excited about the idea. She finally agreed and before we knew it Dorothy, her husband Charles, and I were off to New York. Dorothy had never watched Letterman before, and when she did her comment was, "Oh my!"*

On the day of the show Dorothy was very nervous and Charles was nervous for her. We finally got her to eat a little sherbet before we were picked up and taken to the studio in a limousine. Charles and I waited in the green room while Dorothy charmed David on stage. Far too quickly, Dorothy's part was over and we were flying back to Pittsburgh. Charles said it best when he remarked how very wonderful all this had been for her. He told me that for years she had stayed at home taking care of the children while he was finding success in his career. He said that it was now Dorothy's time to shine.

Creativity has been described as a complex of traits, skills, and capacities, including the ability to work autonomously, curiosity, unconventional thinking, openness to experience, and tolerance of ambiguity. There are a number of misconceptions about creativity: that it is limited to only a few, declines seriously with age, and is associated primarily with uniqueness or innovation or artists. However, research shows that creative thinking is a universal ability that does not decline with age and it is increasingly in demand in the workplace.

Psychologists have been studying the creative lives of older people and how creativity can enhance the aging process. In a range of studies, they've found that being creative can add richness to the aging process. Those who followed their creative passions throughout life are more likely to be happier and satisfied. Creative people keep evolving as they age and many creative people develop new creative styles in old age.

Creative activity is correlated with psychological and physical well-being. Creative expression fosters positive feelings that prompt a positive outlook and a sense of well-being. Artists who remained creative into old age suggest that involvement in creative activity had a positive, therapeutic effect on their lives. Creativity can contribute to productivity and invention.

Learning, tapping into one's potential, and creativity continue independently of age, but many older people first experience an awakening of their creative capacity only in later life. Many retirees tap into old skills and interests they neglected while they were working and raising a family; others learn new skills. The capacities and creative accomplishments of new cohorts of older adults are surpassing earlier older cohorts, because older adults today are physically aging far better than earlier older cohorts, and they are better educated.

Research on adult creativity typically depicts a bell curve, with a peak in the 30s and 40s and a noticeable drop afterward, which leads to stereotypes of decline and deterioration in later life. Such views limit expectations about what is possible in later life and inhibit motivation for seeking novel experiences or new approaches for problem solving. There are numerous exceptions and variations and the quantity of creative output may decline, but not the quality. Individual differences in creative potential outweigh age differences as some adults attain creative peaks at later ages. In one study, more than half of the participants started their most creative period around age 50, some after retirement. Late-life creativity reflects aspects of late-life thinking: synthesis, reflection, and wisdom.

Negative perceptions and stereotypes about aging are so pervasive that even experts in a given field fail to develop an accurate picture of the potential for their own members as those members age. New research into the capacity for learning and creative development in the second half of life has shown that when the mind is challenged, the brain biologically responds in positive ways, regardless of age. The brain responds physically and chemically to environmental challenge. Brain cells involved in thinking and memory communicate with one another in two fundamental ways: through branchlike extensions known as dendrites and through the release of chemical messengers between the branches. Science has shown that a stimulating environment results in the sprouting of new dendritic branches by individual brain cells and an increased production within the brain of acetylcholine, the chemical messenger most involved in memory and thinking functions. The latest research reveal that from an individual's early 50s through late 70s, there is actually an increase in the length and extent of the dendritic branches, which compensates for brain-cell loss that can occur over time.

A recent study at the University of Nebraska-Lincoln found that thinking and acting creatively can help people adapt to the aging process and find meaning in life. Study participants included a mix of nonartists and artists ages 60 and older. Participants said that being creative enhanced their life satisfaction and made their old age more successful and enjoyable. In addition, the study found that creativity can lead to greater cognitive flexibility. Sixty percent of the study participants said they've become even more creative as they've gotten older. Of the remaining 40%, half said they'd remained consistently creative throughout their lives. If people exercise creativity throughout their lives, it should be no different in old age. People with creative potential keep on creating even in old age.

Dean Keith Simonton, PhD, professor of psychology at the University of California-Davis, has studied the career trajectories of composers, writers, and artists. Simonton found that creativity does not decline with age, though it may change in form as creative people often change strategies in old age.

Erik Erikson described a "summing up" phase that typically occurs in one's 70s and 80s, characterized by a looking back and summing up of one's life. The process helps one appreciate what has been gained in life, leading one to want to give back. "Giving back" is reflected in increased sharing of the lessons from life experience through storytelling and autobiography, which noticeably increase in frequency in later life. Volunteerism and philanthropy, both of which weigh in strongly in later life, also reflect this desire to give back. The summing-up process can also result in an accounting of unfulfilled dreams and unfinished business that can lead to a new creative burst to complete a missing chapter in one's life story. The potential is there, but it needs to be recognized and nurtured.

The increased tendency to want to sum up one's life work, ideas, and discoveries and to share them with one's family or society is seen with increasing age and across all fields of human endeavor. The desire to do it late in life is driven by varied feelings—wanting to complete one's life work, needing to give back after having received much in life, sensing that there may not be much time left. Opportunities for creative sharing and expression can result. For example, autobiography becomes one of the most enduring ways of passing on knowledge about an area to the next generation. Leaders in virtually all fields have shown a tendency to write or convey their autobiographies in their later years. Autobiography builds upon the natural tendency with aging to reminisce and elaborate on personal stories. Such expression can be in oral, written, or visual form.

Related to the process of summing up late in life is that of the swan song, the last act or final creative work of a person before retirement or death. The swan song reflects a creative late-life developmental pressure to make a final statement in life, through expression or action.

Gene Cohen describes creativity as "empowering . . . the energy that allows us to think a different thought, express ourselves in a novel way . . . to view life as an opportunity for exploration, discovery, and an expanding sense of self." Cohen describes four developmental phases that shape the way creative energy develops and the way it is expressed in the later years. There can be significant variation in the timing, duration, sequence, and expression of each phase. Each phase is defined by a combination of chronological age, history, and circumstances.

1. *Reevaluation phase.* Creative expression is intensified by a sense of crisis or quest as adults search for ways to make their life and work more gratifying and meaningful.

2. *Liberation phase.* In this phase, typically from a person's 60s to their 70s, creative endeavors are charged with the added energy of a new degree of personal freedom that comes psychologically from within and from a change from full-time to retirement or part-time work. People tend to feel comfortable about themselves by this stage, knowing that if they make a mistake it won't undo the image others have of them and, more important, won't undo their image of themselves. Creative expression in this phase often includes translating a feeling of "if not now, when?" into action. This provides a new context for experimentation, which is liberating and adds to the richness of life.

3. *Summing-Up phase.* In this phase, from the 70s on, older people desire to find a larger meaning in their lives through a process of looking back, summing up, and contributing back whatever was gained in wisdom and wealth. Creative expression in this phase often includes autobiography and personal storytelling, philanthropy, community activism, and volunteerism.

4. *Encore phase.* This phase, featuring adults 80 years or older, reflects the energy of advancing age, in which creative expression is shaped by the desire to make further contributions on a personal or community level: to affirm life, to take care of unfinished business, and to celebrate one's place in family, community, and even in the spiritual realm.

Cohen believes that awareness of these phases can help close the gap between recognizing one's potential and harnessing it and increase an individual's incentive to work at seizing the moment. These phases can set the stage for the creative expression that commences in the second half of life; they can precipitate a change in the direction of one's creative expression; they can provide new energy to promote a continuation of one's ongoing creative work; and they can enable one to become creative in response to loss.

Research on aging has shown that in middle age, a profound experiential event typically occurs. For the first time, one begins to think about how much time is left, as opposed to how much time has gone by. When individuals begin to contemplate the concept of their own mortality, angst can result. Such angst can lead to crisis—as in "midlife crisis"—or it can be transformed into a quest to reevaluate one's life. Either crisis or quest can lead to tapping into unknown human potential in the second half of life and unleash new creative expression that affirms life.

For many, retirement provides more free time for trying new things and pursuing creative endeavors. The downside of retirement historically has been overemphasized with negative myths. Research shows that those at risk for not doing well in retirement are individuals who typically do not want to retire or who are forced to do so because of poor health, or who experience a significant decline in their style of living because of reduced social and economic supports. Most people do fine in retirement, and most have the opportunity for new creative endeavors as a result of retirement's liberating qualities. The feeling of freedom allows older individuals to experiment, to take a risk, to try something new. By age 65, people are comfortable with themselves. If they make a mistake while trying something new, it will not change who they are or how they appear to other people. Hence, older people are less concerned with looking stupid and may even be more receptive to personal experimentation. When risk-taking is appropriate and the potential outcomes of taking a risk are important, studies show that older adults can be just as venturesome as their younger counterparts. The combined, liberating experience of having more time and an increased sense of freedom enhances creativity in later life.

Creativity research has focused on the personality traits of creative individuals. This emphasis has led to the assumptions that creativity is largely innate and creative people are distinct from noncreative people. Recently, more attention is being paid to social, cultural, and environmental factors that influence creativity. Newer definitions describe creativity as the confluence of cognitive processes, education, thinking style, personality, motivation, and social and environmental influences over the life span. For some people, creativity is an outlet, an innovative response to distress such as the death of a loved one, whereas in other people the coping mechanisms might be substance abuse, depression, or withdrawal.

Environmental factors affect the creativity of men and women in different ways. For many women, creative expression is limited by their education and training, culture, lack of social support, family-related chores, gender discrimination, and traditional gender expectations. As parents, men preserve a space of their own but women cede this space to family demands. Social environment, role models, and cultural values, attitudes, and practices also inhibit or nurture creative impulses. Creativity is also inhibited by working under surveillance, restrictive choices, working for inappropriate extrinsic rewards; fear of failure, judgment, or appearing foolish; having to find the "right answer"; being evaluated, working under time pressure, and competing. Cognitive, sensory, or physical impairments may hinder creative expression.

Five levels of creativity have been described. The first three levels of creativity can be attained with motivation and persistence. The last two may be unattainable to all but the inspired or the naturally creative genius.

1.   The first level, primitive and intuitive expression, incorporates the primitive and intuitive expression found in children and in adults who have not been trained in art. The artist creates for the joy of it.

2.   The second level of creativity is the academic and technical level. At this level the artist learns skills and techniques and develops creative expression.

3.   Level 3 is the inventive level. Many artists experiment with their craft, exploring different ways of using familiar tools and medium, becoming increasingly adventurous and experimental.

4.   At the level of innovation, the artist, writer, musician, inventor, thinker is more original. Materials and methods that are extra-ordinary are introduced.

5.   The fifth level of creativity is characterized as genius, individuals whose ideas and accomplishments in art and science defy explanation. It may be the one level of creativity that an individual is born with.

ENHANCING OLDER ADULTS' CREATIVE POTENTIAL

Creativity can be nurtured or heightened as everyone is, or has the potential to be, creative. Senior centers can help older people develop their creative potential and identify and provide recognition for the creative work or ideas of older persons. The Mannsman's Gallery at Vintage is a small gallery dedicated to the artwork of older adults. Six shows are curated each year and have included watercolor, quilting, woodcarving, oil painting, and poetry exhibits to name just a few. Each show begins with an opening celebration.

The organizational climate of the senior center should facilitate the creative process by

- providing the right environment
- providing opportunities to create
- encouraging ideas
- providing challenges
- helping older adults not to be afraid to fail
- providing time and resources
- developing expertise
- providing positive, constructive feedback
- encouraging a spirit of play and experimentation
- providing opportunities for group interaction
- providing a safe place for risk-taking
- offering rewards that recognize achievement
- providing opportunities for brainstorming ideas
- helping older adults develop thinking patterns to create new ideas
- stimulating all of the senses
- providing opportunities to recognize and display the creative work of older people

BIBLIOGRAPHY

Adams-Price, C. E. (Ed.). (1998). *Creativity and successful aging.* New York: Springer.

Cohen, G. D. (1999, November). Aging and peaking. *American Journal of Geriatric Psychiatry, 7,* 275–278.

Cohen, G. D. (1999, May). The aging brain vs. the aging body. *American Journal of Geriatric Psychiatry, 7,* 93–95.

Cohen, G. D. (1998, August). The magic bullets are blanks. Purported shortcuts to improving the aging mind. *American Journal of Geriatric Psychiatry, 6,* 185–195.

Cohen, G. (2000, March/April). C = ME2. *Modern Maturity.* [On-line]. Available: www.aarp.org/mmaturity/mar-apr00/equation.html

Cohen, G. D. (2001, February). The course of unfulfilled dreams and unfinished business with aging. *American Journal of Geriatric Psychiatry, 9,* 1–5.

Kerka, S. (1999). Creativity in adulthood. *ERIC Digest No. 204.* [On-line]. Available: ericacve.org

Margoshes, P. (1995, May). Creative spark lives on, can increase with age. *APA Monitor*. [On-line]. Available: www.apa.org/http://www.apa.org//cgi-bin/ wais2_monitor.pl/cgi-bin/wais2 _monitor.pl

Taylor, A. (1959). The nature of creative process. In P. Smith (Ed.), *Creativity*. New York: Hastings House.

RESOURCES

The Creativity Discovery Corps
Center on Aging, Health & Humanities
The George Washington University Medical Center
10225 Montgomery Avenue
Kensington, MD 20895
202-895-0230
The Creativity Discovery Corps disseminate the best practices of programs, groups, and individuals in the community who provide creative opportunities for older persons.

PART FOUR

Activities

CHAPTER EIGHT

The Arts and Aging

PAULINE

At one time in the history of Vintage we hosted the Vintage Craft and Gift Showcase. This event gave senior adults an opportunity to sell homemade crafts and to be part of a juried show. Each participant in the showcase was required to enter at least one item in the juried show. Categories ranged from woodcrafts to needlework. The day before the opening of the juried event, the participants would bring their items labeled with their name and, if the item was for sale, the cost of the item. With well over 100 artists, one can only imagine the task that lay ahead for staff and volunteers, in light of the 24-hour deadline until the judges arrived to jury the show.

Enter Pauline. Pauline had been coming to Vintage for about 10 years at the time of the showcase. A retired milliner from a major downtown department store, Pauline was very active in the watercolor and oil-painting classes at Vintage. When she heard about the Vintage Craft and Showcase she immediately volunteered to help with the setup. Pauline had such an eye for color and design that I often wonder how we would have ever gotten along without her. While the rest of the staff and volunteers piled items on the tables by category (wood, painting, crafts), Pauline was busy pulling out browns, oranges, and greens for a fall display. When it came to the actual setup, Pauline could make even the most unattractive item take on a pleasing appearance, as she found just the right angle or special way to display it. As I watched her at work it was easy to imagine her as a milliner, matching a feather or flower on a made-to-order hat for someone in Pittsburgh.

Pauline still comes to Vintage to take part in the watercolor class, which meets every Thursday. Age has slowed her walk, but certainly not her creative spirit. The current teacher, Nicole, is a young artist. Nicole will tell you how much the senior adults have taught her, while at the same time the students, including Pauline, have grown immeasurably under her guidance. Nicole recently opened her own art gallery. In the spring of 2002, the Vintage watercolor class, along with other senior artists in the Pittsburgh area, will have their own show in her gallery.

Just as Pauline's lovely royal-blue beret is a perfect match for her eyes, so has Pauline been a perfect match for Vintage. We have been the beneficiaries of her immense talent while she has had an opportunity to develop and expand her creative potential.

MICHAEL

According to the dictionary, a prima donna is an extremely sensitive, vain, and undisciplined person. Michael is a prima donna. I have known him for almost 15 years and it can be said that no participant can play the piano like Michael. He has played for more receptions and programs than any of us can remember, and as an agency we are grateful for his willingness to share his talent and music with us.

When Michael first came to Vintage, he was with a much older woman named Josephine, who was the founder and director of the theater group. They were of mixed race, and she was legally blind. Michael was, at least in part, her caregiver. For Michael she was a surrogate mother and she kept him "in line." Although they did not live together, she had purchased a car for him and he became her chauffeur. I have no idea how they met, although one could suppose her interest in the theater and his musical ability had something to do with it. Josephine had other members in her theater group, but Michael was clearly the favorite. He often composed original songs for her productions. Together they were a team who expected special favors from time to time from Vintage staff. This led to minor irritations, which quickly blew over.

Michael and Josephine would also have disagreements and Michael would come storming into Vintage announcing he was finished with her. The next day they would arrive together at the center and life would go on until the next falling out.

Josephine's health began to deteriorate in the early 1990s, and when she died Michael was without the anchor she provided and the privileges that came with being her caregiver. Michael continued to come to Vintage every day and took over the leadership of the theater group, but I don't think life has been the same for him without Josephine. In recent years he has had medical and financial problems. He was supposed to have a one-

man concert this summer, but he declined, saying his hands would not permit him to play to the standards he had set for himself. The wellness coordinator has worked with Michael, addressing his medical health as well as personal issues. She reports that until Michael is ready to make some changes in his life there is not much she can do to help him.

Michael has given a lot of himself to Vintage—perhaps someday he will be ready to let us repay the favor by helping him.

RUTH

She described herself as painfully shy when she first came to Vintage and I would have to agree with her. My first remembrance of Ruth was when she showed up for the weekly line-dancing class. I would never have noticed her except that at the time I shared my office with a number of activities, including the line dancers. I remember thinking that she was a very good dancer, and she was there every single week.

Ruth had been coming to Vintage for about six months when another staff person saw a letter to the editor in our major newspaper, written by Ruth, addressing the needs of seniors and praising the activities and services one could receive at Vintage. We were looking for someone to edit our monthly newsletter at the time, and Ruth seemed like the perfect choice. Following the line-dancing class one afternoon I asked if I could speak with her. Her face turned red and I could tell she was very uncomfortable with any attention. I suppose she was even more embarrassed when I told her we had seen her letter to the editor and were wondering if she would be interested in volunteering to edit our newspaper. She immediately declined the offer, explaining that she was the caregiver for her husband and only had time to run to Vintage for the dancing and hurry home.

As the weeks went by we understood her time commitment as a caregiver, but the ice was broken and we would frequently talk for a few minutes when she ran in each Wednesday. At one point I asked if she would write a little Halloween skit for the staff and she immediately agreed to this idea. On the very next Wednesday she came in with the entire skit completed. When I read it I knew at once that behind the exterior shyness was a woman with a tremendous sense of humor. All she needed was an avenue to express it. Ruth continued to write skits from home and come to Vintage once a week. It was about this time that her husband needed to be hospitalized and Vintage was able to assist her with some problems related to his care. Her husband passed away shortly after the hospitalization, and soon Ruth was coming to Vintage for dancing and for the creative writing class.

When the women came together to produce "The Celebration of Women," a first-person presentation of 18 important women in history, I asked Ruth if she would write the introduction and perhaps new words to some old standard tunes. In typical fashion she was at Vintage the very next day with the work completed. When she handed it to me, I was hopeful she would be willing to make the next step and take the part of the narrator in the production. She would say I "sweet-talked" her into this role, but once she started, the actress was suddenly born. Ruth has now written and acted in numerous plays for the drama group, and she has performed many times in the community with the line dancers as well as a one-woman comedy act. Additionally, she has been elected twice to serve on the Advisory Board. As they say, "She's come a long way, baby."

When I asked what she would say about her years at Vintage, this is what she wrote: "After eighty years of living, instead of thinking about checking out, I'm at Vintage every day checking in. It is the best prescription for whatever ails me."

The population revolution presents opportunities and challenges for arts organizations, artists, senior centers, and other aging organizations to meet the creative needs of older adults through dance, music, theater, and the visual arts. Arts and aging organizations can expect older adults to need and participate in arts programming as they are increasingly becoming consumers and users of services. The benefits of the arts are many including the following:

- They can help us understand and define aging. Creative writing, painting, music, theater, and dance can be used as vehicles to explore what it means to grow old.
- The arts help older adults age creatively and with dignity.
- They provide an opportunity for self-expression and achievement.
- Artistic expression provides a sense of self-worth.
- The arts provide opportunities for lifelong learning and service to others.
- They can benefit from older people's contributions and resources. Older adults can share the wisdom they have gained through a lifetime of experience as creators, mentors, teachers, and advisors. As role models, they can show younger generations how to age creatively by sharing their unique perspectives on life.
- The arts can provide older adults with positive feelings of a healthy aging process, rather than a feeling of being aged.

- Art is a bridge across generations. Sharing one another's arts, stories, song, dance, and music is a way to connect the generations within families and communities.
- The arts can relieve isolation through opportunities for engagement with others.
- Creativity and expression through the arts are vital to health and well-being through all stages of life.
- The arts can intensify a student's motivation to learn.
- They reflect our diversity and can improve multicultural understanding.

The National Endowment for the Arts (NEA) works to ensure the continued involvement of older adults as artists, teachers, mentors, students, volunteers, patrons, and consumers of the arts. The arts and humanities were a focus of an interagency initiative developed in 1995 by the NEA with the National Endowment for the Humanities, the Administration on Aging, and the White House Conference on Aging. Their goal was to make quality arts and humanities opportunities more responsive and available to older adults and to increase the sensitivity of professionals and practitioners in the field of aging to the potential of cultural programs involving older persons, ensuring that the arts and humanities were on the agenda as a quality-of-life issue. On the federal, state, and local levels, it was recommended that the arts and humanities become more inclusive on a cross-generational basis. Bob Blancato, director of the 1995 White House Conference on Aging, suggests involving organizations such as the Office of Aging, senior centers, nursing homes, mental health associations, boards of education, universities, American Association for Retired Persons (AARP), the National Council on the Aging (NCOA), Council of Senior Centers, Alzheimer's Association, Generations United, state-wide intergenerational coalitions and networks, and the Administration on Aging to create a task force on arts and aging within the community.

The National Council on the Aging also recommends that the NEA encourage programs that help older Americans discover artistic skills in retirement and that the value of work by older artists should be recognized and encouraged. The NCOA advocates public support for adult education, the arts, and the humanities as an investment in the well-being of older adults and the vitality of our society. It believes the best efforts in these areas require full partnership between federal government, state and local governments, agencies that serve older adults, and older Americans themselves. NCOA's public policy agenda recommends that

- the value of work by older artists, outreach to older audiences, and programs that help older Americans discover artistic skills in retirement be encouraged and recognized;
- planning for lifelong learning programs and new opportunities for older persons in education, recreation, the arts and aging be encouraged;
- federal support for library services to older persons should be strengthened, recognizing that they need not only technology, but also innovative programs that encourage learning and self-expression;
- support be provided to museums and performing arts groups to attract and teach older audiences.

Unfortunately, many organizations serving older adults are unaware of how the arts may benefit their constituents and many art groups are not actively concerned with opening up their programs and reaching out to older adults. The need for increased networking between the arts and aging fields was among the recommendations submitted to the 1995 White House Conference on Aging.

PARTICIPATION IN THE ARTS

The NEA's surveys of public participation in the arts, conducted in 1982, 1992, and 1997, provide important statistics on adult participation in the arts. The surveys document the changing composition of arts audiences in America and they provide a snapshot of audiences for classical music, opera, ballet, musicals, jazz, plays, and art museums. Adult participation in the arts is broken down into seven cohorts named according to the era in which they were born:

Progressives—those born before 1916

Roaring '20s—those born between 1916 and 1925

Depression—those born between 1926 and 1935

World War II—those born between 1936 and 1945

Early boomers—those born between 1946 and 1955

Late boomers—those born between 1956 and 1965

Baby busters—those born between 1966 and 1976, also known as Generation X.

The 1997 survey respondents' replies indicate that half of the U.S. adult (18 and older) population attended at least one of seven arts activities (jazz, classical music, opera, musical plays, nonmusical plays, ballet, or art museums) during the previous 12 months. Thirty-five percent of American adults made at least one visit to an art museum or gallery in 1997. Other arts activities with high participation rates were musical plays (25%), nonmusical plays and classical music (both 16%), and jazz and dance other than ballet (both 12%). Ballet and opera had attendance rates of 6% and 5%, respectively. Related activities such as reading literature (63%) and visiting a historic park or an arts and crafts fair (both about 47%) also had high participation rates.

The highest rates of personal participation in 1997 were in creative photography (17%), painting, drawing, or sculpting (16%), dance other than ballet (13%), creative writing (12%), and classical music (11%). Weaving and other related arts also had high participation rates. The lowest rates were in jazz and opera (both 2%) and in ballet (less than 1%). Data for performing in public demonstrate the popularity of singing in groups. In 1997 more than 10% of the adult population—over 20 million people—sang publicly in a choir, chorus, or other ensemble. Country music, blues and rhythm and blues, and gospel and hymns are the most popular forms of music. Older persons attend all the art forms except jazz more often than do younger people of the same education, gender, marital status, income, and other demographics.

Attendance at classical music performances is highest among those born between 1936 and 1945 and lowest in the oldest and youngest cohorts. The classical music audience is aging faster than the population as a whole. From 1982 to 1997, those over 60 years of age rose from 15.6% to 30.3% of the classical music audience. By 1997, a higher proportion of the classical music audience was over 60 than was the audience for any other performing art form.

Members of older cohorts comprise an even higher proportion of opera audiences. For example, the 1916–1925 cohort has higher rates of participation and operagoers are underrepresented among the youngest adults, suggesting that opera is one art form with a graying audience. From 1982 to 1997, the opera audience who were over 60 rose from 16.6% to 23.5%.

The data reveal that younger cohorts are more likely to be found at ballet performances than at the opera or at classical music concerts. Even the youngest cohorts attend the ballet at rates slightly above the most active arts participants, the 47- to 56-year-olds. Those 60 and over comprised 15.4% of the ballet audience in 1982, and by 1997 had risen to 22%, a change comparable with the one for arts audiences generally.

Those over 60 rose from 16.4% to 22.7% of the musical theater audience from 1982 to 1997. The overall rates of attendance at musicals are high compared to rates of participation in the other art forms, and yet cohort differences follow a pattern much like that observed for classical music, with participation lower in the younger cohorts. There seems to be a genuine cohort effect depressing attendance at musicals starting with the older baby-boom cohort and continuing through the youngest cohorts. The over-60 theater audience rose from 15.5% to 22.8% of the theater audience.

In 1982, the jazz audience was unusually young—only 5% of the 1982 jazz audience was over 60—while for all the other benchmark arts, between 15% and 17% of the audiences was above 60 years of age. By 1997, those over 60 rose from 5% to 15% of the jazz audience. Attendance at jazz performances was much higher among the younger cohorts, those aged 46 and younger. This pattern of higher rates of attendance at jazz concerts for adults born after WW II is very different from the patterns seen for the other art forms. The findings for jazz suggest that as these young cohorts replace older ones, it is expected that overall participation at jazz events will grow.

Attendance at theatrical plays is highest for the 1936–1945 cohort, which has significantly higher attendance rates compared to all other cohorts. All of the cohorts born before 1946 have significantly higher rates of attendance at plays than the youngest adult Americans.

The early boomers, the 1946–1955 cohort, rank first in level of attendance at art museums. Unlike all of the other benchmark arts, the proportion of museumgoers 60 and over has not increased appreciably between 1982 and 1997. Evidence suggests that not as many older people frequent art museums because of their impaired ability to walk and stand for extended periods of time.

Not all arts patrons attend with equal frequency. Observers have suggested that older attendees are likely to buy season tickets while those under 30 buy tickets for single events, as time, money, and inclination dictate, and thus generally attend less frequently. Lack of time, lack of a companion, lack of suitable events, and inaccessibility were the primary deterrents to more frequent attendance. Arts participation tends to rise gradually from the 30s through the 60s and then plummets as one approaches 70 years of age. Age is not in itself a deterrent to arts participation, but rather is often associated with other causal factors such as health, education, and income, which influence arts participation. Life course influences have a direct bearing on how often individuals are able to attend live performances or exhibits, and these effects vary with age. Data indicate that most companions are family members, although dates and friends accompanied the respondents more than 40% of the time.

Regardless of income, there is an overall substantial decline in arts participation for people born prior to 1946. These figures suggest that older adults face barriers to cultural activities. Arts organizations in partnership with community agencies are taking steps to encourage older adults to participate in the arts by addressing potential barriers such as transportation, ticket prices, and time and location of arts programming.

Surveys show that many adults are substituting alternative forms of arts participation, such as television and radio broadcasts or through various recorded media such as videotapes and CDs. The rates of participation on jazz, classical music, and opera were more than twice the rates for live arts events. Although dance and visual art were seen primarily on television, the other art forms attracted large numbers of listeners to radio and recordings. Participants in the arts through media were more evenly distributed by race, age, income, and educational level than were participants who attended live arts events.

Data show that it is the 1936–1945 cohort that attends the core art forms at the highest rates among all adult Americans. As has been true historically, education and income are strong predictors of arts participation. In every cohort, in every art form, those with more education and higher incomes participate at higher rates than those with less. Nonetheless, there is an overall decline in adult arts participation after the cohort born during World War II. The baby boomers, although better educated than their predecessors, have not kept up in terms of active participation in the arts. The studies demonstrate that early boomers attended the arts more often than earlier cohorts but not nearly so often as would be expected given their educational and financial advantages. It may not be the lack of interest in culture or lower incomes that keep baby boomers, especially the younger ones, away from active participation in the arts. They may not have the time or money to attend, even if they have the inclination.

Except for jazz, which more often appeals to the young, late boomers are clearly underrepresented in arts audiences. In marked contrast to late boomers, and contrary to all expectations, early boomers were overrepresented in the audiences of six of seven forms in 1982 and in 1997 as well. Neither early nor late boomers are attending the arts more often as they age, bringing into question the assumption that the boomer and later cohorts will age into arts participation.

The analysis of the demographic composition of personal performers and creators of art shows that for most arts activities, the highest rates of participation are found among minority groups. For example, the rate of jazz playing was highest for African Americans with Hispanics second. Hispanics also had high participation rates in other dance and drawing. American Indians had the highest rates of participation in other dance and photography, and Asians had the highest participation rates in opera, musical plays, ballet, drawing, and writing.

PERFORMING ARTS

All people have the ability to express themselves creatively and the performing arts are unique and important in their ability to communicate to all people, regardless of their age or ability. The performing arts stimulate memory, creativity, and social interaction. In addition, singing, dancing, and acting all help keep participants physically active. For the camera-shy, lighting, prop, costume, or promotional activities provide behind-the-scene opportunities to be involved. Many older adults want to know more about theater, and educational programs have been very well attended.

Participants say that the greatest benefits of theater-based activities are the improved interpersonal connections. Being in a theatrical group helps participants feel needed as others depend on them. Performing for an audience and hearing the applause is also a great thrill and morale booster.

Theatrical groups provide an active, enriching experience whether they offer small-scale performances or full productions with lights, sound, and costumes. Senior theater programs range from oral-history performances, simple readings of dramas, variety shows, intergenerational activities to issue-oriented productions. In some cases they bring their groups and participants considerable success and even fame.

History is central to many senior theater productions. Performance content of everything from improvisational exercises to fully staged productions can also be based on life review, reminiscence, literature, poetry, and life stories. Aging is a common thread for senior theater groups: many other subjects, such as community and personal issues, are also explored.

The play *Ready or Not* aims to sensitize people to the issues of aging and affirm the self-worth of older persons. It takes a comic and poignant look at the joys and fears of growing older, and its purpose is to reduce the prejudice and stereotypes that are prevalent today and inspire each of us to celebrate the aging process. The 60-minute play covers such themes as fall prevention, exercise, nutrition, Alzheimer's disease, sensory impairment, grief and loss. Although Kaiser Permanente no longer tours a production of *Ready or Not*, the script and discussion manual are available for use by community organizations.

Senior theater can even break down stereotypes and lead to intergenerational understanding and friendship. Older participants are invigorated by working with younger people, and younger participants say it puts an end to their biases about aging; for instance, they see that many older adults can in fact memorize very well. StageBridge of Oakland, California, has worked intensively with an intergenerational focus for more than 20 years. Using dramatized children's stories and fairy tales, it presents productions that teach children about aging and related topics.

FOLK ART

Folk and traditional arts are practiced among families, friends, and neighbors throughout the United States. Folk arts are an integral part of the rhythm of community and organizational life, expressing and reflecting shared aesthetics and values, a common ethnic heritage, language, religion, occupation, or geographic region. Folk arts provide an opportunity for the development of multicultural educational programs that promote intergenerational dialogue and understanding, as well as acceptance and appreciation of diverse cultures. This is increasingly important as the 2000 Census reveals that immigrants make up 11% of our country's population, the largest share since the 1930s.

Folk art includes a diverse range of activities, from mariachi music to African American gospel, cowboy poetry, Pueblo pottery, Eastern European embroidery, Southeast Asian dance, and Cajun storytelling. The "Report on the Folk and Traditional Arts in the United States" suggests that involvement and interest in folk-arts and folk culture is significant, pervasive, and increasing in ethnic organizations, museums, libraries, schools, historical societies, folk arts organizations, local arts agencies, community service organizations, festivals, and beyond. A strong network of state folk-arts programs and national organizations exist and have played central roles in the preservation and presentation of folk arts and folk culture.

Three primary perspectives guide the folk arts and traditional cultural activities: (a) discipline-specific interests such as weaving groups, pottery centers, folk music societies, and dance groups; (b) arts or cultural organizations such as local arts agencies, historical societies, historic preservation groups, and cultural tourism organizations that serve the needs and interests of a particular region or locale; and (c) programming that focuses on traditional art or culture as an expression of cultural identity.

A 1991 survey of folk artists found that a majority consider identifying and motivating the next generation of artists to be a priority; 90% perform, exhibit or sell their art in public and most would like to do more. Senior centers can and should be involved in fostering awareness, understanding, and appreciation for the role of traditional art or cultural heritage in the legacies of our communities and the preservation and promotion of traditions.

QUILTING

Quilts are a symbol of the cultural diversity of America and of our national history. For traditional quilt-makers, quilt-making was an integral part of the life of a rural economy. Quilters frequently learned to make quilts from older relatives, using remnants from home sewing and recreating patterns passed down from earlier generations. Quilting experienced a revival in the late twentieth century as quilt-makers, many from urban and professional backgrounds, took up quilting as a leisure activity. Many quilt-makers had done other kinds of sewing and needlework, and they found quilting a natural extension of their skills. A broad spectrum of design styles and construction techniques developed. Asymmetrical designs, pictorial images, and the use of computer-generated or photo-transfer images coexist with new interpretations of traditional design elements. Manufacturers designed fabrics especially for quilt-makers, and contests provided competition and recognition opportunities.

A survey of American quilters conducted in 1994 identified an estimated 15.5 million quilters 18 years of age and older, with an average age of 52. The densest concentration of quilting activity per capita occurs in the middle of the country—the upper Midwest, Plains, south central, and mountain states—but active quilting activity occurs most frequently in the Northeast and Pacific Coast regions. The majority of active quilters consider it a leisure pursuit.

The creation of a quilt may result from the desire to make a gift for a wedding, birthday, birth of a baby, or anniversary or from a need to create in fabric. Once the original idea is refined and materials are collected, a template is created, the design is traced onto fabric, and the fabric is cut with scissors. During this process, the quilter may realize the need to modify the design. The give-and-take between the quilter and the quilt is the part of the process that provides the highest satisfaction for many quilters, who bestow specific titles on their quilts that often reflect the inspiration or purpose for the quilt. Each work is the result of a unique process of inspiration and construction, and each has a story to tell.

A common thread that runs throughout the history of American quilts is that of competition. During the nineteenth century, state and local agricultural fairs regularly included competitive categories for the most beautifully designed and well-made quilts. In the twentieth century, women's magazines invited entries in national quilt competitions. Narratives about winning quilts display a remarkable range of motivations and influences. Some depict personal stories, such as the loss of a loved one, or commemorate a special event. Others make political statements about local, national, or international events and concerns. Quilts can serve as a visual reminder of the intended recipients' lives and interests through pictorial images, actual items of clothing, or symbols of personal significance. Nature is a frequent inspiration to quilt-makers, expressed through the design, pattern, or colors chosen. Quilting provides the challenge of creating in fabric.

The process of creating and sharing a quilt can be a rich and profound experience that achieves many purposes, reflects many and complex meanings and relationships, and meets a creative need. For many, working together around a quilt frame is an enjoyable communal experience. Throughout American history, quilting has been a way for women to express their creativity. Some quilters feel a deep sense of union with their own ancestors, or with generations of past quilt-makers. Making a quilt, particularly a prize-winning quilt, takes time and personal commitment. No matter the impetus for making a particular quilt, the challenge of designing, constructing, and completing their quilts rewards the quilt-maker with a strong sense of achievement.

ART AND MUSIC THERAPY

Art and music therapies are allied health services similar to occupational and physical therapies. They are used to address physical, psychological, cognitive, and social functioning for people who experience illness, trauma, or challenges in living and by people who seek personal development. Programs are based on individual assessment, treatment planning, and ongoing program evaluation. Frequently functioning as members of an interdisciplinary team, therapists implement programs with individuals and groups. Art and music therapy can be incorporated into the senior center to meet the needs of special populations.

Based on the belief that the creative process involved in the making of art is healing and life-enhancing, art therapy is the therapeutic use of art-making within a professional relationship. By creating art and reflecting on the products and processes, people can increase awareness of self and others, cope with symptoms, stress, and traumatic experiences; enhance cognitive abilities; and enjoy the life-affirming pleasures of making art.

Music therapy can include singing, playing instruments, rhythmic movement, improvisation, composing, and listening to music. Research results and clinical experiences attest to the viability of music therapy even in those who are resistive to other treatment approaches. Music is a form of sensory stimulation, which provokes responses due to the familiarity, predictability, and feelings of security associated with it.

Art and music therapy provide

- memory recall, which contributes to reminiscence and satisfaction with life
- a way to explore and understand our own and other cultures
- positive changes in mood and emotional states
- a sense of control over life through successful experiences
- awareness of self and environment that accompanies increased attention
- anxiety and stress reduction
- nonpharmacological management of pain and discomfort

- stimulation, which provokes interest even when no other approach is effective

CREATIVE WRITING

Creative writing helps older adults preserve their cultural and artistic heritage. Senior centers can help ensure that today's older adults have an opportunity to tell their stories and benefit from their own self-expression through the written word.

Creative writing activities foster literary talent and achievement, advance the art of writing, and provide an opportunity to develop confidence in presenting one's own work and critiquing others'. Students can learn about elements of literature from inside their own work, rather than from a text. Their own experiences can be expressed in stories and poems. Creative writing can increase self-confidence, self-awareness, and creativity.

Creative writing classes for older adults should take into consideration the needs of adult learners and the challenges of teaching adults to write. Adult-centered techniques will improve writing instruction and help to motivate adult learners to write. Older adult learners may also need help overcoming writing anxiety.

Writing workshops are an excellent tool for improving writing skills. Writing instruction should focus on empowering students by emphasizing fluency, content, and student decision-making in writing rather than grammar.

Readings or a resident-artist program featuring established writers offers students exposure to a variety of voices and aesthetic approaches. Writer-to-writer mentorships provide emerging writers an opportunity to advance to the next level of their development through feedback and individualized assistance from established writers. Residency programs and mentorships can be offered in topics such as screenwriting, fiction, creative nonfiction, and poetry.

SUGGESTED ACTIVITIES

- poetry
- fiction/non-fiction
- journal writing

- playwriting/screenwriting
- women's writing
- writing from personal experiences

ARTS AND AGING PROGRAMS

The National Endowment for the Arts provides opportunities for everyone to celebrate and participate in their artistic heritage, as well as to experience and appreciate the depth and breadth of the nation's diverse cultural riches. The NEA supports the presentation of artists to the public; the documentation of traditional artists through audio and visual records of artists and their work, including the necessary discovery research that locates and identifies new and unknown artistic resources; education, including support for apprenticeship programs, school programs, and lifelong learning projects in traditional arts; preservation of traditional artworks or skills; and conversation, the gathering of artists to share ideas and issues related to the practice and perpetuation of artistic traditions.

State, regional, and local arts councils also provide major public support for artists. State apprenticeship programs bring older, traditional master artists together with young apprentices for periods of intensive, hands-on instruction to preserve and perpetuate cultural traditions. Apprenticeship programs involve the cooperation of many kinds of organizations, including senior centers to recruit participants. Apprenticeships nationwide have represented a wide variety of cultures and genres, including fiddling of the Athabascan peoples in Alaska, Hispanic santo-carving (a wooden image of a saint) in Colorado, *lauhala*-weaving (with leaves of the hala tree) in Hawaii, African American tap and jazz dance in Missouri, and Okinawan classical dance in California.

The success of the apprenticeship programs can be attributed to their diversity, the appeal of intergenerational teaching and learning, responsiveness to local needs, their value in cultural conservation, and consistent NEA support. Their impact goes beyond apprenticeship and preservation of the art form, given that artists often continue to work together, apprentices have gone on to become professionals, spin-off projects were created, communities have gained well-trained practitioners and in some cases, spin-off organizations. In addition, the master artists have received more honors and gained status from their participation.

There are many examples of arts organizations working with aging organizations to serve older adults.

1. The *Arts Council of Oklahoma City* targeted older adults by offering daytime performances and organizing the Readers' Theater Troupe, with support from the State Arts Council of Oklahoma. The troupe, composed of older adults, perform many of their own stories in the theater and senior centers.

2. The *North Carolina Arts Council* in Raleigh, North Carolina, has two mobile trucks. One of the arts trucks was parked near a senior center, and older adults worked with three artists in wood sculpture, batik, and fiber art for two months.

3. The *CineSol Latino Film Festival* in Harlingen, Texas, works in partnership with the local county aging program, *Amigos Del Valle*, to involve older adults. Amigos Del Valle advertises the festival and furnishes free transportation to older adults. In return, the festival provides free videos of its art to area senior centers.

4. *Appalshop* in Whitesburg, Kentucky, takes its roadside theater into rural areas, bringing together older adults and school children to share stories and pass on cultural traditions.

5. In Batesville, Arkansas, the area Arts Council runs the Forever Young at Heart program, where seven artists work with older adults on a wide variety of projects, including murals for senior centers, theater activities, and a writers' group. In one project with fifth- and sixth-graders, the writers' group conducted research on the dress, music, and art of Argentina that culminated in an intergenerational Argentina festival. This initiative is jointly funded by the Arts Council and the Area Agency on Aging.

6. *Elders Share the Arts* in Brooklyn, New York, has Pearls of Wisdom, a touring ensemble of multicultural older storytellers who create and perform original plays.

7. *Center in the Park*, a multipurpose senior center in Philadelphia, has an ongoing Artist-in-Education program. A mural for the Criminal Justice Center was inspired by members' neighborhood memories.

8. *Museum One* uses the arts to inspire and teach older adults in nursing homes, medical centers, retirement centers, and adult day-care centers. In the courses, parallels are drawn between the lives of the older adults and the lives of artists who created great work while in chronic pain in their later years, including Matisse, who created

from his wheelchair with diminishing vision and severe intestinal disorders, and Monet, who continued painting into his 80s following two cataract operations. Visual arts appreciation leads participants to hands-on art workshops where they can express their individual creativity. Museum One in Alexandria, Virginia, has provided educational materials, such as slides and videos, and independent study courses for activity directors, recreation therapists, and volunteers who work with older adult audiences.

Performing arts groups with older adults or intergenerational casts have also used the arts to address vital health care issues.

1.   *Artswatch*, an artist-in-residence program for elders in Louisville, Kentucky, inspired Eldersprites, a troupe of older women who perform and lead dance and storytelling for older adults. Performance issues that relate to aging are addressed, such as arthritis, alcoholism, and diversity.

2.   *Senior Arts* of Albuquerque, New Mexico, promotes multicultural, traditional and contemporary art forms representing native New Mexican, Native American, Hispanic, and Western traditions, Eastern European, African, Celtic, Central Asian, and Asian Pacific cultures. Activities are free and include performances and workshops by prominent New Mexico artists. In addition to providing 3,000 seniors annually with quality arts experiences, Senior Arts offers recognized and emerging artists the opportunity to reach new audiences. Each year, between 60 and 70 artists participate as teachers and performers. While working for Senior Arts, they earn an appropriate wage and have the opportunity to share their expertise and vision with an appreciative population that is often isolated and underserved. The seniors who spend 8 weeks with an important artist have a chance to gain real insight into the creative process. Many sell their work at galleries or display their work in local venues such as the Spanish Market. Senior Arts was awarded an NEA grant for "Connecting People Through Arts," a series of six collaborative cross-generational events that included workshops, performances, exhibits, and an oral-history project.

3.   *Keepers of the Treasure*, a coalition of tribal representatives and federal agencies, developed strategies for the preservation of the traditions of American Indians, Alaskan Natives, and Native Hawaiians, resulting in federal funding for tribal cultural-heritage programs such as oral-history documentation.

INVOLVING OLDER ADULTS IN THE ARTS

The National Endowment for the Arts developed the following suggestions to involve older adults in the arts:

- Identify local resources.
- Develop program ideas.
- Include older adults in the planning.
- Plan how to have older adults participate in the programs.
- Initiate a dialogue and network with arts organizations in the community.
- Plan staff training in partnership with local arts organizations.
- Include an intergenerational arts focus.
- Conduct age awareness training for each age group for intergenerational programs.
- Research local and national funding sources.
- Publicize the program to arts groups and aging organizations.
- Survey and market to target groups.
- Provide incentives for participation, including receptions and refreshments.

SUGGESTED ACTIVITIES

ARTS AND CRAFTS AND FOLK ARTS

- carving
- wood turning
- jewelry-making
- basketry
- paper arts
- bookbinding
- quilting
- knitting, crocheting, and embroidery
- stained glass
- blacksmithing
- tatting
- tinsmithing
- wearable art

- weaving
- printmaking
- silk-screening

CULTURAL OUTINGS AND EVENTS

- field trips to museums, galleries, and exhibits
- cultural performances
- experiential programs with art partners
- behind-the-scene tours

DANCE AND FOLK DANCING

- dance workshops taught by specialists focusing on topics such as ethnic music and dance, clogging, and turning dances
- family folk dances for people of all ages
- beginning, intermediate, and experienced folk dancing
- line dancing
- country-and-western dance
- swing dance
- ballroom dance
- jazz and tap dance

MUSIC

- ensemble and solo musical instrument performance
- choral groups
- musical performances
- musical theater
- interactive lecture and listening experience

THEATRE

- drama, games, and improvisation—develop scenes, characters, and monologues spontaneously

- fundamentals of acting—work on scenes and monologues from popular plays and learn acting skills
- storytelling—techniques for telling personal, folk, and fairy tales in community and school settings
- first-person presentations

VISUAL ARTS

- ceramics and pottery
- drawing
- painting
- photography
- media arts
- graphic design
- sculpture

EDUCATIONAL PROGRAMS

- art appreciation
- local architecture
- famous artists and their work
- theater
- understanding and appreciating music

BIBLIOGRAPHY

Alexander, J. (2001). *Foreword. The arts and older Americans.* Washington, DC: National Endowment for the Arts. [On-line]. Available: www.arts.endow.gov/partner/Accessibility/Monograph/Alexander.html

American Music Therapy Association. (2001). What is music therapy? [On-line]. Available: www.musictherapy.org/factsheets/olderadults.html

Becker, C. (1999). *Literature: Report from the director.* Washington, DC: National Endowment for the Arts.

Holstein, J. (1995). Discovering the dedicated quilter. *Quilt Journal, 4*(1), 14–16.

Horton, L. (1999). *Speaking of quilts: Voices from the late twentieth century.* [On-line]. Available: www.memory.loc.gov/ammem/qlthtml/qltov.html

McConnell, J. (2001). Teaching the elders: Senior Arts, Inc. *The Arts and Older Americans.* Washington, DC: National Endowment for the Arts. [On-line]. Available: www.arts.endow.gov/artforms/Multi/SeniorArts.html

National Endowment for the Arts. (1997). *Age and arts participation: With a focus on the Baby Boom cohort. Executive summary.* Research Report #34.Washington, DC: Author.

National Endowment for the Arts. (1997). *Age and arts participation, 1982–1997. Executive Summary.* Research Report #42. Washington, DC: Author.

National Endowment for the Arts. (2001). Step by step programming: How to begin involving older adults in the arts. *The Arts and older Americans.* Washington, DC: Author. [On-line]. Available: www.arts.endow.gov/partner/Accessibility/Monograph/OlderStep.html

National Endowment for the Arts. (1997). *Survey of public participation in the arts: Summary report.* Washington, DC: Author.

Peelen, C. A. (1993). The writing workshop and the adult learner. *ERIC Digest No. ED369975.* [On-line]. Available: ericacve.org

Peterson, E. (1996). *The changing faces of tradition. A report on the folk and traditional arts in the United States.* Research Division Report #38. Washington, DC: National Endowment for the Arts.

Potera, C. (2000, August). *Theater groups help seniors shine brighter.* [On-line]. Available: www.cnn.com/2000/HEALTH/aging/08/01/seniors.theater.wmd/

Sherman, A. (2001). Arts and health care for older adults. *The Arts and Older Americans.* Washington, DC: National Endowment for the Arts. [On-line]. Available: www.arts.endow.gov/partner/Accessibility/Monograph/Sherman2.html

Sherman, A. (2001). Arts participation: The graying of America. *The Arts and Older Americans.* Washington, DC: National Endowment for the Arts. [On-line]. Available: www.arts.endow.gov/partner/Accessibility/Monograph/Sherman.html

Sommer, R. F. (1989). Teaching writing to adults: Strategies and concepts for improving learner performance. *ERIC Digest No. ED313997.* [On-line]. Available: ericacve.org

Terry, P. (2001). Opening doors to lifelong learning in the arts. *The Arts and Older Americans.* Washington, DC: National Endowment for the Arts. [On-line]. Available: www.arts.endow.gov/partner/Accessibility/Monograph/Terry.html

Vornberg, B. L. (2001). *Break a leg: Growth of senior theater generates directory.* American Society on Aging. [On-line]. Available: www.asaging.org/at/at-211/Seniors.html

RESOURCES

American Art Therapy Association (AATA)
1202 Allanson Road
Mundelein, IL 60060-3808
888-290-0878
http://www.arttherapy.org
The American Art Therapy Association, Inc. is an organization of professionals dedicated to the belief that the creative process involved in the making of art is healing and life enhancing. AATA provides standards

of professional competence, and develops and promotes knowledge of the field of art therapy.

American Folklife Center
Library of Congress
101 Independence Avenue SE
Washington, DC 20540
202-707-5510
http://www.lcweb.loc.gov/folklife
The American Folklife Center at the Library of Congress was created by Congress to preserve and present American Folklife. The Center and its collections encompass all aspects of folklore and folklife from this country and around the world.

American Music Therapy Association, Inc. (AMTA)
8455 Colesville Road, Suite 1000
Silver Spring, MD 20912
301-589-3300
http://www.musictherapy.org/
The American Music Therapy Association's mission is the progressive development of the therapeutic use of music in rehabilitation, special education, and community settings. It publishes the *Journal of Music Therapy*. The American Music Therapy Association is a new organization resulting from the unification of the American Association for Music Therapy and the National Association for Music Therapy.

Americans for the Arts
1000 Vermont Avenue NW, 12th Floor
Washington, DC 20005
202-371-2830
http://www.artsusa.org
American's for the Arts is an arts information clearinghouse and arts advocacy organization dedicated to representing and serving local communities and creating opportunities for every American to participate in and appreciate all forms of the arts.

Amigos del Valle
PO Box 4057
Fairview, NM 87533
505-753-4115

Appalshop
91 Madison Avenue
Whitesburg, KY 41858
606-633-0108
http://ns.appalshop.org/
Appalshop is a media arts and cultural center located in the heart of
the Central Appalachian Coalfields. Appalshop produces and presents
work that celebrates the culture and voices the concerns of people
living in the Appalachian Mountains.

ArtAge Publications
PO Box 12271
Portland, OR 97212-0271
503-249-1137 or 800-858-4998
ArtAge Publications' mission is to connect seniors in the arts with infor-
mation, education & inspiration. Produced *Senior Theatre Connections:
The First Directory of Senior Theatre Performing Groups, Professionals, and
Resources.*

Art & Humanities Resource Center for Older Adults (AHRC)
644 Linn Avenue, Suite 1010
Cincinnati, OH 45203
513-579-1074
The Art & Humanities Resource Center for Older Adults designs and
presents mentally stimulating programs for older adults. AHRC's programs channel older people's personal perspectives and memories of
historic events into original songs, dances, theatrical performances, and
visual artwork, often incorporating musical elements with help from
the Cincinnati Opera Outreach Program, symphony musicians, jazz
artists, and other professional musicians.

The Arts Council of Oklahoma City
400 West California
Oklahoma City, OK 73102
405-270-4848
http://www.artscouncilokc.com/index.html
The Arts Council of Oklahoma City supports the spirit of community
in Oklahoma City by presenting visual and performing arts in a lively,
accessible way.

Arts for the Aging, Inc. (AFTA)
697 Arlington Avenue, Suite 352

Bethesda, MD 20814
301-718-4990
http://www.aftaarts.org
Arts for the Aging, Inc. is dedicated to enhancing the lives of older adults by providing them with access to the arts. AFTA organizes monthly arts workshops in mediums such as painting, drawing, printmaking, sculpture, bookmaking, dance movement, music, and theater for older individuals. AFTA has also offered intergenerational programs. Through AFTA's senior dance troupe *Quicksilver* and art exhibitions, participants are invited to showcase their talents for others.

Artswatch
2337 Franfort Avenue
Louisville, KY 40206-2467
502-893-9661
http://www.artswatch.org
Artswatch promotes innovative arts programming and runs an artist-in-residence program for older adults. Its female acting troupe, *Elderspirites*, performs throughout the community, confronting issues such as arthritis, alcoholism, and diversity.

Arts Midwest
2908 Hennepin Avenue, Suite 200
Minneapolis, MN 55408-1954
612-341-0755 or 612-341-0901
http://artsmidwest.org
Arts Midwest connects the arts to audiences throughout a 9 state region.

Associated Writing Programs
Tallwood House MSN 1E3
George Mason University
Fairfax, VA 22030
703-993-4301
http://awpwriter.org/
Associated Writing Programs is a national, nonprofit literary organization dedicated to serving writers, teachers, and writing programs.

Batesville Area Arts Council
246 E. Main Street, Suite 207
Batesville, AR 72501

870-793-3382
http://batesville.dina.org/recreation/baac.ht ml
The Batesville Area Arts Council exists to promote and champion the
arts in Batesville and surrounding communities.

Canadian Association for Music Therapy
Wilfrid Laurier University
75 University Avenue West
Waterloo, Ontario, N2L 3C5
800-996-CAMT or 519-884-1970 ext. 6828
http://www.musictherapy.ca
The Canadian Association for Music Therapy promotes the use and
development of music therapy in the treatment, education, training,
and rehabilitation of children and adults.

Center in the Park
5818 Germantown Avenue
Philadelphia, PA 19144
215-848-7722
Email: ctrpark@libertynet.org
Center in the Park is a multi-purpose senior center located in an inner-
city community.

City Lore: The New York Center for Urban Folk Culture
72 East First Street #1
New York, NY 10003
212-529-1955
http://www.citylore.org/
City Lore is a cultural organization whose mission is to document,
preserve and present the living cultural heritage of New York and
other cities

Consortium for Pacific Arts & Cultures
2141C Atherton Road
Honolulu, HI 96822
808-946-7381
http://www.pixi.com/~cpac/
CPAC is a private, nonprofit regional arts organization perpetuating
the traditional arts and cultures of the Pacific.

Elders Share the Arts (ESTA)
Center for Creative Aging
72 East First Street
New York, NY 10003
http://elderssharethearts.org
Elders Share the Arts is a nationally recognized arts organization dedicated to bridging generational divides and generating a sense of community through the arts.

Folk Art Society of America
Box 17041
Richmond, VA 23226
804-285-4532 or 800-527-3655
http://www.folkart.org
The Folk Art Society of America advocates the discovery, study, documentation, preservation and exhibition of folk art, folk artists and folk art environments.

GRACE (Grass Roots Art and Community Efforts)
PO Box 960
Hardwick, VT 05843
802-472-6857
http://www.graceart.org
GRACE is dedicated to the development and promotion of visual art produced primarily by older, self-taught artists of rural Vermont. GRACE recruits professional artists to hold instructional training and workshops at nursing homes, senior-meal sites, mental health centers, and hospitals. Provides touring exhibitions, lectures, media documentation, and publications like *States of GRACE: Grass Roots Art and Community Efforts.*

International Society for the Performing Arts Foundation (ISPA)
17 Purdy Avenue
PO Box 909
Rye, NY 10580
914-921-1550
http://www.ispa.org/
The International Society for the Performing Arts Foundation develops, nurtures, energizes and educates an international network of arts leaders and professionals who are dedicated to advancing the field of the performing arts.

The International Quilt Study Center
Department of Textiles, Clothing and Design
University of Nebraska-Lincoln
234 Home Economics Building
Lincoln, NE 68583-0802
402-472-2911
The International Quilt Study Center was created to encourage the interdisciplinary study of all aspects of quiltmaking traditions and to foster preservation of this tradition through the collection, conservation and exhibition of quilts and related materials.

Kaiser Permanente's Educational Theater Programs
5410 Lancaster Drive
Cleveland, OH 44131
216-778-6140
http://www.kaiserpermanente.org/locations/oh/about/theater/aging.html
Ready or Not play script and discussion manual are available for use by community organizations.

Keepers of the Treasures-Cultural Council of American Indians, Alaska Natives and Native Hawaiians
PO Box 28237
Washington, DC 20038-8237
405-382-5194 or 202-208-5732
http://www.keepersofthetreasures.org/
The Keepers of the Treasures is a cultural council of American Indians, Alaska Natives and Native Hawaiians who preserve, affirm, and celebrate their cultures through traditions and programs that maintain their native languages and lifeways. The Keepers protect and conserve places that are historic and sacred to peoples who are indigenous to the United States. The Keepers provide technical assistance and seek to identify funding from private and public sources for these purposes. The Keepers advocate and assist programs that educate and create respect for native lifeways and history.

Liz Lerman Dance Exchange
7117 Maple Avenue
Takoma Park, MD 20912
301-270-6700

E-mail: artsource@compuserve.com
Liz Lerman Dance is composed of dancers whose ages span six decades. These dancers perform, rehearse, teach, plan residencies, choreograph, assist in fundraising and administrative activities, act as spokespeople for the organization, and serve on the board of directors. Programs for older adults include dance classes at senior centers and nursing homes, community performance events, studio dance incentives for older adults, and training in the art of making dance in community settings.

Mid-America Arts Alliance
912 Baltimore Avenue, Suite 700
Kansas City, MO 64105
816-421-1388
The Mid-America Arts Alliance is a regional arts organization serving the states of Arkansas, Kansas, Missouri, Nebraska, Oklahoma and Texas. Its activities encompass regional, national, and international divisions and programs, including performing arts touring, international artists exchange, commissioning, traveling exhibitions, earned-income ventures and partnerships, individual artist fellowships, residency programs, and a diverse range of community, educational, consultative, and technical services to the field and funders.

Mill Street Loft
455 Maple Street
Poughkeepsie, NY 12601
845-471-7477
http://www.millstreetloft.org
Mill Street Loft, a nationally recognized multi arts educational center, is committed to bringing creative educational and culturally enriching programs to children and older adults through the Hudson River Valley region. Its intergenerational programs, including *Seniors Go to Art Camp*, the *Intergenerational Chorus*, *Life Stage Theater*, *Oral Histories*, *Connections*, *Building Bridges*, *Totems*, and *Project ABLE* (Arts for Basic Education, Life Skills, and Entrepreneurship), promote meaningful communication and interdependence between generations. Participants in these programs explore community, economic, and age-related issues through the common ground of music, creative movement, drama, storytelling, or the visual arts.

Museum One, Inc.
7823 Yorktown Drive

Alexandria, VA 22308
800-524-1730
http://www.museumoneinc.org
Museum One is an arts and educational outreach service which brings art appreciation and other art forms such as music, dance, and poetry to the community, with a special emphasis on older adults. Museum One educational programs using slide programs, manuals, and books, are designed specifically for leading older adult participants at senior sites.

Museum One's Creating for Life workshop takes participants step by step through the different expressions of the arts, beginning with visual art, then music and creative movement. The workshop begins with the appreciation of the visual arts or the understanding of artists and their paintings, followed by hands-on art that focuses on helping older adults express themselves on paper or canvas. Specific techniques and guidelines are demonstrated for working with older adults in hands-on art during the workshop. The next phase of the Creating for Life workshop centers on music and creative movement. The group members are taught how to listen to and feel music, and how to move the body creatively to rhythms.

Mid Atlantic Arts Foundation
22 Light Street, #300
Baltimore, MD 21202
410-539-6656
http://www.midatlanticarts.org
The Mid Atlantic Arts Foundation encourages development of the arts and supports arts programs on a regional basis.

National Assembly of State Arts Agencies (NASAA)
1029 Vermont Avenue, NW, 2nd Floor
Washington, DC 20005
202-347-6352
http://www.nasaa-arts.org/
The National Assembly of State Arts Agencies is the membership organization of the nation's state and jurisdictional arts agencies. NASAA's mission is to advance and promote a meaningful role for the arts in the lives of individuals, families and communities.

National Council for the Traditional Arts
1320 Fenwick Lane, Suite 200

Silver Spring, MD 20910
301-565-0654
http://www.ncta.net/
The National Council for the Traditional Arts is dedicated to the presentation and documentation of folk and traditional arts.

National Endowment for the Arts
1100 Pennsylvania Avenue NW
Washington, DC 20506
202-682-5400
http://www.arts.endow.gov/
The National Endowment for the Arts nurtures the expression of human creativity, supports the cultivation of community spirit, and fosters the recognition and appreciation of the excellence and diversity of the nation's artistic accomplishments.

National Quilting Association, Inc.
PO Box 393
Ellicott City, MD 21041-0393
410-461-5733
http://www.nqaquilts.org/
The National Quilting Association is a non-profit organization run by quilters for quilters, was established to create, stimulate, maintain and record an interest in all matters pertaining to the making, collecting, and preserving of quilts, and to establish and promote educational and philanthropic endeavors through quilts.

New England Foundation for the Arts (NEFA)
266 Summer Street, 2nd floor
Boston, MA 02210
617-951-0010
http://www.nefa.org/
The New England Foundation for the Arts connects the people of New England with the power of art to shape their lives and improve their communities.

North Carolina Arts Council
Department of Cultural Resources
4632 Mail Service Center
Raleigh, NC 27699-4632

919-733-2111
http://www.ncarts.org/home.html
The North Carolina Arts Council enriches the cultural life of the state by nurturing and supporting excellence in the arts and by providing opportunities for every North Carolinian to experience the arts.

North Carolina Center for Creative Retirement (NCCCR)
University of North Carolina at Asheville
116 Rhodes Hall
Asheville, NC 28804-3299
828-251-6140
http://www.unca.edu/ncccr
The North Carolina Center for Creative Retirement promotes lifelong learning, leadership, and community service opportunities for retirement-aged individuals. In hopes of contributing to the development of an age-integrated society, it encourages creative intergenerational activities on campus and in the community. In addition to supporting a College for Seniors program, NCCCR organizes trips to theaters, museum tours, and line dancing for older adults.

Poetry Society of America
15 Gramercy Park
New York, NY 10003
212-254-9628
http://www.poetrysociety.org/
The Poetry Society of America has readings, seminars, and competitions intended to challenge and inspire.

Poets & Writers
72 Spring Street
New York, NY 10012
212-226-3586
http://www.pw.org/
Poets & Writers, Inc. provides support and exposure to writers at all stages of development. assisting authors in their search for career-related information, outlets for their work, opportunities for professional advancement, and community with other writers.

Quilt Heritage Foundation
PO Box 19452

Omaha, NE 68119
402-551-0386
800-599-0094
http://www.quiltheritage.com/
The Quilt Heritage Foundation is a private, non-profit organization
that serves as the umbrella organization for The Crazy Quilt Society,
The Quilt Restoration Conference, The Dead Quilt Society, The Quilt
Rescue Squad and traveling exhibits.

SASE: The Write Place
711 West Lake Street, Suite 211
Minneapolis, MN 55408
612-822-2500
http://www.mtn.org/sase/
The mission of SASE: The Write Place is to provide affordable, quality
programming, developed and administered by a diverse group of people, for writers of all backgrounds to develop their craft and present
or publish their works.

Senior Adult Theater Program
University of Nevada-Las Vegas
Department of Gerontology
505 Maryland Parkway
Las Vegas, NV 89154
The Senior Adult Theater program encourages older adults to pursue
their diverse interests in subjects like design, acting, and promotions
through theater courses. Students of all ages and from many states can
enroll in the program to learn about senior theater.

Senior Arts
PO Box 12897
Albuquerque, NM 87195
505-877-6615
Senior Arts invites New Mexico's finest artists to participate in a culturally diverse and challenging arts program for Albuquerque's senior
citizens. The program consists of workshops and performances in the
disciplines of music, dance, theater, literature, and visual arts held in
all of Albuquerque's public senior centers as well as a number of satellite
and residential sites. These workshops and performances, which have
covered topics like Spanish tinworking, Polish paper-cutting, bilingual

poetry, Pueblo ceramic-sculpting, Indian hoopdancing, and African-American storytelling, reflect Senior Arts' commitment to developing both traditional and contemporary art forms.

Southeast Florida Center on Aging
Florida International University
3000 Northeast 151st Street, ACI-234
North Miami, FL 33181
305-940-5550
http://www.fpeca.usf.edu/
The Southeast Florida Center on Aging and the Jazz Studies Program of Florida International University have been working together on a pilot Intergenerational Jazz Masters Project. The project is designed to recognize the lifetime achievements and continuing contributions of older jazz artists and to insure that the wisdom, knowledge, and skills of these artists are passed onto future generations. The Center also includes an Elders Institute that provides continuing education for older learners in areas including drawing, art history, decorative arts, and jewelry making.

Southern Arts Federation
Traditional Artists Technical Assistance Project
1401 Peachtree Street NE, Suite 460
Atlanta, GA 30309
404-874-7244
http://www.southarts.org/
The Southern Arts Federation promotes and supports the arts regionally, nationally, and internationally and enhances the artistic excellence and professionalism of Southern arts organizations and artists so that they successfully connect with citizens and their communities.

The Stagebridge Theater
2501 Harrison Street
Oakland, CA 94612
510-444-4755
http://www.stagebridge.org
Stagebridge uses performance as a means of bridging generations through issues such as street crime, depression, volunteering, stereotypes, technology, love and sex. *Stagebridge* coordinates classes in acting, improv, and scene study, as well as performances of original plays about

aging. Storybridge, is an intergenerational arts and literacy project that enables low-income older adults and at-risk children to interact and learn through storytelling programs.

Tribal Preservation Program
Heritage Preservation Services
National Park Service
1849 C Street, NW, NC200
Washington, DC 20240
202-343-9572
http://www2.cr.nps.gov/tribal/tribal_p.htm
The National Park Service Tribal Preservation Program assists Indian tribes in preserving their historic properties and cultural traditions.

United Statewide Community Arts Association (USCAA)
c/o MACAA
PO Box 6015
Columbia, MO 65205
573-874-7519
Many states have statewide membership organizations that are open to local arts agencies and others. The United Statewide Community Arts Association provides professional development and networking services.

University of Massachusetts, Division of Continuing Education
Arts Extension Service
358 North Pleasant Street
Amherst, MA 01003-9296
413-545-2360
http://www.umass.edu/aes/index.html
The Arts Extension Service is a national, nonprofit arts service organization, a program of the Division of Continuing Education, University of Massachusetts Amherst.

VSA ARTS
1300 Connecticut Avenue, NW, Suite 700
Washington, DC 20036
202-628-2800
http://www.vsarts.org
VSA Arts is an International organization that creates learning opportunities through the arts for people with disabilities. VSA Arts has national

and international affiliates; each state has different programs for children and adults with all types of disabilities.

Western States Arts Federation
1543 Champa Street, Suite 220
Denver, CO 80202
303-629-1166
http://www.westaf.org/
The Western States Arts Federation is a non-profit arts service organization dedicated to the creative advancement and preservation of the arts.

Western Folklife Center
PO Box 888
Elko, NV 89803
775-738-7508
http://www.westernfolklife.org/
The Western Folklife Center is dedicated to the preservation and presentation of the cultural traditions of the American West.

CHAPTER NINE

Computers

JERRY

I clearly remember the day in the early 1990s when our executive director received a phone call from a local company asking if we could make use of three computers that they no longer needed. As a staff, we had often discussed how nice it would be if we could offer computer classes to our participants and were somewhat envious of the sophisticated programs for senior adults in California and other states. We quickly sent someone across town to pick up the valuable merchandise.

I sent off notes to several local universities to see if any of their professors would be interested in coming by during their lunch hours to teach a computer class. I must admit I thought it was a long shot, getting someone to give up his or her lunch hour for this worthy cause. Nevertheless, the letters went out and it wasn't long before I received a call from a gentleman who worked in research at a local university and was retiring in a couple months. He saw the letter on the bulletin board and liked the idea of opening up the world of computers to other older adults. He wanted to know if we had found anyone and if not he would like to stop by someday and see our equipment. Thus began our 5-year relationship with Jerry. I have often wondered what he must have thought when he saw those first 3 computers. He never said. Instead he busied himself developing a curriculum and updating those old machines. We often laughed because we would always see Jerry with work sheets in one hand and a bag of tools in the other. Frequently, repairs were needed before classes could begin.

We started out with classes one day a week. In the morning we offered beginning computers and in the afternoon intermediate computers. With only three computers, class size was limited. Still, it wasn't long before Vintagers were composing letters to friends or making special programs for their churches. The word Internet was not part of our vocabulary at that time. Additionally, Jerry began coming to the center during tax season to assist with the VITA (Volunteer Income Tax Assistant) program.

When we moved into our new building in 1994, we were able to purchase tables specially designed for computers. Class size grew, and frequently 10 to 12 participants waited eagerly to have their turn at the computer. We knew it was time to update both the equipment and the space, so the agency sought funding to begin this process. In the spring of 1996, Jerry became ill and the original computer room was closed. It seemed as though the staff was waiting for Jerry to return and were unwilling to seek another volunteer teacher. This was not to be, as Jerry passed away in the winter of 1997.

One year later the computer studio opened with nine computers for the students and one for the instructor. All are connected to the Internet and six teachers rotate to provide classes to the more than 300 students who have taken classes in the past 2 years. Sometimes humble beginnings and a dedicated volunteer like Jerry have a way of growing and developing into a very a successful program.

At the ribbon cutting, the program director recognized funders for their generous gift that made the computer studio possible. He acknowledged the help the staff had given him with the project and finally he remembered Jerry for his effort in bringing the world of technology to Vintage.

Seniors do not want to be left out of training to use computers and the Internet, and they have filled the computer classes at Vintage since the classes were first introduced. Computer technology provides a senior the opportunity to keep up with the times. Affordable access to training, equipment, and learning how to use new computer application programs is more important to usage than fear of technology. Many seniors today are getting their first introduction to computer technology by means of free community access and lower costs for PCs, which is helping to narrow the digital divide. The digital divide refers to the gap between those who can effectively access and use new information and communication tools such as the Internet, and those who cannot. The Internet is the gateway to a vast array of content and applications and is expected to become a primary medium for commerce, education, and entertainment in the twenty-first century. To be on the less fortunate side of the divide means there is less opportunity to take part in the education, training, shopping, entertainment, and communication opportunities that are available on-line.

More Americans are going on-line to conduct day-to-day activities such as business transactions, personal correspondence, research, information gathering, and shopping. Each year, being digitally connected becomes ever more critical to economic, educational, and social advancement. Now that a large number of Americans regularly use the Internet to conduct daily activities, people who lack access to those tools are at a growing disadvantage. Therefore, raising the level of digital inclusion by increasing the number of Americans who use the technology tools of the digital age has become a vitally important national goal.

It is highly unlikely in the foreseeable future that prices will fall to the point where most homes will have computers and Internet access. As a result, the digital divide may continue to exist at home between the information-rich and the information-poor. Given the great advantages accruing to those who have access, a Department of Commerce report indicates that it is not economically or socially prudent to wait until most, if not all, homes can claim connectivity. Part of the short-term answer lies in providing Internet access at community access centers, such as schools, libraries, senior centers, and other public access facilities. These sources tend to be used by groups that lack Internet access at home or at work, including older adults, minorities, people earning lower incomes, those with lower education levels, and the unemployed.

Commerce Department 2000 data show that the overall level of U.S. digital inclusion is rapidly increasing. The share of households with Internet access soared by 58%, from 26% in 1998 to 41% in 2000. Nationally, more than half of all households (51%) have computers and more than 80% of these households have Internet access. If growth continues at the current rate, more than half of all Americans will be using the Internet in 2001.

Groups that traditionally have been digital have-nots are now making dramatic gains:

1.   The gap has narrowed between households in rural areas and households nationwide that access the Internet.

2.   Americans at every income level are connecting at far higher rates from their homes, particularly at the middle-income levels. Today, more than two thirds of all households earning more than $50,000 have Internet connections.

3.   Access to the Internet is also expanding across every education level, particularly for those with some high-school or college education.

4.   Large gaps remain regarding Internet penetration rates among households of different races and ethnic origins. Asian Ameri-

cans and Pacific Islanders have maintained the highest level of home Internet access at 57%. Blacks and Hispanics, at the other end of the spectrum, continue to experience the lowest household Internet penetration rates at 23%. However, Blacks and Hispanics have shown impressive gains in Internet access and are now twice as likely to have home access than they were 2 years ago.

5.   Individuals 50 years of age and older are among the least likely to be Internet users. The Internet use rate for this group was only 29% in 2000. Though still less likely than younger Americans to use the Internet, this group experienced the highest rates of growth in Internet usage of all age groups: 53% from 1998 to 2000, compared to a 35% growth rate for individual Internet usage nationwide.

However, the data show that noticeable divides still exist between those with different levels of income and education, different racial and ethnic groups, old and young, and those with and without disabilities. Persons with a disability are only half as likely to have access to the Internet as those without a disability: 21.6% compared to 42.1%. And although nearly 25% of those without a disability have never used a personal computer, almost 60% of those with a disability fall into that category. Among those with a disability, people who have impaired vision and problems with manual dexterity have even lower rates of Internet access and are less likely to use a computer regularly than people with hearing and mobility problems.

Older Americans with disabilities do not have to be left out, as technological advances are helping to make computers and the Internet more accessible. The nonprofit Alliance for Technology Access offers information about computers and other high-tech tools to those with disabilities. For example, scanners can convert text to a digital format that can read text aloud, and software can convert text into Braille and print it by a special embosser.

Cost prevails as the biggest reason for not having Internet access. For seniors who cannot afford a computer or the Internet at home, the senior center can provide access to computers and the Internet. This is extremely important because many seniors are not able to access computer technology otherwise. For older Americans living on a fixed income, even a relatively inexpensive computer is unaffordable, and Internet access itself is expensive. Although demand is at an all-time high, many senior centers lack the tools to meet this growing need. In a 2000 survey of Oregon senior centers by Senator Ron Wyden, the majority lacked sufficient computer and Internet access, resulting in a shortage of accessible technology for older Oregonians.

Seniors who do have access are embracing computer technology. Forrester Research indicates that retirement gifts of PCs, increased leisure time, and a love of communication (especially with their grand-children) affect seniors' on-line behavior. Seniors with discretionary income sufficient to purchase the equipment and software are achieving computer literacy at the same rate as younger adults. A Packard Bell study conducted in 1995 showed that improvements that made comput-ers easier to use resulted in an increase in purchases and use by seniors in their homes, senior centers, public libraries, and other organizations. Internet appliances that simplify Web access and make e-mail easier to use are being developed constantly. A survey by Dell Computer Corporation found that 78% of those polled would be more inclined to purchase a home computer if they were confident of receiving good technical support to help them along the way. Even when seniors are aware of the advantages of owning and using PCs, service and support concerns prevent many from plugging in. Only one in five people over the age of 70 have used a computer and only 15% can access the Internet.

According to a 2000 AARP survey, about 40% of computer users surveyed rate themselves as novice computer users. Those who classify themselves as novices are older, less educated, and less affluent than more experienced computer users. Novice computer users spend less money than more experienced computer users on both software and hardware upgrades, and they use a much smaller variety of software. Computer users aged 65 and older and less affluent and less educated users are generally less proficient and less confident than those who are younger, more affluent, and more educated. Moreover, a substantial portion of computer users aged 45-plus appear unable or unwilling to spend money for maintenance and upgrade of their systems.

Use of the Internet continues to grow at an unprecedented rate. A company called eMarketer predicts that by 2003, more than a quarter of all Americans who are 55-plus will be active Internet users. Internet use has grown to more than 116 million users, and seniors are the fastest growing group on-line. However, Americans 65 and older are the lowest users of the Internet; only 16% regularly use the Internet, compared to an over all national average of 42%. Only one in five people over the age of 70 has ever used a computer and only 15% can access the Internet. A 1998 survey by SeniorNet, a volunteer nonprofit organization of senior PC users, and Charles Schwab & Co. found that 70% of computer owners aged 55 or older have Internet access at home. One in 10 seniors who do not have Internet access at home or work say they sometimes access the Internet from another location such as a friend's or relative's house or a public library.

Another major barrier to participation for the over-50 population is the challenge of acquiring computer skills. Exposure in work or school usually teaches the basics to even the most computer-resistant person. But trying to teach various software applications and double-clicking to someone who has had no exposure to computing can be very challenging. Older persons often think that there is nothing relevant or of interest to them on the Internet to justify the cost and effort involved. Poorly designed sites and the excessive information generated by an Internet search are also barriers to participation.

A study conducted by the Pew Internet and American Life Project found that seniors and aging baby-boomers are also the most resistant to the Internet. The older a person is, the more likely it is they do not have Internet access. Those not on-line say the Internet is too expensive, they are concerned about privacy, and the on-line world is confusing and hard to negotiate. Those without Internet access are more likely to be minorities, less well-off financially, and have less education. Older people living in rural communities are also less likely to have Internet access. A 1999 Forrester Research report found that only 8% of seniors aged 65 and older have Internet access, compared to 40% of the under-65 population. One major factor is their lack of contact with computers.

However, once older persons go on-line they become enthusiastic Net users, spending an average of 8 hours a week on-line, which is more than any other demographic group. A 2000 Media Metrix study found that older users access the Internet more often, stay on-line longer, and visit more Web sites than younger users. Higher education is the most likely predictor of Internet use, followed by a favorable attitude towards technology, higher income, and having at least one member of the household who works at, or brings work to, the home.

The Internet provides the opportunity to research a variety of topics, including health information, and is fast becoming the preferred method for obtaining news and information. In fact, the Internet has surpassed television and radio as an information resource. Internet users rank e-mail and Web surfing as the most important Web applications.

E-mail is a popular means of communication, with the numbers of messages sent in the United States projected to grow to several trillion in the next few years. It enables older adults to stay connected with their families, many of whom are scattered around the country and the world. According to a 2000 Yankee Group study, e-mail was the top on-line activity for 68% of those polled, with education and learning taking second place. The Department of Commerce 2000 report found that nearly 80% of Internet users reported using e-mail, and on-line shopping and bill paying are seeing the fastest growth.

Research surveys conducted by Packard Bell in 1997 and SeniorNet in 1998, indicates the following breakdown of senior adult PC usage:

- used most often for personal correspondence (e-mail) with family and friends (72%)
- used to research a particular issue or subject (59%)
- used to access news (53%)
- used to try the latest adventure games and CD-ROM puzzles (52%)
- used to research travel or vacation destinations (47%)
- used to obtain weather information (43%)
- used to perform volunteer work for various organizations (25%)

Seniors participating in a survey by Dell would use PCs for many of the same reasons other people do: 46% reported they would e-mail friends and family; 33% would play computer games; 26% would surf the Internet; 29% would pursue hobbies and interests; and 19% would use it to make travel arrangements.

Other popular uses include producing memoirs, monitoring investments, writing legislators, and tracing genealogy. Some seniors have put their knowledge to use to build an electronic community. For example, seniors have developed their own Internet relay-chat forums such as the 65Plus channel.

SeniorNet also looked at how seniors learn their PC skills. The results indicated that 40% of those sampled taught themselves, 21% learned to use computers at work, 17% had taken computer classes, and about 15% learned from a friend. George Breathitt, founder of the Silver Fox Computer Club, found that seniors learn to use computers best when taught by fellow seniors with whom they can identify.

In September 2000, Secretary of Commerce Norman Mineta stressed the importance of getting seniors on-line through a "Digital Inclusion" tour. The tour highlighted examples of creative programs offered throughout the country to bring more people on-line. At the first stop, the Philadelphia Senior Learning Center, Mineta urged children to send their grandparents an e-mail greeting on Grandparents' Day, visited computer classes, and witnessed how to use Generations on Line, a software program that introduces the Internet to seniors. It is designed for use in libraries, retirement centers, and senior centers, where seniors can work at a computer individually or participate in classes.

Generations on Line, a national nonprofit corporation, recognized that the Internet was both a potential opportunity to multigenerational communications and a threat because Internet illiteracy could further marginalize elders from a fast-moving society. Using familiar images and large-type instructions, the program guides older persons who have no computer experience through four basic Internet functions: electronic mail (e-mail), discussion (threaded chat), a multilingual search by AltaVista, and links to other sites. Memories: Generation to Generation is designed to link school children with elders in an oral history and culture exchange.

CHIPS (Computers for Homebound and Isolated Persons) is a nonprofit project aimed at reducing the social isolation of persons who are housebound by providing a computer and free Internet access through KORRnet, which manages the project. Volunteer mentors visit CHIPS participants once a week to provide basic instruction on how to use e-mail and the Internet. This instruction results in the participant's ability to use e-mail to contact families and friends, meet other housebound and isolated persons through the CHIPS listserv, and use the Internet for purposes such as research on health concerns.

In addition to providing access to the Internet, senior centers must respond to the rise in seniors' interest in the Internet by providing communication and information on-line, as senior Internet users will expect centers to have substantial Web services and presence. A Web site provides the opportunity to reinforce printed materials, as there is almost no limit to the amount of information that can be provided there. A presence on the Web allows anyone to find your center, including potential donors.

SUGGESTIONS FOR IMPLEMENTATION

Learning technology provides seniors with new opportunities for informal and lifelong learning, distance learning, mental stimulation, and wellness. Communicating electronically, older adults can keep in touch with family and friends, exchange materials and ideas on a chosen topic, encourage each other to continue learning, and reduce their sense of isolation.

To assist older adults to learn about information technology, senior centers need to address the concerns seniors have and provide equitable computer and multimedia learning opportunities that are user-friendly and that enhance lifelong learning experiences. Older adults do have specific difficulties learning to use computers, but these difficulties can be reduced by strategies such as step-by-step learning, remedial help, self-pacing, frequent breaks, good lighting, small class size, and allotting more time for tasks and repetition. Suggestions to help introduce seniors to information technology from successful senior education programs and a review of the literature include the following:

- Provide support networks for learning and social support.
- Use instructors with the experience and qualifications to teach these classes.
- The curriculum should reflect an understanding of current hardware and software and how people use them. It should offer different strategies for learning how to use computers, both in and outside a class situation.
- Use mentors or peer helpers (older adults or youthful mentors) to provide learning assistance.
- Use equipment that is suitable to the needs of the older adult learner and that is regularly maintained and ergonomically suited to older adults.
- Offer classes in space that is comfortable, accessible, and that creates a friendly, supportive, and welcoming learning environment.
- Keep the length to no more than 1 hour without a stretch break.
- A minimum of two sessions per week is recommended to maintain learning and reinforce concepts.
- Offer instruction in small groups, through a tutor or mentor, and seminars to accommodate various learning styles.
- Computer training should be responsive to the unique experience and learning needs of older adults.
- Standard equipment may be inadequate for some older adults and attention should be given to monitor size and keyboard and mouse design.
- Purchase a good word-processing program.
- Start with games, the Internet, and e-mail.

- Set up a home page and bookmark sites of interest to seniors.
- Provide a help line.
- Develop a resource library.
- Offer open computer-lab time to give students the opportunity to use computer and communications technologies to explore their own interests, to develop skills, and to discover what the technology can do. Open lab-time provides those who are otherwise involved in structured classes with opportunities to practice what they are learning or to branch out into further explorations.
- Provide distance-education capabilities to link with isolated seniors.
- Enlist the involvement of seniors from the beginning, including planning the curriculum.
- Conduct needs assessments, surveys, and ongoing evaluation and feedback.
- Maintain a slow pace with friendly, open exchange.
- Establish a computer club.
- Using older hardware is sometimes less threatening as there is less fear of damaging something, and older hardware is slower, which allows more time and increases comfort levels.
- Setting up computers with a solitaire game and encouraging use of e-mail as a communication tool can help warm them up.
- Provide reference programs such as encyclopedias on CD-ROM.

CTCNet has a wealth of information available on planning, developing, and evaluating technology and computer classes, including recommendations for software and hardware and curriculum design.

SUGGESTED ACTIVITIES

Senior centers can provide classes and instruction on the following topics:

- basic computer skills, using the mouse and keyboard
- word processing
- database and spreadsheet skills
- introduction to e-mail
- basic Internet skills—using e-mail, chatting, search engines, and browsing the World Wide Web
- games such as chess, Go, or backgammon

- communications software
- electronic research (on-line, databases, CD-ROM)
- desktop publishing
- graphics
- Web-page design
- financial management
- how to access, find and use information on advocacy, travel, health care, and other topics and services
- family tree and genealogy programs

BIBLIOGRAPHY

Adler, R. P. (1996). *Older adults and computers: Report of a national survey.* SeniorNet. [On-line]. Available: www.seniornet.org/intute/survey2.html

American Association of Retired Persons. (2000). *A survey of computer users age 45 and older. Executive summary.* AARP National Survey on Consumer Preparedness and E-Commerce.

Arseneault, M. *How to identify and assess the needs of older adults related to learning technologies.* Third Age Centre, St. Thomas University, Resource & Research Centre on Aging.

Breeden, L., Cisler, S., Guilfoy, V., Roberts, M., & Stone, A. (1998). *Computer and communications use in low-income communities: Models for the neighborhood transformation and family development initiative.* Newton, MA: Prepared for the Annie E. Casey Foundation. Education Development Center, Inc.

Card, D., Johnson, M., & Patel, V. (2000, May 24). Assessing the digital divide(s): The Jupiter Internet Population Model, Part II. *Jupiter Communications.*

General Accounting Office. (2001, February). *Characteristics and choices of Internet users.* Washington, DC: Author.

CHIPS. (2001). *Computers for homebound and isolated persons.* [On-line]. Available: www.kornet.org/chips

Dell/Bruskin Goldring. (1999, May 11). *Older Americans and computer use, quick facts.* [On-line]. Available: www.dell.com

Dickerson, J. (1995). Never too old. *Time, 145*(12). [On-line]. Available: www.alliancenet.com/Articles/Never2old.html

Forrester Research Inc. (2000). *UK retirees adapt rapidly online and present vast, untapped opportunity, according to Forrester Research.* [On-line]. Available: www.forrester.com/ER/Press/Release/0,1769,399,FF.html

Haas, B. (1995). Intel Corporation joins with SeniorNet to bring PC power to older adults. *SeniorNet* [On-line]. Available: www.seniornet.org/inside/nr951128.html

King, D. A. (1997, June 1–4). *Coming of age: The virtual older adult learner.* Seniors' Education Centre, University Extension, University of Regina, Saskatchewan. Paper presented at Canadian Association for University Continuing Education conference (CAUCE), Saskatoon, Saskatchewan.

Lenhart, A., Rainie, L., Fox, S., Horrigan, J., & Spooner, T. (2000). *Who's not online: 57% of those without Internet access say they do not plan to log on.* Washington, DC: Pew Internet and American Life Project. [On-line]. Available: www.pewinternet.org

Mazur, B. (2001). *Barriers to participation for older persons.* Washington, DC: American Association of Retired Persons.

National Telecommunications and Information Administration. (1999). *Falling through the Net: Defining the digital divide.* Washington, DC: U.S. Department of Commerce.

National Telecommunications and Information Administration. (2000). *Falling through the Net: Toward digital inclusion.* Washington, DC: U.S. Department of Commerce.

Nua Ltd. (2000). *eMarketer: Senior citizens to embrace the web.* NUA Internet Surveys. [On-line]. Available: www.nua.ie/surveys/index

Nua Ltd. (2000). *Media metrix: Older users take to the Internet in droves.* NUA Internet Surveys. [On-line]. Available: www.nua.ie/surveys/index

Nua Ltd. (1998). *PR newswire: Rising number of over 50s online.* NUA Internet Surveys. [On-line]. Available: www.nua.ie/surveys/index

Packard Bell. (1995). *Computer savvy senior citizens as interested as teens.* [On-line]. Available: www.packardbell.com/gfx/news/survey95/1srvysen.html

Portland State University. (2000). *Too old for computers.* Office of Information Technology. [On-line]. Available: www.web.pdx.edu/~psu01435/tooold.html

Stelter, L. (2001, Spring). Silver surfers. Can you afford to ignore seniors on the Web? *AHP Journal.* Association for Healthcare Philanthropy, 10–12.

Wyden, R. (2000). *Oregon seniors and the digital divide. A survey of senior centers' Internet access in the new millennium.* Portland, Oregon.

RESOURCES

AgeLight LLC
9057 Points Drive NE
Clyde Hill, WA 98004-1611
425-455-8277
http://www.agelight.org
AgeLight.com provides resources to active adults, organizations and business to help bridge the digital and generational divides.

American Association of Retired Persons
601 E. Street NW
Washington, DC 20049
800-424-3410
http://www.aarp.org/comptech

The American Association of Retired Person's computer and technology site, offering software and hardware reviews, tips, featured Web sites and Web instructions.

Alliance for Technology Access
2175 East Francisco Boulevard, Suite L
San Rafael, CA 94901
415-455-4575
http://www.ataccess.org
Alliance for Technology Access helps to connect children and adults with disabilities to technology tools.

Computers for Homebound and Isolated Persons (CHIPS)
Knoxville-Oak Ridge Regional Network
600 Henley Street, Suite 313
Knoxville, TN 37996-4137
423-215-1540
http://www.korrnet.org/chips
CHIPS is a non-profit project aimed at reducing the social isolation of persons who are homebound, by providing a computer and free Internet access.

CTCNet
372 Broadway Street
Cambridge, MA 02139
617-354-0825
http://www.ctcnet.org
CTCNet offers resources to provide technology access and education. The CTCNet evaluation toolkit is available at: http://www.ctcnet. org/evalkit.doc

Closing the Digital Divide
Office of Telecommunications and Information Applications
National Telecommunications and Information Administration
U.S. Department of Commerce
1401 Constitution Avenue, NW, Room 4092
Washington, DC 20230
202-482-2048
http://www.digitaldivide.gov
Closing the Digital Divide is a comprehensive clearinghouse for information about efforts to provide all Americans with access to the Internet

and other information technologies that are crucial to their economic growth and personal advancement.

Generations on Line
108 Ralston House
3615 Chestnut Street
Philadelphia, PA 19104
215-222-6400
http://www.generationsonline.org
Generations on Line promotes Internet technology to enhance the quality of life of older people.

Senior.com.
17500 Redhill Avenue, Suite 220
Irvine, CA 92614
949-784-1600
http://www.senior.com
Senior.com.is an online community for older adults providing free e-mail service and home-page instructions.

Seniornet.com
121 Second Street, seventh floor
San Francisco, CA 94105
415-495-4990
http://www.seniornet.com
Seniornet.com provides older adults with access to and education about computer technology.

CHAPTER TEN

Health Promotion and Physical Fitness

MARGARETTA

She looks great crossing the finish line with a time of 27:37 at the Vintage 5K Masters Race and Walks. Why is this so unusual? After all, it is a masters race for runners who are 40-plus. It is unusual because Margaretta is 72 years old and she just started running 22 years ago. There were 47 runners who finished after her, 42 of whom were younger than she. Margaretta has been ranked among the top 10 American senior female runners by USA Track & Field.

She started to run at age 50 because her daughter, Pat, was running on lonely country roads, and Margaretta nagged her so much that Pat suggested Margaretta come along and walk. It wasn't long before mother and daughter were running partners.

Their first race together was a 10K in a suburb of Pittsburgh. Pat said she knew the course to be steep with lots of turns and figured her mom would hate it, but instead Margaretta got hooked.

They developed a strict training schedule, even running in rain and snow. They also worked out at a gymnasium and skied cross-country. They have been training together for more than two decades and have competed in numerous races, including the Pittsburgh Marathon and the Boston Marathon. A granddaughter has joined the two older women. She is clearly the fastest of the trio, and has broken several records at her high school.

Margaretta is such an unassuming person that unless you knew her racing history, you would never guess her accomplishments. Vintage has been very fortunate to have her in the Vintage race these past 20 years. We always look forward to seeing her streak across the finish line, leaving runners nearly half her age in the dust.

The National Council on the Aging's *Myth and Realities of Aging 2000* showed that in the minds of many, old age begins with a decline in physical or mental ability rather than with the arrival of a specific birthday. People are living longer than at any time in history, and they want to minimize disease and impairment in their later years. In fact, older people want to expand their potential for living well and aging successfully. Today's seniors are much more aware of the benefits of exercise and a healthy lifestyle, and they desire a varied and sophisticated program of activities. Their tremendous interest in physical fitness stems from hearing of studies that demonstrate the enormous health benefits to be obtained from a higher level of fitness. The senior center can add life to years and years to life for older adults, through opportunities for physical fitness, health promotion and education, and disease prevention.

Despite the increased awareness, many seniors are under the mistaken impression that they get adequate exercise from their daily activities. Physical activity can be divided roughly into two major categories: normal physical activity (activity intended to complete normal daily activities) and exercise (activity intended to improve fitness). Normal activities alone often are not enough to prevent some disabilities or diseases that cause disability; hence additional exercise may be required.

Aging is generally accompanied by a progressive decline in the level of physical activity. By age 75, about one in three men and one in two women engage in no physical activity. As individuals retire from employment, they may become more sedentary and often eventually rely on others to assist them in the activities of daily living. Some activities are curtailed voluntarily, whereas others become too difficult because of functional limitations. The reduction in normal activities itself could lead to disability resulting from disuse, muscle atrophy, loss of flexibility, and diminished endurance. This disuse disability perpetuates a further reduction of activity, setting up a vicious cycle of disuse and declining function.

Physical inactivity increases the risk of disability. A cross-sectional study of noninstitutionalized persons aged 65 to 84 years found evidence that being physically inactive increased the odds of being disabled, independent of age. Maintaining continued activity could limit the impact of disuse and slow the onset or reduce the risk of disability. Sustained exercise appears to be an excellent form of primary prevention of disability.

Physical activity can retard a decline in many of the determinants of physical ability, and research has shown that older adults can regain function in old age. Individuals who are frail, even those of very advanced age, have the potential to increase muscle strength. Resistance training, as a secondary prevention, improves function and may translate into declines in the level of disability. The study that proved weight training can reverse muscle loss even in 90-year-olds has researchers questioning other assumptions about normal aging changes. Some decline in physical ability is an inevitable result of the normal processes of advancing age; however, a decline in physical ability as a result of impaired muscle strength cannot be entirely attributed to aging. Loss of muscle mass, memory, and bone mass are no longer considered normal aging. In fact, many problems experienced by older persons are related to disuse. Exercise has been shown to improve strength, endurance, flexibility, and balance in older adults. Increasing the level of physical activity, therefore, might reverse some individuals' disabilities. The potential for improvement in health changes the emphasis to the prevention of disease and disability. Older adults must take a more proactive role in managing their medical problems through exercise, diet, and other lifestyle changes.

Chronic diseases are considered to be a primary cause of disability in middle-aged and older adults. Heart disease, cerebrovascular disease, hypertension, diabetes, osteoporosis, arthritis, visual impairment, and dementia have all been associated with disability. Physical activity plays a role in the prevention of coronary artery disease, stroke, and hip fracture. Exercise can also reduce the severity of hypertension, diabetes, osteoporosis, and osteoarthritis.

Osteoarthritis (degenerative arthritis) is one of the leading causes of disability. Obesity and sports-related injuries have been identified as the most common preventable causes of osteoarthritis. The National Health Interview Survey showed that the rate of persons with arthritis who reported no leisure-time activities was significantly higher than the rate among those without arthritis. However, it is not known if decreased physical activity increases the risk of osteoarthritis or whether persons with arthritis limit their physical activities because of their health. Evidence suggests that persons suffering from osteoarthritis can achieve symptom relief and improvement in function with exercise or a combination of strength and endurance exercises. Walking can also be beneficial.

Fatigue and pain resulting from arthritis, lower back problems, or other ailments cause many older people to become more sedentary, thinking that if they rest they will get better. For many years it was thought that people with arthritis and related conditions shouldn't exercise because it would damage their joints. This vicious cycle of disability and pain causes decreased movement that results in less fitness and a higher level of dysfunction. Today, however, doctors and therapists know that moderate physical activity can improve health without hurting the joints. Older adults with arthritis or osteoporosis who participate in physical activities demonstrated decreased pain and stiffness, increased mobility and muscular strength, and increased bone strength. The PACE® (People with Arthritis Can Exercise) exercise program, developed by the Arthritis Foundation for people with arthritis, is an excellent program that is easily adaptable to the senior center. PACE® uses gentle activities to help increase joint flexibility and range of motion and to help maintain muscle strength.

Another group that could benefit from health promotion and fitness opportunities at the senior center is older adults with mental retardation. Research indicates that as a group, adults with mental retardation often lack strength and have poor fitness levels. Additionally, almost half of all people with mental retardation are overweight. This general lack of fitness and obesity increases the risk for diabetes, hypertension, heart disease, stroke, arthritis, respiratory diseases, cancer, and other disabling conditions as they age and increases the likelihood that many will have health problems beyond those of their nondisabled peers.

MEDICATION MISUSE

Older adults are at greater risk than others for medication-related problems. Although medications are one of the single most important factors in improving the quality of life for older adults, this population remains especially susceptible to medication-related problems. Medication misuse is a complex problem among older populations. Older adults use prescription drugs approximately three times more frequently than the general population, and the use of over-the-counter medications by this group is even more extensive. The disproportionately greater exposure to medications, coupled with age-related physiologic changes, increases the likelihood of medication-related adverse events.

There are many reasons why an older person may misuse prescription or over-the-counter medications. Medication misuse is present when patients consciously or unconsciously consume medications in a manner that deviates from the recommended prescribed dose or instructions.

Misuse may include overuse because of a belief that more is better, as well as underuse due to cost issues or as a way to avoid side effects. Abuse of prescribed or over-the-counter drugs occurs when a patient continues to use the drug even when it is not required for the primary purpose for which it was recommended or when the person takes it in greater than recommended amounts because of its psychotropic effects. Sometimes older people receive medications from multiple prescribers for similar conditions, and polypharmacy is likely to occur.

America's seniors are undertreated for diseases every day. More than three in five Medicare beneficiaries lack access to an outpatient drug benefit and often must risk the health consequences of not receiving potentially beneficial therapies because they cannot afford their medication. Undertreatment of pain, asthma, osteoporosis, depression, and other conditions also have been reported in seniors.

It has been estimated that approximately 50% of people taking drugs do not take them correctly. Improper use of medications can cause problems such as disorientation, dizziness, and poisoning, all of which put older adults at risk of injury and illness, permanent disability, loss of independence, hospitalization, long-term institutionalization, and the loss of home and community. Twenty-five percent of hospital admissions of older people are the result of medication errors, and 25% of nursing home admissions are related to the inability of older persons to take their drugs correctly.

The reasons commonly given by older adults for misusing their medications include the following:

- They thought "more is better" or that a larger dose would make them well sooner.
- They believed the drug was not working so they stopped taking it.
- They felt better so they stopped taking their medication.
- They did not understand or remember instructions.
- They did not hear instructions correctly or misinterpreted the doctor's instructions.
- They didn't get the prescription filled or refilled.
- The medication had an unpleasant taste.
- Forgetfulness resulted in missed or wrong doses.
- Multiple medications or a complex dosage schedule made it difficult to keep track of when and how to take medicines.
- The drugs themselves cause confusion and created problems in taking the correct dose.

- They feared becoming drug-dependent.
- They tried to reduce the high costs of medications by taking old medicine, taking one half the dose, diluting the dose, skipping a day, or not having a prescription filled.
- They accidentally misused, unknowingly mixing a prescription drug with an over-the-counter drug or took medicine with alcohol, producing an undesirable effect.
- Limited mobility made it difficult to get to the pharmacy or store to purchase the medicine or to take the medicine.
- Impaired vision made it difficult to read the label, distinguish medicines, or detect evidence that a drug had deteriorated.
- They could not open the medication container because it was too difficult (childproof).

Senior centers can help by empowering seniors with the knowledge and skills to make healthy decisions. Some topics for discussion include how to provide a good medical history, and how to talk to the doctor or pharmacist about over- and behind-the-counter drugs and prescribed medications. "Brown-bag" medicine workshops can help identify older adults who may be misusing their medications. Older adults are asked to bring in all their medications in a brown paper bag, then a pharmacist or other health care professional screens the contents.

PHYSICAL FITNESS

A good physical fitness level, regardless of the disability, helps older people maintain their quality of life and independence. Older adults can obtain significant health benefits with a moderate amount of physical activity. Additional health benefits can be gained through greater amounts of physical activity, either by increasing the duration, intensity, or frequency. According to the Centers for Disease Control (CDC), physical activity

- helps maintain the ability to live independently and reduces the risk of falling and fracturing bones;
- reduces the risk of dying from coronary heart disease and of developing high blood pressure, colon cancer, and diabetes;
- can help reduce blood pressure in some people with hypertension;
- helps people with chronic, disabling conditions to improve their stamina and muscle strength;

- reduces symptoms of anxiety and depression and fosters improvements in mood and feelings of well-being;
- helps maintain healthy bones, muscles, and joints;
- helps control the joint swelling and pain associated with arthritis.

Between the ages 20 and 70, the average adult loses 30% of muscle mass, which slows metabolism, increases body fat, decreases aerobic capacity, and lowers bone density. This syndrome, called sarcopenia, reduces physical performance and predisposes older persons to diabetes, hypothermia, and osteoporosis. Joint mobility, gait, posture control, and balance, as well as strength, walking speed, and endurance are also affected. The combined effects of stiffer joints, weaker muscles, chronic diseases, and problems with vision or hearing gradually erode an older person's ability to lead a normal, vigorous life.

A sedentary lifestyle increases the risk for hip fracture, just as hip fracture leads to an increasingly sedentary existence. Even moderate exercise such as walking reduces the risk of hip fracture. Exercise has an impact on at least two risk factors for hip fracture—osteoporosis and falling. Among the independent risk factors for falls in older persons are difficulty standing up from a chair and performing a tandem walk. These can be the result of impaired leg strength and balance. Exercise has the potential to limit these impairments.

With advancing age, a gradual loss in bone mass takes place. In addition, the loss accelerates in women after menopause. Weight-bearing exercise and walking can reduce the loss of bone mass, which can reduce the risk of osteoporosis. Some interventions may retard these age-related changes. Exercises to prevent disability include resistance or strength training, endurance or aerobic training, flexibility training, and balance training. A combined program of muscle-strengthening exercise, adequate sleep, and a healthy diet will help prevent or overcome frailty and achieve optimal conditioning. Senior centers can help prevent physical frailty and falls in older persons by

- providing educational programs to help identify and eliminate environmental hazards in the home;
- providing exercise and physical training to preserve muscle and bone integrity (10 weeks of resistance exercise can nearly double leg strength, increase walking speed, improve stair climbing, and increase spontaneous physical activity);
- encouraging walking for exercise;

- teaching older persons to include adequate calcium and protein in their diet.

The literature on rehabilitation and physical activity exercise yields multiple studies that document the positive health outcomes resulting from exercise, fitness, and recreational interventions, including restoration of physical and cognitive functioning; ongoing health maintenance and self-management; prevention; community functioning and reintegration; and psychosocial well-being. Participants in a variety of physical recreation, exercise, and fitness interventions experienced significantly increased cardiovascular fitness, decreased body weight and body fat, decreased blood pressure, and increased flexibility, strength, ambulation, and range of motion. Interventions include organized sports and fitness activities, adventure activities, activities promoting socialization and self-expression, and health and lifestyle education. These interventions address restoration of functioning, health maintenance, reduction of health risk factors, and psychosocial health concerns.

Coronary artery disease promotes disability as a result of myocardial infarction and by its progression to congestive heart failure, which causes significant morbidity by compromising strength and endurance. A sedentary lifestyle is the most prevalent modifiable risk factor for coronary artery disease, far exceeding hypertension, elevated serum cholesterol, and smoking. In the United States, a sedentary lifestyle contributes to more coronary artery disease deaths than any other risk factor. The relationship between a lack of physical activity and the risk of stroke is also significant. Evidence from studies has shown a consistent association between greater physical activity and the reduced rate of coronary artery disease and that the cardiovascular benefits of endurance exercise extend into late life. It has been estimated that sustained exercise in patients with established coronary artery disease reduces the risk of cardiac mortality by 20% to 25%. In addition, the severity of several risk factors for coronary artery disease, hypertension, hyperlipidemia, diabetes, and obesity can be reduced by physical activity.

Participation in various exercise and fitness activities resulted in significant improvements in cardiovascular and respiratory functioning; increased strength, endurance, and coordination; improvement in long-term health status and reduction in health risk factors such as lowered cholesterol levels; reduced heart disease risk; and improved ability to manage chronic pain for persons with disabilities. A study of postmenopausal women athletes found their body fat was 33% lower than that of postmenopausal women in general and they had the cardiovascular function of women 30 years younger. Physically disabled participants in fitness and athletic activities also show improvement in psychosocial health and well-being, including decreased depression, improved body image, and increased acceptance of disability.

Exercise has been advocated as a means of improving mood, reducing the impact of other health risks, reducing the risk of disability, and decreasing the risk of dying prematurely. To obtain the maximum benefit, physical fitness must be maintained for a lifetime. Although a lifetime of fitness is the ideal, the initiation of exercise in adulthood is also beneficial. In one study, unfit men who improved their level of fitness over an average of 5 years reduced their mortality risk by nearly 50%.

The U.S. Preventive Services Task Force has recommended that health care providers counsel sedentary adults to engage in regular moderate physical activity. Although vigorous exercise may provide more cardiovascular benefits, moderate physical activity is nearly as beneficial and carries less risk of injury. Moderate physical activity is defined as activities that can be comfortably sustained for at least 60 minutes.

For healthy individuals, exercise for the primary prevention of disability should include regular sessions of moderate physical activity. Although aerobic activities have substantial cardiovascular benefits, the addition of strength training is required to reduce the risk of loss of function. Light to moderate weight-training that includes relatively lightweight resistance with numerous repetitions of the upper limbs, lower limbs, and torso can maintain the strength needed to continue independence in the activities of daily living. Strength training should be used in addition to endurance exercises, such as walking, biking, and related aerobic activities. Frequent short sessions are recommended for endurance training as they have a better rate of compliance. Flexibility training is also recommended.

For people who already have disabilities, exercise as a secondary prevention offers an opportunity to reduce the burden of impairment and possibly to improve function. Even patients of very advanced age who are frail can improve muscle strength. Improved strength of the lower limbs may increase mobility and decrease the risk of falling.

By minimizing disuse, strengthening muscles and bones, improving performance, and limiting the effects of chronic or disabling illnesses, physical activity has an important role in the prevention of disability.

Although the maintenance of normal, everyday activities may decrease the risk of disability, added exercise seems necessary to slow age-related declines in muscle strength and aerobic capacity.

HEALTH, FITNESS AND SEXUALITY

Marian E. Dunn, PhD, director of the Center for Human Sexuality at the State University of New York in Brooklyn, sees a strong link between health, fitness, and sexuality in older couples. Aging is often blamed for sexual problems that are actually caused by disease. The medications taken for major illness or surgery, as well as the exhaustion and physical and psychological trauma of illness and surgery, affect sexual desire and performance in both women and men.

The American Association of Retired Persons and *Modern Maturity* conducted a sexuality survey of 1,384 adults aged 45 and older in 1999. The mail survey found that midlife and older adults are optimistic about the quality of their lives as they age, and the majority say a satisfying sexual relationship is important to that quality of life. Relationships are even more important than sexual activity per se. Nine in ten say a good relationship with a spouse or partner and close ties to friends and families are important to their quality of life.

The *partner gap* is one of the most obvious factors affecting sexual activity. Though 8 in 10 adults aged 45 to 59 have sexual partners, only 58% of men and 21% of women aged 75 and older have partners. Gender and age influence the sexual attitudes and activity of midlife and older adults, and sexual activity tends to be more important to men than to women. For example, among those aged 45 to 59, 71% of men and 48% of women agree that sexual activity is important to their overall quality of life, but among those who are 75 and older, only 35% of men and 13% of women agree.

Declining health has serious consequences for both sexual activity and sexual satisfaction as people age. The AARP/ *Modern Maturity* sexuality survey shows that many older adults are not being treated for ailments that may be affecting their sex lives. More than half of those who report no major diseases or depression say they engage in sexual intercourse at least once a week, compared to around 3 in 10 of those with either depression or some other major disease.

The most important factors that both men and women believe would improve their sexual satisfaction are better health for themselves, better health for their partners, and less stress. In addition, men also cite more free time and women add finding a partner to the list.

Currently available treatments can help older adults overcome health impediments to sexual satisfaction. However, only a small minority of those with self-described sexual problems are currently availing themselves of these treatments, and large numbers are not even receiving treatment for common ailments that can affect sexual performance, such as arthritis. Senior centers can help by providing education and screening programs and opportunities for individuals to discuss their concerns with a health professional.

HEALTH PROMOTION

The World Health Organization's formulating health as "physical, mental and social well-being, not merely the absence of disease and infirmity" was an important step in elaborating a new concept of health that served as the basis for health promotion. Henry E. Sigerist, a medical historian, described health as "not simply the absence of disease but as something positive, a joyful attitude toward life, and a cheerful acceptance of the responsibilities that life puts upon the individual."

Health-promotion education emphasizes personal motivation and individual responsibility to help older adults develop healthy lifestyles to maintain and enhance their state of well-being. However, according to the President's Commission on Health Needs of the Nation, individual responsibility for health can be fully effective only if access to necessary education, social supports, and professional services is available. Behavior and social networks are increasingly recognized for their relationship to health. Social support from family and friends has been consistently and positively related to regular physical activity. The U.S. government's emphasis on community programs and the evidence linking the positive relationship of behavior and social networks to health makes senior centers a logical choice for promoting health and fitness.

Healthy People 2010 is the prevention agenda for the nation as established by the U.S. government, designed to identify the most significant preventable threats to health and establish goals to reduce these threats. Physical activity, weight, mental health, and access to health care are among the leading health indicators identified by *Healthy People 2010*, reflecting major areas of health concern. The government wants everyone to understand the importance of health promotion and disease prevention and to encourage wide participation in improving health. The goals of *Healthy People 2010* include increasing the quality and years of healthy life and eliminating health disparities through educational and community-based programs, health communication, physical activity, and fitness. Individuals, groups, and organizations are encouraged to integrate *Healthy People 2010* into current programs and health care providers are encouraged to have their patients pursue a healthier life and participate in community-based programs.

Vintage began an affiliation with The Western Pennsylvania Hospital in 1976. This affiliation has included nursing support, health and wellness programming, and active mutual participation in joint health activities. In 1996, the affiliation was formalized into an active partnership. West Penn Hospital's Division of Geriatrics was moved into Vintage's senior center and a physician and nursing office was opened there.

Today, the staffs of West Penn's Senior Health Services program and Vintage join together to continue to provide quality health and wellness programs. The array of programs includes exercise classes, health screenings, on-site nursing support, health and wellness lectures, and individual consultations on a variety of health and wellness issues. A nurse practitioner is available for nursing concerns.

This unique relationship enables physicians to encourage their patients to participate in the programs at Vintage. In 2001, personal wellness profiles were implemented to help identify seniors who are the best candidates for a successful lifestyle change. Assessment data and health enhancement recommendations are built from senior-specific research. The program provides each participant with an individual report that leads them to a thorough understanding of their health status. Progress and group summary reports illustrate the impact of wellness programs.

The CDC recommends community-based physical activity programs that offer aerobic, strengthening, and flexibility components specifically designed for older adults and community activities that include opportunities for older adults to be physically active. Community-based senior centers provide the perfect venue that is affordable and accessible to create healthy older adults in cooperation with governmental and health care partners.

Collaborations can provide unique opportunities that build on the strength of participating organizations. Young at Heart was a 12-week exercise and wellness program designed to encourage seniors to participate in cardiovascular, weight, strength, and resistance exercises under the supervision of trained fitness and health professionals. Made possible by a collaboration among The Western Pennsylvania Hospital, the YMCA, and Highmark Blue Cross Blue Shield, Young at Heart also contained health education and health promotion components to help seniors become more active participants in their health care. The Joslin Diabetes Center of The Western Pennsylvania Hospital, in collaboration with the Allegheny County Health Department, provides diabetes screening and nutrition education to area senior centers.

Wellness Works is a comprehensive health promotion effort of the Milwaukee County Department on Aging and the University of Wisconsin-Milwaukee to conduct research on factors that motivate older adults to change health-related behaviors.

The National Council on the Aging's public policy agenda for 1999–2000 recommended that increased attention be focused on actions and techniques intended to prevent illness or disability, because it is easier to prevent disease than it is to cure it. Disease prevention—including access to health promotion activities, protocols, and regimens for older and disabled persons—should be an essential component throughout the continuum of care. Health promotion fosters physical, mental, emotional, and spiritual well-being that is vital for older adults and helps prevent costly medical care.

The Health Promotion Institute of the National Council on Aging produced *Best Practices: Health Promotion and Aging,* a manual featuring programs such as the Get Fit-Stay Fit Challenge series from Phoenix, Arizona, as a best-practice health-promotion program. The series aims to help people develop, maintain, or increase their commitment to regular physical activity by employing goal setting, progress recording, and positive feedback with a community focus that emphasizes participation as part of a community effort. Another featured program is Positive Adults Taking Health Seriously (PATHS), which is an interdisciplinary wellness program that provides health promotion to older adults at senior centers from three vantage points: (a) the biology of aging and physical health education, (b) mental health and coping skills, and (c) exercise.

Practicing healthy behaviors such as avoiding tobacco, eating nutritious foods, and exercising regularly will help dispel the myth that disease and disability are inevitable with age. Good health habits can preserve and even improve function and prevent disability. Yet healthy aging is much more than preventing disease and disability. Continuing to be a productive member of society, maintaining friendships, remaining mentally active, and developing interests and skills are also very important in health promotion. The senior center is uniquely qualified to meet all those needs.

A University of Chicago Medical School study of older men with diabetes found that those who learn self-care techniques and participate in member-run support groups 2 years later are less depressed, less stressed, gain more knowledge, and rate the quality of their lives higher than those who didn't take such actions. Self-help groups make significant contributions to positive outcomes for persons affected by mental and behavioral disorders. Former Surgeon General C. Everett Koop's experience as a medical practitioner taught him the importance of self-help groups in assisting their members in dealing with problems, stress, hardship, pain, isolation, powerlessness, and alienation. Self-help groups are a powerful and constructive means for people to help themselves and one another.

COMPLEMENTARY AND ALTERNATIVE MEDICINE

Complementary and alternative medicine cover a broad range of healing philosophies, approaches, and therapies that conventional medicine does not commonly use, accept, study, understand, or make available. These include the use of acupuncture, herbs, homeopathy, therapeutic massage, and traditional Oriental medicine to promote well-being or treat health conditions. Therapies may be used alone, as an alternative to conventional therapies, or in addition to conventional, mainstream therapies, in what is referred to as a complementary or integrative approach. Many complementary and alternative medicine therapies are considered holistic as they consider the whole person, including physical, mental, emotional, and spiritual aspects.

Recent studies have reported that one third of older adults use at least one form of complementary and alternative medicine and baby boomers are particularly interested. This figure is projected to grow, particularly as the government, insurers, and medical schools continue to embrace these approaches. Herbal medicine, massage, megavitamins, self-help groups, folk remedies, energy healing, and homeopathy are the most popular forms of complementary and alternative medicine. People used complementary and alternative medicine not only because they were dissatisfied with conventional medicine, but because these health care alternatives mirrored their own values, beliefs, and philosophical orientations toward health and life. Despite the broad use of alternative therapies, older adults need more information to use them effectively and safely. Senior centers can help older adults understand the types of available complementary and alternative medicine modalities and develop empowering health programs and services for them.

SPORTS AND FITNESS

Today, senior athletes are challenging old ideas about fitness after 50. Older athletes are breaking records, including some of their own. They are participating in team sports such as softball, baseball, and hockey. Golf is one sport in which participation increases with age, and golfers actually play more as they get older because they have more time to play. Some begin playing sports to combat health problems such as high blood pressure or for therapy. Others are returning to the athletic sport they excelled in as youths or are discovering the fun of friendly competition they missed the first time around in high school.

Many senior centers sponsor team sports, sport clubs, and athletic events. Vintage sponsors the Vintage 5K Masters Race and Walk, which began in 1981 as a vehicle to promote positive aging during Older Americans' month. The Penn Hills Senior Center in western Pennsylvania was one of the original sites to sponsor a senior softball team. Today six teams of 100 older men participate in the local intramural league. The Penn Hills Center also hosts the Western Pennsylvania Softball League and the National Senior Softball League, which leads to the Senior Softball World Series. They also host a women's softball league, in which the oldest participant is 75 years old. Pittsburgh's Citiparks Senior Centers recruit participants for Pennsylvania's Senior Games. More than 10,000 senior athletes participate in senior game competitions every year. The local senior games feed into state senior games that feed into the National Senior Games—the Senior Olympics.

Physical changes that accompany aging can affect the ability to enjoy sports. Because the human body is not designed to withstand the stresses of some professional and amateur sports, participation can cause physical damage. The most common sports injuries are ankle sprains, shoulder and rotator-cuff problems, shin splints, Achilles tendonitis, pain in the front of the knee, elbow problems, and low back pain. Though the body is very good at repairing itself, the aging body takes longer to recover. Senior athletes can benefit from injury prevention programs.

Another way to help prevent injury is by cross-training, which combines two or more types of exercise into a physical activity routine. It can alleviate boredom and help prevent injury from overworking the same muscles. Cross-training increases the likelihood of incorporating the four building components of fitness (endurance, strength, flexibility, and balance) into an exercise routine, especially if the activities are varied. It also can help the older adult become a more versatile athlete, learn new and different skills, build more flexibility into the workout routine, and improve overall athletic performance. Activities in each of the major exercise categories include the following:

ENDURANCE

- swimming
- running, jogging, walking
- dancing
- cycling
- jumping rope
- rowing
- skiing
- cross-country skiing
- stair climbing
- court or team sports (volleyball, tennis, racquetball)

STRENGTH

- free weights
- weight machines, circuit training
- bands and tubes
- calisthenics (push-ups, pull-ups)
- aquatics
- stair climbing
- skating

FLEXIBILITY

- yoga
- Pilates method of conditioning
- other stretching exercises

Balance

- tai chi
- leg-strengthening exercises (machines, weights, chair exercises, stair climbing)
- dancing

SUGGESTED ACTIVITIES (IN ADDITION TO THE ACTIVITIES SUGGESTED ABOVE)

Activities

- aerobics
- aquatics, water aerobics
- golf and bowling leagues
- balance training
- People with Arthritis Can Exercise (PACE®)

Educational Programs

- therapeutic massage for stress relief and relaxation
- meditation
- chi kung for health and vitality
- "brown-bag" medication workshops
- smoking cessation
- depression information
- mental fitness
- falls prevention, flexible fitness
- nutrition education, healthful eating
- cooking light
- sexuality
- health screenings
- sports injury prevention
- health promotion education
- chronic disease self-management (such as diabetes and arthritis) workshops and self-help groups
- complementary and alternative medicine

BIBLIOGRAPHY

American Association of Retired Persons. (1999). *AARP/Modern Maturity sexuality survey. Summary of findings.* [On-line]. Available: www.research.aarp.org/health/ mmsexsurvey_1.html

American Association of Retired Persons. (2000). *Cross training for optimal fun and fitness.* [On-line]. Available: www.aarp.org/confacts/fitness/crosstrain.html

American Society of Consultant Pharmacists. (2001). *America's seniors. The most to gain, the most to lose.* [On-line]. Available: www.ascp.com/public/ga/quality/

American Society of Consultant Pharmacists. (2001). *ASCP's prescription for quality care. Preventing medication-related problems among older Americans.* [On-line]. Available: www.ascp.com/public/ga/quality/

Breslow, L. (1999, March 17). From disease prevention to health promotion. *Journal of the American Medical Association, 281*(11), 1030–1033.

Butler, R. N. (2000, February). Fighting frailty—Prescription for healthier aging includes exercise, nutrition, safety, and research. *Geriatrics.*

Butwin, D. (1999, July/August). Living to the max. *Modern Maturity.* [On-line]. Available: www.aarp.org/mmaturity/jul_aug99/livingmax.html

Carlson, J. E. (1999, January 1). Disability in older adults 2: Physical activity as prevention. *Behavioral Medicine, 24*(4), 157.

Centers for Disease Control and Prevention. (2000). *A report of the Surgeon General on physical activity and health.* National Center for Chronic Disease Prevention and Health Promotion. Atlanta, GA: Author.

Gilden, J., et al. (1990, January). Diabetes support groups improve health of older diabetic patients. *Journal of the American Geriatrics Society, 40,* 147–150.

Koop, C. E. (1992). *Self-help: Concepts and applications.* Philadelphia: Charles Press.

Mamula, K. (2001, March). How old is old? *Pitt Magazine,* 20–25.

National Council on the Aging. (1999). *Best practices. Health promotion and aging.* Washington, DC: Author.

National Council on the Aging. (2000). *Myths and realities of aging 2000.* Washington, DC: Author.

National Council on the Aging. (2001). *NCOA's 1999–2000 public policy agenda.* Washington, DC: Author. [On-line]. Available: www.ncoa.org

National Council on the Aging. (1999, October/November). Staying fit in Phoenix. *Innovations: The Journal of the National Council on the Aging.* [On-line]. Available at: www.ncoa.org/news/get_fit.html

Ohio State University Extension. (2001). *Medication misuse among older adults.* Senior Series. SS-128-97. [On-line]. Available: www.ohioline.ag.ohio-state.edu/ss-fact/ 0128.html

Patterson, T., Lacro, J., & Jeste, D. (1999, April). Abuse and misuse of medications in the elderly. *Psychiatric Times, 16*(4). [On-line]. Available: www.psychiatrictimes. com/p990454.html

President's Commission on Health Needs of the Nation. (1952). *Building America's health.* Washington, DC: U.S. Government Printing Office.

Rimmer, J. H. (1997). *Aging, mental retardation and physical fitness.* Chicago: University of Illinois Chicago Center on Health Promotion Research for Persons with

Disabilities, Rehabilitation, Research and Training Center on Aging with Mental Retardation, Institute on Disability and Human Development.

Raasch, W. G. (2000, March 14). *Advice for the aging athlete.* Medical College of Wisconsin and Froedtert Hospital. [On-line]. Available: www.healthlink. mcw.edu/article/953058816.html

Temple University. (1991). *Benefits of therapeutic recreation: A consensus view.* Philadelphia: Author.

U.S. Department of Health and Human Services. (2000). *Healthy people 2010.* Washington, DC: Office of Disease Prevention and Health Promotion, United States Department of Health and Human Services. [On-line]. Available: www.health. gov./healthypeople.

U.S. Department of Health and Human Services. (1991). *Healthy people 2000: National health promotion and disease prevention objectives.* Washington, DC: Author.

Wellness Walks, Milwaukee, WI. (2002). National Council on the Aging. [On-line]. Available: www.ncoa.org/men/bp_wellness.htm

World Health Organization. (1985). *Basic documents, 35th edition.* Geneva, Switzerland: Author.

RESOURCES

The Arthritis Foundation

1330 West Peachtree Street
Atlanta, GA 30309
404-872-7100
www.arthritis.org
The Arthritis Foundation is a national organization that supports the more than 100 types of arthritis and related conditions with advocacy, programs, services and research.

Centers for Disease Control and Prevention (CDC)

1600 Clifton Road
Atlanta, GA 30333
404-639-3311
http://www.cdc.gov
The Centers for Disease Control and Prevention is the lead federal agency for protecting the health and safety of people. The CDC serves as the national focus for developing and applying disease prevention and control, environmental health, and health promotion and education activities designed to improve the health of the people of the United States.

Department of Health and Human Services
Office of Disease Prevention and Health Promotion
Hubert H. Humphrey Building, Room 738G
200 Independence Avenue, SW.
Washington, DC 20201
http://odphp.osophs.dhhs.gov/
The Office of Disease Prevention and Health Promotion works to strengthen the disease prevention and health promotion priorities of the Department of Health and Human Services.

Fifty-Plus Fitness Association
PO Box 20230
Stanford, CA 94309
650-323-6160
http://www.50plus.org/
Fifty-Plus is an international organization devoted to information about, motivation toward, and participation in exercise and fitness while aging.

International Association of Physical Activity, Aging and Sports (IAPAAS)
706 Madison Ave.
Albany, NY 12208
518-465-6927
http://www.rit.edu/~pjr0120/csa/iapaas/
The International Association of Physical Activity, Aging and Sports is a membership division of the Center for the Study of Aging of Albany, NY.

National Council on the Aging (NCOA)
Health Promotion Institute
409 Third Street
Washington, DC 20024
202-479-1200
www.ncoa.org/hpi
The Health Promotion Institute of NCOA is devoted to promoting optimal quality of life including good physical, mental and emotional health, and social and spiritual well-being for older adults.

National Center for Complementary and Alternative Medicine
PO Box 8218
Silver Spring, MD 20907-8218

301-231-7537
http://nccam.nih.gov/
The National Center for Complementary and Alternative Medicine at the National Institutes of Health stimulates, develops, and supports research on complementary and alternative medicine.

National Senior Games Association
3032 Old Forge Drive
Baton Rouge, LA 70808
225-925-5678
http://www.nsga.com/
The National Senior Games Association promotes a healthy lifestyles for seniors through education, fitness and sports. The National Senior Games spearheads the senior games movement, sanctioning and coordinating the efforts of senior games organizations across the country.

Penn Hills Senior Center
147 Jefferson Street
Penn Hills, PA 15235
412-244-3400
Penn Hills Senior Center hosts local, regional, and national senior softball games.

Self-Help Clearinghouse
100 Hanover Ave., Suite 202
Cedar Knolls, NJ 07927
973-625-3037
www.selfhelpgroups.org
Publications include *Self-Help Sourcebook* and the national self-help group database. This searchable database includes information on approximately 700+ self-help support groups, ideas for starting groups, and opportunities to link with others to develop needed new national or international groups.

U.S. Department of Health and Human Services
200 Independence Avenue, SW
Washington, DC 20201
202-619-0257
http://www.os.dhhs.gov/

The Department of Health and Human Services is the United States government's principal agency for protecting the health of all Americans and providing essential human services.
National Institutes of Health (NIH)
http://www.nih.gov/
Comprised of 27 separate Institutes and Centers, the National Institute of Health is one of eight health agencies that is part of the U.S. Department of Health and Human Services.

Wellsource, Inc.
Health assessment and prevention programs
15431 SE 82nd Drive
Clackamas, OR 97015
503-656-7446
http://www.wellsource.com
Wellsource provides a portfolio of tools that help organizations develop successful health management programs.

West Penn~Vintage Community Care for Seniors
Senior Health Services
401 N. Highland Avenue
Pittsburgh, PA 15206
412-362-1480
http://www.seniorhealthservices.com/
The West Penn Hospital-Vintage Community Care for Seniors office is a primary care physician practice located at the Vintage Senior Center. The staffs of West Penn Hospital's Senior Health Services program and Vintage join together to provide quality health and wellness programs.

CHAPTER ELEVEN

Horticulture

FELIX

Sometime around the middle of April, Felix shows up at my office door with a plastic bag containing a beautiful rhododendron flower. As the gardening season progresses we usually receive lilies, but an orchid may appear at any time during the year. Felix does not grow ordinary run-of-the-mill plants, only special varieties that would be the envy of any gardener. Recently he gave me a lovely cream-colored blossom that looked like a lily, but when I asked him about it, he told me it was a Peruvian daffodil.

At 72 years of age, Felix is a walking encyclopedia on plants and gardening. He was lucky because he got a very early start when he was adopted as a gardening buddy by the landlord of the apartment building in Atlanta where Felix lived with his parents. Felix and the landlord and his wife searched the local nursery each spring where they traveled the fields, choosing the perfect specimens.

When they returned home, Felix helped plant their purchases in a large backyard, all the while receiving instructions on how to place them in the ground as well as valuable plant information that has remained with him to this day.

When the family moved to Pittsburgh, Felix will tell you that gardening was put on the back burner until around 1943 when he remembered building a flower box for his sister who was at college. He planted gladiolus in the box, but his sister did not appreciate his work at all. He agreed that his choice of flowers for a window box was not the best. When he saw an ad in Mechanics Illustrated *advertising a correspondence course in growing orchids, his father agreed he could take the course.*

Felix remembered receiving some orchids along with the written material and says they never grew but his interest in orchids clearly did. He describes his love of them as an "infectious disease." Over the years his collection has grown to the point where he now has a greenhouse in which to grow his many plants.

Felix has shared his love and knowledge of gardening with the Vintage staff and the participants. He has offered seminars on gardening as well as helping with a garden at Vintage. Felix also volunteers as a mentor in the computer studio.

When asked what this lifelong interest in plants and gardening has meant to him, he said, "It has made it possible for me to live as long as I have because it has given me an outlet. It is therapeutic and challenging. Additionally, it has given me an opportunity to travel and to increase my knowledge."

Felix is an example of someone who brings a new dimension to a senior center. His knowledge of gardening is remarkable and his willingness to share this knowledge is appreciated by Vintage. At 72, Felix remains a vibrant man, due in part to his continued interest in horticulture.

Horticulture is the science and art of growing fruits, vegetables, flowers, or ornamental plants. A horticulture program can be of great value in any therapeutic, educational, or recreational setting, offering opportunities for developing skills, creativity, and self-esteem. People have a natural affinity for gardens and gardening as food, medicine, relaxation, and as a creative outlet. The end results—fresh vegetables and herbs and beautiful flowers and plants—provide a sense of pride and achievement.

Gardening is the number one outdoor leisure activity in America, with 84% of households involved in at least one form of gardening activity, a source of personal satisfaction providing esthetic pleasure and relief from stress. With a little planning and creativity, it can be available to everyone. Horticulture programs provide many older adults with the opportunity to use existing skills derived from a lifetime of gardening experience. Older adults who have never gardened can acquire a new and rewarding hobby.

It is not necessary to have expensive facilities or a large garden to initiate a successful horticulture program. Even the most limited facilities can be modified to accommodate horticultural activities. If there is no greenhouse available, use a sunny window. If there is no window, special lights can be used for growing plants. If there is no place for a garden, plant in containers and terrariums. In fact, an increasing number of gardeners are discovering the advantages of gardening in planters, containers, and raised beds. Containers and raised beds make it easier for disabled and older gardeners and for those who lack adequate space. With the appropriate modifications, gardeners who have lost physical ability can continue this valuable activity.

HORTICULTURE THERAPY

Horticultural therapy is a process that utilizes plants and horticultural activities to improve the social, educational, psychological, and physical adjustment of persons while increasing recreational and leisure options. It has proven to be beneficial for older adults and people who are physically disabled or mentally ill; hospital patients and those who are developmentally disabled; substance abusers, public offenders, and those who are socially disadvantaged. A major therapeutic aspect of horticulture therapy is the benefit to be derived from nurturing living plants. Beyond that, the type of horticultural activity depends on the abilities and needs of the participants. Therapeutic goals include sensory stimulation; social interaction and integration; feelings of belonging; engagement with others; development of self-esteem and self-worth; positive, enjoyable experiences; and integration into everyday community life.

Three groups of individuals are involved in implementing horticultural therapy programs:

1. professional horticultural therapists who conduct programs that focus on horticulture as the treatment method
2. allied professionals, including occupational therapists, physical therapists, recreation therapists, activity specialists, nurses, and rehabilitation specialists
3. volunteers who are knowledgeable about horticulture and wish to help others

Horticultural therapy activities are meaningful, motivational, productive, nonthreatening, and extremely rewarding to participants. They can enhance self-esteem, alleviate depression, improve motor skills, feed the imagination, encourage social interactions and communication, educate people about an important aspect of life, and teach certain marketable horticultural and business skills. Participants can be involved in all phases of gardening, including selling the produce and plants they grow. A horticultural therapy program can even support itself through sales of the end product.

Horticultural therapy is validated by research and complements other forms of therapy. It is an increasingly popular health-promotion activity. Several studies illustrate the physical value of gardening, reporting that you can burn as many calories in 45 minutes of gardening as in 30 minutes of aerobics. One hour of weeding burns 300 calories (the same as walking or bicycling at a moderate pace), and manual mowing of the lawn burns 500 calories per hour (the same rate as playing tennis).

Studies conducted over the last 50 years confirm that the relationship between people, plants, and their habitats are critically important to the health of the individual, the community, and the environment. Nurturing living plants places the participant in the caregiving role, providing confidence and a sense of purpose and self worth.

Surveys of gardeners revealed that the most beneficial aspect of growing plants is achieving a sense of peace and tranquillity. Simply looking at trees and vegetation reduces stress, lowers blood pressure, and relieves muscle tension. Gardening can produce endorphin highs similar to those experienced when jogging and cycling. Other benefits of horticultural activities include the following:

INTELLECTUAL BENEFITS

1. Attainment of new skills: The student gains many new abilities such as plant propagation, gardening, and flower arranging.
2. Improved vocabulary and communication skills: Participants in the program learn new terms and new concepts.
3. Aroused sense of curiosity: Plants are interesting; they generate questions and offer opportunities for experimentation.
4. Increased power of observation from watching the interaction between plants, people, and animals.
5. Vocational and prevocational training: Participants may pursue horticulture-related jobs after completion of a horticulture program.
6. Stimulation of sensory perceptions: Vision, hearing, touch, taste, and smell all play an important role in gaining the full benefit from a horticultural therapy program. Sensitivity to one's surroundings increases the perception of details.
7. Stimulation of an understanding of abstract concepts such as time management, coping with change, worry, stress management, and grief.

SOCIAL BENEFITS

1. Provides interaction within the group. The members of a group learn to relate to one another in a more meaningful way as they work together toward a common goal.

2. Provides opportunities for interaction outside of the group at garden clubs, flower shows, and on field trips. Helps participants feel they are productive members of society when they can share the products of their own effort with others.

EMOTIONAL GROWTH

1. Improves confidence and self-esteem and enhances well-being. Pride in the completed project and a sense of responsibility and accomplishment all lead to an improved self-concept.

2. Relieves aggression in a socially acceptable manner. Horticultural therapy program provides many outlets for aggression, leading to improved self-control through redirection of aggressive drives. (A study of residences for Alzheimer's patients showed that at residences with gardens, the rate of violent incidents declined by 19% over 2 years. At the residences without gardens, the violent incidents increased by 680%.)

3. Promotes interest and enthusiasm for the future. This is an important aspect for older persons and individuals who are emotionally disturbed who have lost interest in the future, providing an opportunity to participate in the creation of life and the anticipation of its growth.

4. Satisfies creative drives. Creativity and self-expression are evident in flower arranging, landscaping, and many other aspects of horticulture.

5. Provides an opportunity to have some control over, and make a positive impact on, the immediate surroundings.

6. Provides a distraction from pain or compulsive behavior.

PHYSICAL BENEFITS

1. Development and improvement of basic motor skills, manual dexterity, and muscle strength. Specific activities can be used to improve muscle coordination and to train unused muscles.

2. Increased outdoor activities. Flower and vegetable gardens and landscape maintenance provide many opportunities for meaningful outdoor activities.

SUGGESTIONS FOR IMPLEMENTATION

Once the decision has been made to incorporate horticulture into the program of the senior center, three areas must be given thoughtful consideration: (a) the individuals who will participate in the program, (b) the specific goals toward which the program is directed, and (c) the techniques for implementing the program. Some of the factors to be considered include the following:

- Each individual should work according to his or her needs and abilities.
- Design the project so that participants can manage most of the work themselves.
- Not all members of the group will have equal interest in plants. Encourage participation in related activities such as building birdhouses.
- Every activity should have a definite function and be an integral part of the entire program.
- Present information about plants that will increase the enjoyment of gardening and encourage further activity. Avoid too scientific or complex an approach to horticulture.
- Incorporate projects to show the interrelationships among various aspects of nature, including plants, people, and animals.
- Participate in flower shows and other exhibits to give participants an opportunity to display their talents.
- Public and private parks, gardens, arboreta, and greenhouses can be sites for field trips.
- In planning a vegetable or herb garden, consider how the produce will be used (consumed on the premises or elsewhere, sold, given away) and what facilities are available to handle it after harvest.

SUGGESTED ACTIVITIES

A full range of activities are available, making it possible to plan a year-round program of activities.

ARTS AND CRAFTS

- model gardens
- artificial flowers and arrangements
- needlework projects such as decorating aprons for yard work, cross-stitching flowers, etc.
- jewelry-making from seeds, cones, and dried flowers
- weaving with materials from the garden
- wall plaques such as seed mosaics, seedpod pictures, and pressed and dried flowers
- stationery and note cards using techniques such as leaf and flower prints, potato block prints, and pressed flowers
- sachet and potpourri
- building and decorating planters
- dried and pressed flowers
- holiday crafts such as ornaments from pinecones, wreaths, corsages, holiday cards, etc.
- garden sculpture
- bird and butterfly attractors (i.e., feeding stations, houses, baths, etc.)
- floral design
- herbal vinegars and oils

GROUP ACTIVITIES

- games (garden bingo, flower quizzes)
- movies and slide shows (many available through libraries, arboreta, and garden clubs)
- excursions to arboreta, gardens, flower shows, nurseries, greenhouses, orchards, and parks
- collecting trips for crafts—rocks, insects, weeds, wildflowers, cones, tree flowers, seeds and seedpods, mosses, and terrarium plants
- horticultural exhibit
- garden tours
- garden club
- intergenerational activities
- plant identification
- arboriculture studies
- nutrition through gardening
- ecology

Support Groups

Horticultural therapy activities have included support groups as an additional resource for healing and support to individuals, their caregivers, and other family members dealing with a chronic illness. By focusing on the person and not the disease, the support group encourages the individual's ability to participate in self-nurturance for his or her own healing. Each session can include an issue for discussion, such as relaxation techniques, and a hands-on plant-related activity such as planting container gardens or plant propagation. Through horticultural activities and discussion, connections are made between natural life processes and the healing journey.

Indoor Plants

- flower arranging
- corsage making
- dish gardens, terrariums, and other containers
- culture, identification, and propagation of houseplants
- forcing of bulbs
- bonsai
- potting plants

Outdoor Activities

- landscaping and garden design
- activities with birds and animals in the garden
- plant propagation
- organic, vegetable, flower, or herb gardening
- raised-bed gardening
- container gardening and hanging planters
- water gardening
- pruning
- community garden

ADAPTATIONS

Millions of individuals with disabilities garden or would garden if given greater accessibility to tools and techniques that would facilitate this hobby. Numerous books and articles have been published that are targeted to gardeners with disabilities, as this is a growing area of opportunity.

Several arboreta and botanical gardens have developed accessible demonstration gardens to assist individuals with disabilities in developing home gardens. The scope of their existing educational programs has been expanded to make them of interest and value to special populations.

The most common difficulties experienced by older persons while they are gardening are difficulty in bending, poor balance, weak grip, impaired vision, and decreased arm span. Gardening can be used in a therapeutic way to address the issues of aging and disability. Some modifications can be made in gardening practices and tools to improve accessibility:

- Paint tools a bright color.
- Use larger seed, seed tape or seed pellets to make it easier to see and grasp the seeds.
- Grow plants with more tactile and olfactory stimulation.
- Provide smooth surfaced paths.
- Use raised beds and other containers to reduce the need for bending or kneeling and provide a place to sit while gardening.
- Watering wands and lightweight watering cans make watering plants easier.
- Adaptive tools such as elongated and padded handles provide better leverage and improved grip.
- Garden stools and kneeling cushions help make it easier for older adults to raise and lower themselves to the ground.
- Use plants that trigger memories, such as roses.
- Allow plenty of time for gardening activities, keeping the pace leisurely and projects simple.

COMMUNITY GARDENS

Research has shown that people prefer scenes of nature over urban scenes with buildings and manufactured features. Among urban scenes, those with vegetation are preferred to those without views of nature and they have a positive physiological impact on individuals whether or not they are consciously aware of them. These effects include lower blood pressure, reduced muscle tension, lower skin conductance, and faster recovery from stress. In one study of college students under stress from an exam, views of plants increased positive feelings and reduced fear and anger. Parklands tend to be among the most highly preferred kinds of settings. Trees and forested areas, water, good maintenance, and peace and quiet were among the most preferred features of urban parks. Workers with a view of natural elements, such as trees and flowers, experienced less job pressure, were more satisfied with their jobs, and reported fewer ailments and headaches than those who either had no outside view or could only see buildings from their windows. Just knowing that the view was available was important to employees, even if they did not take advantage of it.

The physical condition of an area, whether it is a neighborhood or a senior center, provides a measure of the self-worth of the area, defines the value of the individuals within that area, and projects that definition to outsiders. Thus, if an area is dilapidated or vandalized, has trash-filled vacant lots, or is sterile concrete, it sends a message that those in charge (the government, the owner, the organization, or the employer) do not place value on the area and the people who live and work there. It implies that the people have no control over their environment, and it sends a message to others that this is not a good place to live or be. Plants are the fastest, most cost-effective agents for changing negative perceptions of an area and creating a positive community atmosphere.

The strongest indicator of residential satisfaction is the ease of access to nature, which is an important factor in life satisfaction. The availability of nature elements in the surrounding area strongly affected neighborhood satisfaction, especially the availability of trees, well-landscaped grounds, and places for taking walks. Among residents of retirement communities, pleasant, landscaped grounds were either important or essential to 99% of the residents. A window view of green, landscaped grounds was 3 times as important as a view of activity areas. The configuration and natural elements of the grounds were given as the most important reasons for selecting a particular retirement community.

Perceived security and personal safety also play a role in neighborhood satisfaction. Studies have documented the importance of design and maintenance in perceived security. In a study of urban parking lots, security was rated high only when vegetation was well maintained and appeared to be part of the landscape design. Unkempt, densely wooded areas often elicit concern of physical danger.

Matthew Dumont, a community psychiatrist, has looked at cities to try to understand them in terms of the mental health needs of the city dweller. He found that the city dweller has a need for stimulation to break the monotony of daily life, for a sense of community, and for a sense of mastery of the environment. Community gardening, landscaping, and tree-planting projects can meet these needs.

Residents in apartments, townhouses, and other sites without access to private garden space benefit from community gardens. Community gardens are particularly important to elderly, disabled, and disadvantaged individuals in urban areas. The community garden is frequently developed under the leadership of a neighborhood group or other not-for-profit association that is interested in horticulture and uses it to improve the quality of life, increase involvement in the community, and improve the appearance of the community. Community gardens have been established in order to improve the nutrition of the people who are gardening, to develop leadership skills among these people, and to help them improve their communities. Organizations like the American Community Gardening Association have resources available for assistance in establishing community gardens.

Working together on tree plantings, community gardens, and beautification projects, people get to know one another and help in creating a community whose inhabitants have a sense of loyalty to and responsibility for their surroundings. Plants provide a positive physical environment in which it is more comfortable to live and work by purifying the air, moderating temperatures with shade or windbreaks, reducing glare and noise, removing pollutants from the air, screening unattractive sights, and increasing relative humidity. There is a need also to teach children an appreciation of plants and nature through active participation in gardening, which provides an opportunity for an intergenerational activity.

BIBLIOGRAPHY

Beisgen, B. (1989). *Life-enhancing activities for mentally impaired elders. A practical guide.* New York: Springer.

Kerrigan, J. (2001). Gardening with the elderly. *Ohio State University Extension Fact Sheet.* HYG-1642-94. Columbus, OH: Ohio State University, Horticulture and Crop Science. [On-line]. Available: www.ag.ohio-state.edu/~ohioline/hygfact/1000/1642.html

McDonald, J. (2001).Why is horticulture a good medium for work with people with special needs? *Horticulture for all.* [On-line]. Available: www.ourworld.compuserve.com/homepages/Jane_Stoneham/jmcd.htm

Relf, D. (1995). *Gardeners and individuals with physical disabilities.* Publication 426-020. Blacksburg, VA: Virginia Polytechnic Institute and State University.
Relf, D. Horticulture: A therapeutic tool. *Journal of Rehabilitation, 39*(1), 27–29. [Online]. Available: www.hort.vt.edu/human/ht5a.html
Relf, D., & Dorn, S. (1987). *Horticulture: Meeting the needs of special populations.* [Online]. Available: www.hort.vt.edu/human/HortTher1.html#sd
Relf, D. (1992, April/June). Human issues in horticulture. *Hort Technology, 2*(2).
Ulrich, R. S. (1979). Visual landscapes and psychological well-being. *Landscape Research, 4*(1), 17–23.

RESOURCES

The American Horticultural Society
7931 East Boulevard Drive
Alexandria, VA 22308
703-768-5700
http://www.ahs.org/
The American Horticultural Society is a national gardening organization that provides gardeners with high quality gardening and horticultural education with the help of a network of experts.

American Horticultural Therapy Association
909 York Street
Denver, CO 80206
720-865-3616
http://www.ahta.org/
The American Horticultural Therapy Association promotes therapy and rehabilitation through horticulture.

American Community Gardening Association
100 N. 20th Street, 5th Floor
Philadelphia, PA 19103-1495
215-988-8785
http://communitygarden.org
The American Community Gardening Association is a membership organization supporting the idea of community gardening for urban and rural dwellers who don't have their own land.

Canadian Horticultural Therapy Association (CHTA)
80 Westmount Road

Guelph, Ontario, Canada
N1H 5H8
519-822-9842
http://www.chta.ca/
The Canadian Horticultural Therapy Association promotes the use and awareness of horticulture as a therapeutic modality.

Chicago Botanic Garden
1000 Lake Cook Road
Glencoe, IL 60022
847-835-5440
http://www.chicago-botanic.org/
The Chicago Botanic Garden publishes a range of resources, including fact sheets, articles and activity guides for planning horticultural therapy programs. The Enabling Garden at the Chicago Botanic Garden has received worldwide recognition for its innovations in barrier-free gardening techniques.

City Farmer, Canada's Office of Urban Agriculture
#801-318 Homer St.
Vancouver, BC V6B 2V3 Canada
http://www.cityfarmer.org/
City Farmer promotes urban food production and environmental conservation. City Farmer produced a handbook and Web information about gardening with people with disabilities.

Denver Botanic Garden
909 York Street
Denver, CO 80206
Christine Kramer
(303) 370-8190
http://www.botanicgardens.org/
The Denver Botanic Garden's mission is to connect people with plants, especially plants from the Rocky Mountain Region.

National Gardening Association
180 Flynn Ave.
Burlington, VT 05401
802-863-1308
http://www.garden.org

The National Gardening Association helps gardeners and helps people through gardening. The NGA is focused primarily on children and the ways that gardening enhances education and helps build environmentally responsible adults.

People Plant Council
Virginia Polytechnic Institute and State University
Office of Environmental Horticulture, Saunders 407
Blacksburg, VA 24061-0327
540-231-6254
http://www.hort.vt.edu/human/PPC.html
People Plant Council is a national clearinghouse of academic research being conducted in the area of the benefits and effectiveness of horticulture therapy.

CHAPTER TWELVE

Humanities

ALBAN

In November of 1997, Vintage hosted "A Conversation on Democracy in America," based on the book by Alexis de Tocqueville. C-Span was recreating the voyage that the French statesman made 160 years earlier. Because Pittsburgh was one of the cities that de Tocqueville visited, the Vintage staff thought it would be interesting to build a program around it.

Vintage has hosted numerous humanities programs, from conversations about the rivers of America to ones about our local Italian American community. For the de Tocqueville program we decided to do a five-part discussion series using Democracy in America as the text. We were fortunate to receive funding for this program, which enabled us to engage the services of five local scholars. We covered five topics: women and the family, race, government, religion, and the media. The 20 individuals who took part in the discussion included students from public and private schools, members of the community, and Vintage participants.

Alban joined the group as a Vintage participant. This may have been the first humanities discussion he had ever taken part in, but his contributions were unique due to his multicultural experiences. One needs to know Alban to understand this. Born in Germany in 1910, he immigrated to America in 1938. He shared pictures of his home in Germany and family photos with the staff. During the de Tocqueville discussions and for sometime following the series, it was clear that Alban was reflecting privately about his own life. He brought more family photos to Vintage for everyone to see.

When he came to America he married, and with his wife raised three daughters and one son. He served in World War II, and worked as a salesman after the war.

When he first came to Vintage Alban was already suffering the effects of Parkinson's disease. At first he managed to get along with a cane, then

189

a walker, and eventually a motorized scooter. We often saw him playing chess, and anyone will tell you he is a good chess player. Alban also sings with a group at Vintage and still treats us to a favorite German melody, sung in German of course. When I asked him to join the Tocqueville conversation, he was very willing and eager to receive text so he could begin the assigned reading.

Alexis de Tocqueville's visit to Pittsburgh was unremarkable. He had just traveled over the Allegheny Mountains in the middle of November and was looking forward to boarding the steamboat in Pittsburgh and continuing his trip to Wheeling, West Virginia. As a result, C-Span had very little to film on their stop in Pittsburgh, thus Vintage was able to convince them to tape our discussions. They taped three of the five conversations and on the evening of November 25, 1997, 160 years to the date of de Tocqueville's visit to Pittsburgh, C-Span broadcast live from Ellis School. Richard Johnson, PhD from California State Polytechnic University, traveled to Pittsburgh to do a presentation of de Tocqueville with a question-and-answer session to follow. It was a very exciting evening for everyone, but especially for Alban. He was dressed in a dark suit, a white shirt, and a red bow tie. He spoke to me that evening of his life in Germany, his immigration to America, and now of being on national television, discussing the writing of a French writer—he was very proud that evening.

The humanities give all of us an opportunity to examine our feelings and to contribute to conversations based on our own life experiences. Alban's experiences were different than most: His thoughts and ideas were invaluable to the conversations and at the same time validated his life experiences.

The humanities disciplines are concerned primarily with heritage, including history, culture, and folklore. They have the capacity to illuminate how individuals relate to society, history, literature, art, and geography. The act that established the National Endowment for the Humanities (NEH) says "the term humanities includes, but is not limited to, the study of language; linguistics; literature; history; jurisprudence; philosophy; archaeology; comparative religion; ethics; the history, criticism and theory of the arts; those aspects of social sciences which have humanistic content and employ humanistic methods; and the study and application of the humanities to the human environment with particular attention to reflecting our diverse heritage, traditions, and history and to the relevance of the humanities to the current conditions of national life." The NEH and its partners, the state humanities councils, have supported a variety of projects and initiatives.

A recent study funded by the NEH called *The Presence of the Past: Popular Uses of History in American Life*, found abundant evidence of a widely felt connection to America's traditions, stories, and places. Americans' compile photo albums, collect antiques, visit historic sites, keep diaries, plan annual family gatherings, make patchwork quilts, and record oral histories to preserve their heritage. The ideas and questions addressed by the humanities remain important throughout a person's life, not just during the years of formal education. The National Endowment for the Humanities supports public programs in the humanities that help to sustain a continuum of lifelong learning opportunities for individuals of all age groups. The NEH also targets nontraditional and underserved audiences including older adults, youth who are at risk, and rural residents. As a result, millions of adults who are working or retired and no longer engaged in formal education can find cultural enrichment in libraries and museums, at historical sites, on television, or in the communities where they live.

The NEH has long supported regionally oriented projects, including initiatives under the theme of *Rediscovering America Through Place and Region*. Region refers as much to variations in daily life and differences in cultural characteristics as it does to geography. Regional diversity is a source of intellectual interest as well as national pride. Interest in the study of regional cultures, genealogy, and local history is high among public audiences. Studies show that people of all ages are interviewing their parents and grandparents, constructing family trees, reviewing family photographs, going to family reunions, or traveling back to the country or town of their ancestors. The NEH initiative *My History Is America's History* was designed to help Americans' preserve and share family histories and deepen their understanding of how their families fit into the context of their communities, their regions, and the nation. A family-history kit and Web site provide advice and models on how to save family stories; guidelines on conducting oral histories; resources for history, genealogy, and oral history; a timeline and links to the nation's history to explore how historical events relate to an individual's family history; and a place to exchange stories.

Historical and cultural sites in the United States have become popular travel destinations because they help Americans make a tangible connection with the past. Museum attendance is one of the most popular recreational activities, and the American Association of Museums reports that more people go to museums annually than attend sporting events. Public libraries are the primary resource for cultural enrichment and lifelong learning opportunities in many communities; nearly 9 out of 10 libraries offer some form of cultural activity.

Public television and radio have presented award-winning, NEH-funded programs such as *The Great War* and the *Shaping of the 20th Century, Liberty! The American Revolution,* and *Divided Highways: The Interstates and the Transformation of American Life. I'll Make Me a World: A Century of African American Arts,* a three-part series on the contributions of African American writers, poets, painters, filmmakers, and other artists, was broadcast nationally in 1999 at the same time that schools, museums, libraries, and community centers in 11 cities hosted local events that brought young people and adult artists together for performances, oral history interviews, and other activities.

Digital technology is a useful tool in the humanities classroom, offering an enhanced, interactive content. Educators have found that the use of digital resources is having a highly positive effect on humanities teaching and learning in the classroom, promoting greater interactivity with the content and access to sources of information. Web sites make it possible for people who are unable to attend an exhibition to experience it in their own homes, senior center, or other community site. However, there are also many obstacles to the use of digital technology: inequality of access, inaccurate and inappropriate materials on the Web, and a large number of humanities teachers who lack adequate time, training, preparation, and equipment to take advantage of the best digital tools available to enrich their curriculum. NEH has helped propel advances in digital technologies for education, having contributed to the development of Web sites, CD-ROMs, and a meta-Web site called EDSITEment, which features selected sites that are excellent in content, design, and usefulness in the classroom. Digital technology is an important feature of NEH's new projects, such as *My History Is America's History.* The site includes learning guides and step-by-step lesson plans that are keyed to subject areas and skills acquisition. Many state humanities councils also support a variety of digital projects that facilitate lifelong learning opportunities.

The National Endowment for the Humanities is developing the potential of the new digital technology to promote knowledge in the humanities. Exciting opportunities are emerging to create enhanced humanities content that utilizes the converging capabilities of the Internet and broadcast radio and television. Digital television will make multicasting possible, whereby broadcasters can simultaneously transmit four or more channels of programming, providing additional airtime for thematically linked program series and program strands for specific audiences. Digital television will also include datacasting that offers the potential for enriched humanities programs with the simultaneous distribution of additional content such as curriculum materials, interview transcripts, and interactive games. Digital enhancements of broadcast program content (enhanced television) offers the opportunity to engage audiences, including teachers and students, with significant interactivity and user choice of how to engage audiences with interactive games and simulations, alternative content, and dialogues with scholars and other viewers. Multicasting, datacasting, and enhanced television will enable the NEH to connect public television programs to the classroom with curriculum materials, contribute to teacher development and enrichment, localize national content, create a wider range of age-based content, and facilitate distance learning. More services of enhanced educational value will be accessible to more and diverse audiences at the same time.

The NEH has a variety of grant programs to enable professional staff at smaller institutions or those new to humanities programs to consult with humanities scholars, curators, film producers, and others who can help them explore their ideas or collections through the humanities and provide on-site consultation visits. Institutions of higher learning have shown an increased interest in becoming more involved with their communities.

SUGGESTED ACTIVITIES

- reading and discussion groups
- oral-history project
- participation in NEH projects such as *My History Is America's History*
- lecture series on the humanities
- local history
- folklore
- art history
- traveling exhibitions
- field trips
- programs to commemorate national and special events

BIBLIOGRAPHY

National Endowment for the Humanities. (2001). *My history is America's history.* Washington, DC: Author. [On-line]. Available: http://www.myhistory.org/

National Endowment for the Humanities. (2000). *Report of the humanities, science and technology working group.* Washington, DC: Author.
National Endowment for the Humanities. (1999). *Report of the regional studies working group.* Washington, DC: Author.
National Endowment for the Humanities. (2000). *Report of the teaching and learning working group.* Washington, DC: Author.
National Endowment for the Humanities. (2000). *Research opportunities through centers for advanced study and international research organizations.* Washington, DC: Author.
Rosenzweig, R., & Thelen, D. (1998). *The presence of the past: Popular uses of history in American life.* New York: Columbia University Press.

RESOURCES

American Antiquarian Society
185 Salisbury Street
Worcester, MA 01609-1634
508-755-5221
www.americanantiquarian.org
The American Antiquarian Society maintains a major research library in American history, literature and culture through 1876.

Association for the Study of African American Life and History
7961 Eastern Ave. Suite 301
Silver Spring, MD 20910
301-587-5900
http://www.artnoir.com/asalh/
The Association for the Study of African American Life and History supports the study of African American history and sets the annual theme for National African American History Month and kit; sponsors specialized professional development curriculum workshops and seminars; and supports diversity through dialogue and public education.

The John Carter Brown Library
Box 1894
Providence, Rhode Island 02912
401-863-2725
http://www.JCBL.org
The John Carter Brown Library Center for advanced study in history and the humanities is located on the campus of Brown University.

The Center on Aging, Health & Humanities
The George Washington University Medical Center

425 Aldemarle Street
Washington, DC 20016
202-895-0230
The Center on Aging, Health & Humanities stimulates, coordinates, and conducts sponsored research on both the problems and potentials of aging, with the goal of improving the quality of life for older adults and their families. Particular attention is paid to understanding and tapping creative potential in later life and to creative problem solving for social and health challenges associated with aging.

H-Net
Michigan State University
310 Auditorium Building
East Lansing, MI 48824
517-355-9300
http://www2.h-net.msu.edu/
H-Net is an international interdisciplinary organization of scholars and teachers dedicated to developing the enormous educational potential of the Internet and the World Wide Web.

National Council on the Aging, Inc.
409 Third Street SW, Suite 200
Washington, DC
202-479-6688
http://www.ncoa.org/
Developed the reading and discussion series, *Discovery Through the Humanities*. Topics include *A Family Album: The American Family in Literature and History*, *Work and Life*, *We Got There on the Train: Railroads in the Lives of the American People*, *Portraits and Pathways*, *Remembering World War II*, *Roll on River*, *The Search for Meaning*, *Words and Music*, *Exploring Values*, and *Imagenes de la Vejez en la Literatura*. Each topic comes with a booklet for every participant and a discussion leaders guide.

National Endowment for the Humanities
1100 Pennsylvania Avenue, NW
Washington, DC 20506
202-606-8400
http://www.neh.gov/
National Endowment for the Humanities is an independent grant-making agency of the United States government dedicated to supporting research, education, and public programs in the humanities.

- Directory of State Humanities Councils: http://www.neh.gov/state/states.html
- EDSITEment offers a gateway for searching for high-quality material on the Internet in the subject areas of literature and language arts, foreign languages, art and culture, and history and social studies. EDSITEment: http://edsitement.neh.gov/

National Humanities Institute
214 Massachusetts Avenue NE, Suite 303
Washington, DC 20002
202-544-3158
http://www.nhinet.org/
The National Humanities Institute promotes research, publishing, and teaching in the humanities.

The Newberry Library
60 West Walton Street
Chicago, IL 60610
312-943-9090
http://www.newberry.org
The Newberry Library is an independent research library dedicated primarily to study in the humanities.

The Omohundro Institute of Early American History and Culture
PO Box 8781
Williamsburg, VA 23187-8781
757-221-1114
http://www.wm.edu.oieahc
The Omohundro Institute of Early American History and Culture supports study and publication in early American history.

Schomburg Center for Research in Black Culture
515 Malcolm X Boulevard
New York, NY 10037-1801
212-491-2228
http://www.nypl.org/research/sc/scholars /index.html
The Schomburg Center for Research in Black Culture is a research unit of the New York Public Library devoted to collecting, preserving, and providing access to research resources on black heritage.

CHAPTER THIRTEEN

Intergenerational Programs

MILLIE

There was just something about Millie that drew children to her. I can't tell you what it was, I can only tell you that it happened. A tall, graceful African American woman, Millie started coming to Vintage in the late 1980s. Initially we knew her from the trips she enjoyed taking as part of the Vintage program.

I got to know her better when she took the part of Madam C. J. Walker in the Celebration of Women *production. She was great in that part. It was easy to see the actress in her and she was very convincing in the role. Following that program, Vintage had an opportunity to be involved in several intergenerational projects. Millie enjoyed the company of young people and told me she would like to be part of it.*

Intergenerational programming is something that evolves. When the students first arrive at the center, the seniors almost always sit on one side of the room, and the children on the other, each sizing up the other.

Millie was involved in two projects. The first was an after-school program with "at-risk" middle-school students, the Vintage photographers, and a handful of Vintage participants. The purpose of the program was for the students to interview the participants and ask questions about their life histories. After several hours of interviewing the seniors, the students were to write biographical sketches of their candidates and then work with the photographers to create a portrait photograph to go with their writing.

An attractive redheaded student chose Millie, and to say the girl was disruptive during the first session would be an understatement. She made fun of the project and interrupted the teachers and Vintage staff while the project was being explained to everyone. The second time they came together her unruly behavior continued, and I wondered how we would accomplish anything, because many of the students were beginning to imitate her behavior. Near the end of the second session I noticed Millie and the student sitting in the atrium. After the students left, Millie came to me and explained that she had started talking to the student about her own life as a young woman. When the girl heard that Millie's life had been far from perfect, she settled down and listened. She told Millie her parents had just been divorced, and she was not happy. At the third session, many of the students gathered around Millie. Somehow she got the students to trust her. This small step was enough for the students to trust the other Vintage members and they were able to finish the project. The final result was a display of their essays and photographs in the Mansmann Gallery at Vintage. At the opening reception Millie and her red-haired friend stood proudly beside their work, greeting friends and family—a real testament to how a bridge across generations can be built.

The second project was a musical production with a local elementary school. The theme of the show was the weather and Millie sang "Stormy Weather." A cancer that had been in remission for years had returned and frequently Millie felt miserable. It was not her nature to complain, and in the tradition of the stage, "the show must go on." The students were never told that Millie wasn't feeling well, they just knew. The love and affection they showed her during the rehearsals and the actual program was remarkable: young people saving her seat and acting on cue to take her arm as part of the program was very touching for those of us backstage.

Intergenerational programming is an opportunity for the young and the old to come together to make a difference in one another's lives. It was clear that Millie made a difference in a young girl's life and that a group of elementary students made a difference in hers.

Historically, the extended family helped maintain and support its members, families lived closer together, and senior adults were an important part of the family. Changes in society and the family have greatly influenced intergenerational relationships. Over the course of the last century, America has become highly segregated by age, and family functions have been assumed by a range of age-specific institutions. Children attend age-segregated schools, adults work in environments where there are no children or adults over 65, older adults live in age-segregated housing, and children and older persons are cared for by age-segregated services. Age segregation—marked by geographic distance between parents', children's, and grandchildren's residences and attitudes that promote social and physical separation—result in few genuine opportunities for interaction among the generations. As a result, the old do not have relationships with the young, and the young do not understand their elders or the aging process. The myths and stereotypes that result from separating the generations, in combination with shrinking resources, fosters tension between the generations. These trends suggest a need for increased communication and interaction across generations.

Intergenerational relations refer to any informal interaction between youth and older adults, and senior centers can encourage this interaction through intergenerational programs. These programs are an important vehicle for linking generations and cultures and can be used to assist with critical social issues such as illiteracy, violence, education, social isolation, and health and wellness, particularly in a time of diminishing economic resources for the social and educational needs of young and old alike. Through intergenerational programs, people of different generations share their talents and resources and support each other in relationships that benefit the individual and the community. Young and old learn, share experiences, practice new skills, cooperate, gain respect, and practice teamwork as they solve problems together. These programs have proven particularly effective because they provide opportunities for individuals, families, and communities to again enjoy and benefit from the richness of an age-integrated society, and they are cost-effective.

THE BENEFITS OF INTERGENERATIONAL PROGRAMMING

Although the outcomes of any given program will be unique, certain benefits can be anticipated from a well-planned program. Intergenerational programs help prevent unnatural age segregation; facilitate community collaboration, pooling of resources, and cooperative problem-solving; and increase community awareness about issues that affect both young and old. The strengths of one generation can be applied to meet the needs of the other.

Intergenerational programs provide opportunities for interaction among people of diverse backgrounds and ages; for sharing of the experience of family life, ethnic origin, occupation, religious beliefs, stage of life, and recreation; and for promoting appreciation of cultural heritage, traditions, and histories and understanding of shared values. The traditional knowledge and skills required to plant a garden, season foods, decorate homes, weave a blanket, or make a quilt can be exchanged or learned by imitation. It is not simply skills that are transferred in such interactions, but a sense of identity, belonging, and purpose.

Older adults are often able to give an unconditional love that contributes to the development of children's self-esteem. Grandparents and other older adults are not required to be responsible for children in the same way that parents are. This freedom from responsibility allows them to accept children as they are. Older adults may be less hurried, thus able to give children additional time and attention. Children of employed parents may especially benefit from interaction with an older person who can tell or read a story, play games, or just listen. Other benefits of intergenerational programs for children include

- promoting personal relationships with elders
- developing positive social behaviors
- fostering positive attitudes toward aging and the life cycle
- increasing empathy
- unconditional acceptance and emotional support
- promoting understanding of physical disabilities
- the opportunity to learn skills and wisdom from another generation
- helping children feel connected to the past when older adults explain historical events and share past experiences
- providing mentors, role models

Older adults, even with limited resources, are able to give love and time to young children. This has been found to be important in maintaining the morale of older people and can provide the adult a purpose for living. Additionally, intergenerational relations

- promote positive, fulfilling use of retirement time
- expand the support network for the older adult
- reduce isolation and loneliness through social contact
- encourage the older adult that another generation will carry on
- provide enjoyment
- stimulate the senses
- provide unconditional acceptance and emotional support
- improve self-esteem
- offer the opportunity to share a lifetime of experience and skills
- provide opportunities for reminiscence

- provide access to assistance from younger, more able-bodied people
- can inspire the older adult to be more adventuresome

As individuals learn more about each other, stereotypes and barriers to interaction disappear, resulting in improved relations between the generations. Additional benefits to the community include

- increased community awareness about issues that affect young and old
- greater utilization of resources and experiences in community
- increased communication among segments of the community
- improved image of children and of older people
- recognition of needs of all age levels
- preservation of historical and cultural traditions
- partnerships among community organizations and individuals
- organizations and individuals united to take action on public policy issues that address human needs across generations
- closing of gaps in services
- enhanced community spirit

IMPLEMENTATION

Intergenerational programs should be publicly supported because they have benefits that reach beyond the needs and interests of the very young and the very old. Dr. Rick Moody and Dr. Robert Disch from the Brookdale Center on Aging contend that in order to gain public support, these programs must demonstrate that they fulfill a public purpose by strengthening the community at large. When intergenerational programs are conceived as vehicles for strengthening communities they garner public support and demonstrate the common stake that different generations have in one another. Doctors Moody and Disch suggest the following strategies:

1. Structure programs so they not only provide a specific service such as tutoring, but also meet critical community needs such as improving support for public education and overcoming racial and ethnic tensions.
2. Include an educational component and opportunities for reflection for young and old so participants understand that their

activities and personal interactions are part of a larger community effort.

3. Form or join coalitions or networks.
4. Hold public forums or events to raise awareness about issues such as crime prevention, access to health care, healthy lifestyles, homelessness, hunger, the need for child care and elder care and other family supports, and the community stake in public schools.
5. Work with the media to promote the intergenerational program and the impact that it has on the community.
6. Invite local businesses, foundations, employers, agencies, and organizations to visit the program and learn about its impact on the community.

Developing intergenerational programs requires building partnerships between the senior center and groups such as child care agencies, schools, youth organizations, parent groups, service groups, religious institutions, cultural and ethnic organizations, and other community-based organizations. It is important to look for partners that complement the capabilities of the senior center and enhance leadership. Partnerships require bringing all who are involved to the table and maintaining communication. Administrators and program coordinators from both agencies must be involved in the planning process. Intergenerational programs run smoothly when there is one lead organization and the lines of accountability and responsibility are clear. As the success of the program depends on careful planning, each organization's responsibilities should be specified. A needs assessment will help determine what program components will best meet the needs of the participants and the community. A designated coordinator who is responsible for intergenerational activities, staff training, and sharing among program components has been found to be essential to the success of the program.

Key components found in successful intergenerational programs include

- competent, committed leadership
- designated staff to coordinate the program
- needs assessment
- measurable goals and objectives
- monitoring and evaluation plan
- collaboration between organizations representing participants

- realistic program design and budget
- policies and procedures
- marketing and outreach plan
- adequate funding, equipment, and supplies
- recruitment, selection, and matching of participants
- training of staff, volunteers, and participants
- cross-training for staff and volunteers on child development, aging, and specific issues of concern
- orientation to the program
- program supervision
- recognition of those involved
- pleasant, consistent, and supportive environments
- respectful and helping relationships

An ongoing evaluation of the program to determine the accomplishments, challenges, needs, and benefits is another key to success. An evaluation that determines outcomes and demonstrates program effectiveness provides the basis for future planning and support for the program. Areas for evaluation include cost-effectiveness, impact on and satisfaction of the participants and their families, staff effectiveness, procedures, success of the intergenerational relationships, and the degree to which the program is meeting participant and community needs.

Intergenerational programs enjoy very positive press, and this can be capitalized on to help ensure their future success. Raise awareness of any intergenerational activities by continuously informing the media and inviting the community to attend celebrations and special events. Consistently bring the program to the attention of current and potential funders. Almost all programs have multiple sources of funding that may include foundations, corporations, support from local businesses, service organizations such as the Rotary, Area Agency on Aging, school districts, private donations, and fee for service.

Another approach to intergenerational programs and a growing trend are Intergenerational Shared Site (IGSS) programs in which multiple generations receive ongoing services or program at the same site. Collaborative approaches to delivering services have become an effective strategy in many communities with limited public resources. Although IGSS programs are colocated, the degree of integration varies greatly. The most common IGSS programs involving senior centers offer early childhood programs and before- and after-school programs. Some senior centers are located in schools or youth organizations, providing seniors the opportunity to serve as mentors or tutors.

MENTORS

Mentoring is the process of encouraging, teaching, sponsoring, and guiding the development of another individual. The concept of mentoring has expanded from that of a professional training relationship (preparing an individual for a career or job) to include a supportive relationship with a family, friend, or child. Mentoring provides a supportive environment for children and adults to address challenging issues together, such as birth, death, divorce, moving, and change in health or economic status. Everyone needs someone who cares. Adapting to life's challenges requires families to explore a variety of resources, and mentoring can assist in the development of individuals and families.

An important part of the intergenerational movement is America's population of at-risk youth. They crave adult attention and approval but often lack any positive social influences. Mentoring is a valuable tool in working with this population. Mentoring involves an older person who takes a genuine interest in a young person. The older person guides the younger person and provides opportunities to help the younger person prosper and gain an increased sense of self-esteem and independence. Mentoring is an experience that rewards individuals with increased productivity, increased respect for diversity, and a new outlook on life events. A child's need for nurturing, self-identity, self-worth, positive role models, learning, security, acceptance, and knowledge of history can be met through a mentoring relationship. Conversely, the older adult's need to nurture and pass on cultural traditions, skills, and knowledge can also be met.

MODEL INTERGENERATIONAL PROGRAMS

The number and variety of intergenerational programs involving older adults and children continues to grow. They are most frequently found in schools, child and adult day-care programs, community centers, senior centers, and with civic organizations and youth groups. Music, dance, theater, horticulture, art, storytelling, animals, crafts, sports, games, language, history, and computers are just some of the tools that are well suited to intergenerational activities. Some examples of successful intergenerational programs follow.

THE BROOKDALE CENTER ON AGING

Intergenerational Language Learning. This project recruited and trained older adults who were native speakers of foreign languages for the purpose of helping Hunter College undergraduates improve their ability to speak and understand foreign languages.

Intergenerational World War II Veterans Project. This project linked veterans of World War II with undergraduates and high-school students for the purpose of helping the students gain a better understanding of the period both in the military and on the home front.

Intergenerational "Remembering Old New York" Project. This project linked high-school students with retired working-class people who had lived most of their lives in New York City. The goals were to help students see how the city has changed, how people in working-class jobs survived the Depression and World War II, and how social classes and ethic groups related to each other through the decades.

CORNELL UNIVERSITY APPLIED GERONTOLOGY RESEARCH INSTITUTE

Grandparents as Parents. Cornell Cooperative Extension educators lead community education activities and serve as a resource for other extension educators throughout the state. Efforts include workshops, newsletters, support groups, and collaborations.

Horticultural Intergenerational Learning as Therapy (HILT). A program designed to use horticulture service learning to bring young and old people together. A manual called *Using Plants to Bridge the Generations* gives step-by-step instructions for instituting a HILT program.

Project EASE (Exploring Aging through Shared Experiences). A model for developing intergenerational programs, its goal is to bring groups of early adolescents together with older adults for joint service, shared group activity, or one-on-one matching. Course materials consist of a leader's guide and member's guide.

Project GUIDE (Growth and Understanding of Intergenerational Programming through Distance Education). A learning experience that trains youth-development educators and other human-service practitioners to learn about and create intergenerational programs uniquely suited for their own communities. Participants interact in a 4-week on-line course, gaining knowledge about intergenerational program models and Internet resources. As they interact in the course, learners build a network of colleagues for ongoing support of their programs as implementation unfolds.

DOROT

DOROT's mission is to enhance the lives of older residents of New York City through a dynamic partnership of volunteers, professionals, and elders; to foster mutually beneficial interaction between the generations; and to provide education, guidance and leadership in developing national and international volunteer-based programs for older individuals. The Family Circle program matches families with elders whom they visit at home for holidays and special occasions. Holiday workshops give children and parents the opportunity to socialize and to create special gifts and holiday treats for their adopted seniors. The Department of Youth Volunteer offers intergenerational classroom programs. There are many opportunities for preteens, teenagers, and college students to serve, interact with, learn from, and socialize with seniors. Students run errands, document elders' lives on audio- or videotape, help with DOROT cultural or social events, and read to or visit with elders. DOROT also developed two multigenerational, multiethnic music programs.

ELDERS SHARE THE ARTS: CENTER FOR CREATIVE AGING/ELDERS SHARE THE ARTS

Elders Share the Arts (ESTA) is an arts organization dedicated to bridging generational divides and generating a sense of community through the arts. The staff of professional artists works with young and old in underserved communities to transform their life stories into dramatic, literary, and visual presentations that explore social issues, shed light on neighborhood history, and draw from their imaginations answers to community issues and conflicts.

Living History Arts. These are life-review workshops based on participants' oral histories, which are transformed into theater, dance, storytelling, and literary presentations.

Living History Classroom. These interactive workshops introduce life-cycle awareness, deal with age stereotypes, and redefine concepts of family. Through techniques that combine oral history and the creative arts, students engage in activities such as community mapping and family interviews.

Living History and Creative Movement. Participants experience oral-history interviewing and storytelling while uncovering the history of their communities. Memories and experiences are transformed into creative movement and dances are created. As the process unfolds, issues such as life-cycle awareness and age stereotypes are addressed.

Living History Theater. Training in acting and various theater techniques allow participants to transform oral history and storytelling into original theater pieces.

Living History Visual Arts. Techniques such as sculpture, painting, collage, and puppet-making are used to transform life stories from the verbal to the visual.

Living History as the Written Word. Oral histories are reinterpreted by budding writers nurtured and guided by ESTA artists.

Pearls of Wisdom. "Story swapping" provides the students with a hands-on opportunity to experience the art of storytelling. Students learn to craft original stories of life and imagination to swap with members of Pearls of Wisdom, a multicultural community-based ensemble of touring elder storytellers. They also perform stories of heritage, humor, courage, and strength.

Conflict Resolution and Conflict Mediation Theater. These problem-solving and leadership-training theater programs for intergenerational groups use theater as a means of addressing complex social problems. Groups emphasize the role of citizenship, action, and leadership.

Professional Training and Consultation (Staff Development). ESTA provides training in planning and managing intergenerational and youth arts programs. Using a hands-on approach the artists delve into areas such as oral history, life review, reminiscence theory, intergenerational arts, and cultural diversity.

Legacy Art Works. Living Legends is a project of ESTA's Discoveries' program, which pairs renowned elder artists with young people who are disadvantaged so they may pass on artistic legacies and arts skills.

INTERGENERATIONAL ENTREPRENEURSHIP DEMONSTRATION PROJECT: HOWE-TO INDUSTRIES

The AARP Andrus Foundation funded the Intergenerational Entrepreneurship Demonstration Project (IEDP), the first project of the Retirement and Intergenerational Studies Laboratory of the Strom Thurmond Institute. The efforts of the institute and the Department of Parks, Recreation, and Tourism at Clemson University allowed for the expansion of an existing Enterprise Market Program at the John de la Howe School in McCormick, South Carolina. IEDP is a mentoring project where elders teach business skills to at-risk youth so that they may successfully operate a small business and function as productive adults once they leave de la Howe. Sharing lifetime skills and experiences, retirees help the youth operate their own country market out of a renovated dairy barn at the school, known as Howe-To Industries.

PENN STATE COOPERATIVE EXTENSION AND OUTREACH: GENERATION CELEBRATION

Designed to help students develop communication skills and to foster positive attitudes about older persons, this awareness program uses a variety of activities including family history, simulation, heritage crafts and household skills, shared recreation, and visits in a variety of settings. Local adaptations by communities include Generation Connections, through which teams of high-school youth work with an Area Agency on Aging to provide regular telephone reassurance to a vulnerable older person. The program has available a 4-H juried curriculum guide.

SPELLBINDERS

Spellbinders supports and nurtures the age-old tradition of storytelling. Spellbinders' mission is to help establish programs in communities across the nation.

TEXAS AGRICULTURAL EXTENSION SERVICE: YOUTH EXCHANGING
WITH SENIORS (YES)

YES promotes positive intergenerational relationships between youths
and seniors by training 4-H Club and Future Homemakers of America
volunteers to provide assisted-living services that enhance independent
lifestyles of older persons in rural communities. The youth provide
housekeeping, lawn care, and minor home and auto repair services for
the older participants, who reciprocate by sharing their time and talent
with the youths; the youth in turn learn about the aging process, communicating between generations, and career opportunities in family and
consumer sciences, health and social services. The program has available
a training manual, a youth service provider workbook, and video
cassettes.

UNIVERSITY OF MINNESOTA EXTENSION SERVICE: ELDER'S
WISDOM, CHILDREN'S SONG: COMMUNITY CELEBRATION OF PLACE

School children listen to oral histories of local elders and with the
assistance of a troubadour create songs, recitations, and art based on
the personal stories. The program culminates in a community-wide
celebration honoring the elders that is recorded on audio- and videotape and in an original songbook illustrated by the students. Communities are taught how to continue and expand this process for
intergenerational learning.

BIBLIOGRAPHY

Administration on Aging, National Aging Information Center. (2001). *Intergenerational programs.* Washington, DC: Author. [On-line]. Available: http://www.aoa.
dhhs.gov/naic/notes/intergenerational.html
American Association of Retired Persons. (1994). *Connecting the generations: A guide
to intergenerational resources. An overview of intergenerational programming and selected
listing of books, manuals and media resources.* A cooperative project of Generations
Together, Generations United, National Council on the Aging, Temple Univer-
sity and American Association of Retired Persons. Funded by a grant from the
Administration on Aging, United States Department of Health and Human
Services. Washington, DC: Author.
Fowler, L. K. (2001). *Families meeting the challenge.* Ohio State University Extension
Fact Sheet, HYG-5168-96, Family and Consumer Sciences, Ohio State University:

Columbus, Ohio. [On-line]. Available: http://www.ag.ohio-state.edu/~ohioline/hyg-fact/5000/5168.html

Goyer, A. (1998). *Intergenerational shared site project. Practitioner's guide.* Washington, DC: American Association of Retired Persons.

Intergenerational Community Service: Moving Beyond Good Feelings. (2001). [On-line]. Available: http://www.gu.org/progservice.htm

Intergenerational Programming. (2001). Senior Series. Ohio State University Extension, SS-142-98. [On-line]. Available: http://ohioline.ag.ohio-state.edu/ss-fact/0142.html

Linking Young and Old Through Intergenerational Programs. (2001). [On-line]. Available: http://www.gu.org/proglinky&o.htm

Perlstein, S. (2001). *The arts and older Americans. Arts programs uniting generations.* National Endowment for the Arts. [On-line]. Available: http://arts.endow.gov/partner/Accessibility/Monograph/Perlstein.html

Rubin, R. J. (1999). *Benefits of intergenerational programs.* [On-line]. Available: www.ala.org/olos/ig_benefits.html

U.S. Department of Agriculture. (2001). *Into the 21st century: Intergenerational programming.* Washington, DC: Author. [On-line]. Available: www.reeusda.gov/4h/ip/intergenerational.htm

RESOURCES

American Library Association
Office for Literacy and Outreach Services (OLOS)
Intergenerational Subcommittee
50 East Huron Street
Chicago, Illinois 60611
800-545-2433 #4294
http://www.ala.org/olos/intergenerational.html
The Intergenerational Subcommittee of the Office for Literacy & Outreach Services Advisory Committee recommends, supports and develops projects which encourage mutually beneficial, mutually enjoyable library programs linking generations and provide a forum for the exchange of information and ideas regarding intergenerational library programs.

Brookdale Center on Aging of Hunter College
Intergenerational Program
1114 Avenue of the Americas, 40th floor
New York, NY 10036
646-366-1000

http://www.brookdale.org/intergen/
The Brookdale Center on Aging of Hunter College is the largest university-based gerontology center in the Northeast. The Brookdale Center provides training and technical assistance to staff at all levels within the aging network.

CYFERnet
612-626-1111
http://www.cyfernet.org/
CYFERnet is a national network of Land Grant university faculty and county Extension educators working to support community-based educational programs for children, youth, parents and families. CYFERnet is coordinated by the University of Kentucky (Program), University of Arizona (Evaluation) and the University of Minnesota (Technology).

DOROT
171 W. 85th Street
New York, NY 10024
212-769-2850
http://www.dorotusa.org/
DOROT's mission is to enhance the lives of Jewish and other elderly in the Greater New York City Metropolitan area through a dynamic partnership of volunteers, professionals, and elders; to foster mutually beneficial interaction between the generations; and to provide education, guidance and leadership in developing volunteer-based programs for the elderly nationally and internationally.

Elderhostel
11 Avenue de Lafayette
Boston, MA 02111-1746
877-426-8056
http://www.elderhostel.org
Elderhostel is a non-profit organization that provides high-quality educational adventures for adults, age 55 and older. Elderhostel's intergenerational programs are designed for hostelers and children.

Elders Share the Arts (ESTA)
Center for Creative Aging
72 East First Street
New York, NY 10003

http://elderssharethearts.org
Elders Share the Arts (ESTA) is a nationally recognized arts organization
dedicated to bridging generational divides and generating a sense of
community through the arts.

The Generation Connection Society (GCS)
1085 West Seventh Avenue
Vancouver, BC V6H 1B2
604-731-5399
http://www.genconn.ca/
The Generation Connection Society is a volunteer non-profit society
whose purpose is to develop educational programs and resources that
foster positive intergenerational communication. GCS produced a series
of documentary videos covering a wide range of intergenerational issues,
and workshops in collaboration with schools, senior centers and other
community organizations.

Generations Together
University Center for Social and Urban Research
University of Pittsburgh
121 University Place, Suite 300
Pittsburgh, PA 15260-5907
412-648-7150
http://www.pitt.edu/~gti/
Generations Together promotes mutually beneficial interaction between young and old through community outreach, education, research, and dissemination of knowledge.

Generations United
122 C Street, NW, Suite 820
Washington, DC 20001
202-638-1263
http://www.gu.org/
Generations United is a national coalition promoting intergenerational
strategies, programs, and policies and dedicated to fostering linkages
between organizations and people of different ages to improve the
quality of life for individuals and their communities.

Iowa State University Extension
Iowa State University

Ames, Iowa 50011
515-294-4111
http://www.extension.iastate.edu/
The Iowa State University Extension creates public and staff access to information on community aging resources, extension resources, ISU aging courses, related Web sites, interactive learning and the Shared Stories project.

Intergeneration Day
Intergeneration Foundation
430 N. Tejon, Suite 300
Colorado Springs, CO 80903
719-471-2910
http://www.intergenerationday.org/
Intergeneration Foundation's role in combating age-segregation is the sponsorship of Intergeneration Day, culminating Intergeneration Activities Week. Intergeneration Day is celebrated on the first Sunday of October.

Intergenerational Innovations
3200 NE 25th Street, Suite #
Seattle, WA 98125
206-525-8181
http://www.intergenerate.org/
Intergenerational Innovations is a non-profit organization that develops and implements creative programs and activities that bring children, youth, and elders together in volunteer service to each other and to the community through tutoring, mentoring, service learning, and computer activities. The Resource Center houses a large collection of books, manuals, and videos on a wide variety of intergenerational programs.

LinkAge 2000
http://library.thinkquest.org/10120/core.html
A Web site created to provide students (ages 12–18) from around the world with the opportunity to interactively learn about aging and older adults. In addition, LinkAge 2000 serves as a resource for teachers and educators who want to incorporate the study of aging into the curriculum.

New York State Intergenerational Network (NYSIgN)
Brookdale Center on Aging of Hunter College

425 East 25th Street
New York, NY 10010
212-222-5164
http://www.nysign.org
Database of intergenerational programs in New York and best practices material.

The Pennsylvania State University
Agricultural and Extension Education
323 Agricultural Administration
University Park, PA 16802
814-865-1688
http://agexted.cas.psu.edu/FCS/mk/menu.html
Penn State University, through its Cooperative Extension System, develops intergenerational initiatives and studies their impact on program participants and surrounding communities, and provides leadership and resource support for organizations interested in establishing intergenerational programs.

Spellbinders
Office of Community Partnerships
900 Grant Street #110
Denver, CO 80203
http://www.spellbinders.org
Spellbinders support volunteers interested in storytelling.

Strom Thurmond Institute of Government and Public Affairs
Retirement and Intergenerational Studies Laboratory
Clemson University
Perimeter Road
Clemson, SC 29634-0125
864-656-4700
http://www.strom.clemson.edu/teams/risl/index.html
Implements intergenerational projects, and helps others implement projects, project evaluation, and school program evaluation.

- The Retirement and Intergenerational Studies Laboratory focuses on implementing intergenerational projects, helping others implementing projects, project evaluation, school program evaluation, and consulting on issues related to children or retirement/old age.

Developed the manual *Preparing Participants for Intergenerational. Interaction: Training for Success.* http://www.strom.clemson.edu/teams/risl/

- The intergenerational enterprise market program at the John de la Howe School in McCormick, SC, is known as Howe-To Industries. http://www.strom.clemson.edu/teams/risl/howe-to.html

Temple University
Center for Intergenerational Learning
1601 North Broad Street, Room 206
Philadelphia, PA 19122
http://www.temple.edu/cil/
The Center serves as a national resource for intergenerational programming through the development of innovative cross-age programs, such as the Full Circle Theater Troupe; the provision of training and technical assistance; and the dissemination of materials.

Texas Tech University
College of Home Economics
Youth Exchanging With Seniors (YES) Project
Box 4170
Lubbock, TX 79409-1162
806-742-3189
http://coa.kumc.edu/RIT/models/no_46.htm
The YES intergenerational program assists older adults with minor help around the house; transportation for shopping, medical appointments; and social or civic activities to remain independent, while building mutually beneficial relationships between seniors and teenagers.

U.S. Administration on Aging, Region VIII
1961 Stout Street
Denver, Colorado 80924
303-844-2951
http://www.aoa.dhhs.gov/regionviii/default.htm
The Administration on Aging, Region VIII worked in partnership with The Administration for Children and Families, Region VIII in the development of a document titled *Cyberspace Resources for Intergenerational Partnerships.* http://www.aoa.dhhs.gov/regionviii/cyberig.htm

University of Maryland
Adult Health & Development Program (AHDP)

International Network for Intergenerational Health
301-405-2528
http://www.inform.umd.edu/EdRes/Colleges/HLHP/AHDP/
History.html
The Adult Health & Development Program at the University of Maryland is the model for the National Network for Intergenerational Health. It was the first multi-ethnic, interracial, intergenerational health promotion and rehabilitation program in the country.

University of Minnesota
University of Minnesota Extension Service
240 Coffey Hall, 1420 Eckles Avenue
St. Paul, MN 55108-6070
612-624-5329
http://www.extension.umn.edu/
Elder's Wisdom, Children's Song: Community Celebration of Place
http://www.extension.umn.edu/projects/grants/internal/collegiate/
AF1021.html

University of Southern California
Intergenerational Health Research Team
http://uscnurse.usc.edu/healthcom/index3.htm
The Intergenerational Health Communications Team, (IHRT) is concerned that older adults may have lost credibility with the advent of the information deluge. The team is engaged in exploring the extent to which older adults share information and advice with younger members of their family. The goal is to design an intervention to bring families together to share information and wisdom across generations. The first stage of the study looks at Korean, Chinese, and Latino families.

Worchester State College
Intergeneration Urban Institute
Worcester State College
486 Chandler Street
Worcester, MA 01602
508-793-8000 ext. 8900 or 8629
http://www.cpn.org/sections/affiliates/intergen_urbaninstitute.html
The Mission of the Intergenerational Urban Institute at Worcester State College is to harness the combined talents of college students of all

ages to meet the urgent challenges facing the urban environment. The Intergenerational Urban Institute offers a Teen Parent Support Program; debates and forums on intergenerational issues; pre-retirement planning and outreach; and arts collaborative including intergenerational theater, chorus, dance and media projects.

Travel

SHIRLEY

A postcard from Shirley dated August 7, 2000, from Whidbey Island, Washington, reads:

"Hi Marilyn, Had a choice of a ferry boat from Puget Sound or a 3 1/2 hour bus ride over Deception Pass and I chose the scenic bus this time. Mary and I worked at the Western Gear Works during WWII making gears for the bombardier doors on Boeing's B-52's. Our other worker, Margaret, is arriving tomorrow from Tulsa. Mary lives at the end of Penn Cove and I am only three yards away from the ebbing tide, which is leaving mussels, clamshells and sometimes colored starfish on the beach. Down a little further are mussel rafts and when the crew isn't harvesting, the seals do their sun bathing and eating. We may go kayaking this afternoon. We just had clam chowder Mary made from the clams her neighbor dug right in front of us. On a clear day you can see Mt. Baker across the cove. I'll send you a lengthy letter later.

Shirley in Paradise (Card #5, about 65 to go)

At age 79 nothing stops Shirley and indeed 3 days later, a letter arrived detailing her trip from Pittsburgh to the state of Washington and her reunion with her "war buddies." I have a small bundle of postcards and letters from Shirley, sharing with me her wonderful adventures. When I read her correspondences, something as simple as a trip to the airport can seem like an exciting challenge. She writes, "It was cold this morning. I caught the bus from Aspinwall, wheeling my baggage five blocks to catch the bus into town (6:30 a.m.), then I got the 28x bus to the airport as I had a 9:40 a.m. flight with a change in Detroit arriving Ft. Meyers at 3:30 p.m." You absolutely have to love her determination.

Until she had a stroke a couple of years ago, she drove her 1987 Cadillac across the country alone to visit friends and family in the Midwest. Shirley takes at least two and sometimes more trips a year. She doesn't go in for group outings, preferring to make her own arrangements and be independent. The money she earns from house-sitting and respite care for a few older clients sustains her "traveling habit." She is so knowledgeable about interesting places to go and how to make all the necessary arrangements that about 3 years ago we offered her the position of trip coordinator. She did a great job, but resigned after 6 months because it curtailed her own traveling.

Shirley has been coming to Vintage for about 6 years. She enjoys line-dancing and is a member of STAR, a group of older adults who visit local schools to read stories to the children. Additionally, she has a great Connie Francis act that she performs at Vintage and other centers.

It is wonderful that Shirley still has the wanderlust and that she is willing to share all of her adventures with her many friends. I count myself lucky to be #5 of 65 and continue to look forward to her cards and letters.

Travel ranks among the top leisure activities for men and women who are 50 and older. Today's Americans are retiring earlier, have more disposable income and leisure time, a longer life span, and better health to pursue their travel interests. The travel industry also provides senior discounts, making travel more affordable.

Statistics from the last 5 years show a 23% increase in travel in the U.S. Much of that increase is associated with people aged 55 and over who have increased their travel by almost 40%.

Older vacationers travel more frequently than their younger counterparts and their stays tend to be longer. In a study conducted for *Modern Maturity* magazine, adults who are 50-plus identified travel abroad, the beach, a cruise or other waterside vacations, and the mountains, theme parks, or resorts as their top vacation destinations. Baby boomers are redefining the tourism industry with a quest for vacations of significance, such as ecotourism, heritage tours, and educational tours. Ecotourism, the hottest segment of the travel industry, is described by the Ecotourism Society as "responsible travel to natural areas, which conserves the environment and sustains the well-being of local people." Ecotourists want to interact with the natural environment, experience the local culture, and learn things from qualified experts, and the typical ecotourist is a baby boomer with a college degree. Ecotourism suits baby boomers so well because of four generational traits: they are interested in the environment, enjoy hands-on involvement, love learning, and are interested in their own culture.

The Internet is another phenomenon affecting the popularity of senior travel, providing convenient travel information and e-tickets for any computer user with access to the Internet. Most mature vacationers prefer booking their own travel arrangements rather than going on a package tour.

Many seniors who would like to travel but can't afford to have found creative ways to do so. For example, some seniors have found employment and outdoor recreational opportunities at our national parks. In Yellowstone National Park, Hamilton Stores recruits retirees who are "interested in a summer of adventure, of exploration, meeting new people, and making new friends." A majority of their employees are retirees in their 50s and 60s. Employees can room and board in the employee dormitory or reserve an RV site for a nominal fee. On their off days, they can participate in a variety of activities at the park, including walking, hiking, fishing, horseback riding, boating, and observing nature. It is a great experience for the seniors and young people who work there.

Take Jack and Kay from Florida. Jack took an early retirement and they immediately headed south from Ohio to Florida. When they heard about the summer work in Yellowstone, they applied over the Internet and both were accepted, so they purchased an RV and drove across the country. They now work adjoining counters at one of the Hamilton Stores. Jack is such a hit that customers, especially those with children, will wait until seats are available at his counter. He makes eating fun, and the kids love him.

This is their third year there. They love working around vacationers and the younger staff. During a conversation with Kay, she briefly excused herself to have a farewell picture taken with one of the younger people who was heading back to college. Working part-time gives them plenty of time to hike, fish, or just hang out at a campfire with the younger people. Kay told us they had pretty much saved their summer earnings this year and planned to use it to take a cruise this winter. She said that you never get burned out because the season is not that long and there is always something fun to do on your days off.

Ninety-three-year-old Myrtle sent a letter addressed to "Summer Jobs, Yellowstone National Park" and she got a job—her first *paying* job since she retired 30 years ago. She plans to be back next year. Myrtle lives in the dormitory with other seniors and college students and admitted that she was a bit tired on the day we met because some of the students had taken her out the previous night to the local pub.

Field trips to museums, zoos, nature centers, science centers, aquariums, conservatories, and other similar institutions provide opportunities for learning about the natural world when you can't visit the great outdoors. Adults want experiential activities—they want to experience something physically through their senses, rather than read or hear about it. Field trips also introduce visitors to art, ideas, history, nature, environmental issues, and knowledge. Field trips have the potential to create interest and inspire further involvement. Learning and understanding can be enhanced with guidance and facilitation through learning opportunities from educators. However, it is important to keep in mind that not all visitors attend field trips for the purpose of learning—many visitors attend primarily for social reasons.

SUGGESTED ACTIVITIES

In addition to senior-center-sponsored trips, the following activities can be offered to center participants who are interested in travel:

- travel club to share tips and information and plan trips
- travel resource center
- travelogues
- cooperative programs with museums, conservatories, zoos, etc.
- information on employment opportunities at parks and resorts

BIBLIOGRAPHY

American Association of Retired Persons. (1992). *Mature America in the 1990s. A special report from Modern Maturity Magazine and the Roper organization.* Washington, DC: Author.

Berger, S. (2001). *Grown-up gallivanting* [On-line]. Available: www.aarp.com/comptech/features/feature039.html

Carpenter, D. (2001, August 8). *You can rest when you are at home.* Chicago: The Associated Press, Pittsburgh Post Gazette.

Foot, D. K. (1998). *Boom, bust and echo 2000. Profiting from the demographic shift in the new millennium.* Toronto: Macfarlane, Walter & Ross.

Hamilton Stores, Inc. (2001). *Employment opportunities with Hamilton Stores, Inc.* West Yellowstone and Bozeman, MT: Author. [On-line]. Available: www.hamiltonstores.com/employment

Heimlich, J., Diem, J., & Farell, E. (1996). Adult learning in non-formal institutions. *ERIC Digest No. 173.* [On-line]. Available: ericacve.org

RESOURCES

Access-Able Travel Source, LLC
PO Box 1796
Wheat Ridge, CO 80034
303-232-2979
http://www.access-able.com/
Access-Able Travel Source is dedicated to aiding travelers with disabilities and the mature traveler by providing information on transportation, accommodations, attractions, adventures, and travel resources.

Society for Accessible Travel & Hospitality (SATH)
347 Fifth Avenue, Suite 610
New York, NY 10016
212-447-7284
http://www.sath.org
The Society for Accessible Travel & Hospitality provides travel tips, access information, articles from Open World Magazine, useful links, and information on upcoming events.

PART FIVE

Meeting Special Needs

CHAPTER FIFTEEN

Information and Referral Programs

CHERYL

It's 9:00 a.m. and Cheryl is writing her name on the sign-in sheet at Vintage. She is carrying her usual assortment of bags, including a black leather attaché, a canvas tote, and a large purse. Sticking out of one is the Pittsburgh Post-Gazette, *the local morning newspaper. She will not find time to look at it until much later in the day, when she peruses the paper for any news about seniors in the community, and of course checks the obituaries. Until then, it will sit on the corner of her desk amid a collection of other papers. Cheryl is a pack rat and this is a good thing for Vintage. The rest of the staff knows they can always count on her to find a newsletter article from the late 1980s, or a brochure from the agency when it first opened its doors in 1973.*

Cheryl is the Information and Referral Specialist. She has held this position for 22 years. We all say she has more information in her head than is contained in all the papers she has managed to collect over the years. The staff dreaded when she took time off to give birth to her two daughters.

On this particular day she spends a few minutes talking to the receptionist who is about to take her vacation. It is Cheryl's responsibility to make sure the desk is covered when the receptionist is away. When she heads for her office near the main entrance, someone is waiting with a question even as she unlocks her door and unloads her many bags. It is Cheryl's cheerful nature to welcome the person, put her newspaper and lunch on the desk and the rest of her stuff on the floor before asking the person how she can help. There are many days when the lunch never makes it to the refrigerator in the kitchen.

Cheryl has done everything from assisting a participant in selling their home and moving into an assisted-living facility, to helping an older woman figure out her bra size. Many staff still chuckle when we remember

Cheryl with a tape measure in hand, closing her office door so she could measure Mabel.

Life is often complicated for older adults, especially those who find themselves alone and bombarded with forms for insurance, taxes, and a variety of other problems. Some rely on Cheryl to read their mail, and she is perfect for this job. No question is considered stupid, and everyone who enters her office is greeted with a smile. There is no way we will ever know how many people she has helped, but it surely numbers in the hundreds of thousands.

On a recent day I asked her to log the issues she had been called on to answer that day and this is what she told me:

- *Answered a call about our adult day care and referred the caller to our downtown facility.*
- *Received a call from a family looking for an assisted-living facility and put information in the mail to them.*
- *Filled out a new membership for a young retiree and gave her a tour of Vintage, explaining its services.*
- *Ordered new Allegheny County Area Agency on Aging consumer identification cards, showing a person is registered, and a voter registration card for someone who lost her wallet.*
- *Renewed five Vintage memberships (no tour necessary).*
- *Answered 15 inquiries about vouchers for the Farmers' Market (a statewide program that gives vouchers worth $20 to seniors, allowing them to purchase fresh fruits and vegetables).*
- *Registered a participant for Access, a senior citizen bus pass, and OPT (Older Person's Transportation) so that the person can get to doctor appointments and attend recreational activities, including the center.*
- *Answered an inquiry about handicapped parking spaces at our facility.*
- *Set up an interview with a local TV station and participants concerning safe driving and seniors.*

Cheryl's day almost never ends at 5:00. Frequently, it is only after the building becomes quiet that she has time to get to the many reports required of her. She knows her first responsibility is to the people who make their way to her door with the question that in the participant's mind needs to be answered immediately.

The other day we were talking about age and Cheryl said she is 46. I commented she has some time before retirement. Vintage will indeed be fortunate if she decides to spend the second 22 years of her career with us.

In 1973, amendments to the federal Older Americans' Act required state and area agencies on aging to develop information and referral (I&R) services accessible to all older Americans. Many of these services are located in senior centers. The National Association of State Units on Aging established the National Aging I&R Support Center in 1990 to provide training and technical assistance to support state and area agencies on aging and local I&R providers. The National Aging I&R Support Center adopted the Alliance for Information and Referral System's (AIRS) standards for professional I&R as the measure of quality to be used by the aging network.

The National Aging Support Center and AIRS have developed an aging I&R specialist-certification program. The aging I&R specialist needs to be aware of emerging issues for both the older population and the aging services network, understand the special needs of older persons and their caregivers, and be knowledgeable about the services available in the community. The aging I&R specialist is a professional with a comprehensive understanding of the human service delivery system and a holistic view of older people's needs and wants.

Information and referral programs have been the traditional point of contact for people in the community who require information about, or linkage with, human-services providers to meet their needs. Information and referral programs for older adults receive about 3 million calls a year and simplify access through the maze of social service programs that frequently exist. I&R programs in senior centers serve as the entry point for many older adults who need to access aging-network services, including senior-center programs. The services provided through I&R are an essential component of the senior center and contribute to the center's vitality.

The main functions of the I&R program include

- developing and maintaining a comprehensive resource file or database about the organizations that provide human services in the community
- providing information to people who need it
- providing problem-solving assistance and advocacy to ensure access to services

- following-up with inquirers and providers to ensure that needed services were received
- collecting information regarding requests for service and identifying service gaps
- participating in education activities regarding community resources

I&R can help older adults learn about and access benefits they are entitled to. In most states, there are as many as 40 to 60 different benefits that are available to older adults. According to the National Council on Aging:

- More than 1 million seniors are eligible for and not receiving supplemental income checks of $300 or more per month.
- An estimated 3 million seniors are missing out on Medicaid benefits that could help pay hospital, doctor, prescription drug, and other medical expenses.
- More than 3.7 million seniors are eligible for and not receiving food stamp benefits that could be used to purchase food.
- Most state pharmaceutical programs that help seniors pay for prescription drugs are greatly underutilized, as are state property-tax-relief benefits.

Other benefits that are underutilized include federal and state veterans' benefits, health insurance counseling services, weatherization programs that provide free home-energy repairs and services that can lower energy bills, and congregate and home-delivered meals.

The I&R program may also make its information and services available to the community in a variety of other ways including establishing a presence at other sites in the community; compiling and distributing a resource directory; allowing the public to access the resource files and database; and making all or a portion of its database available on community-based kiosks or on the Internet.

Information must be relevant, accessible, and reliable. People need to be able to obtain necessary information in a way that is meaningful to them, regardless of their technological sophistication, language, income, or other factors. Computer and telecommunications technology promises to give the average person instant interactive access to a vast and potentially overwhelming array of information. However, even the most user-friendly computer will be of no benefit to the person who has no idea where to begin. Direct access to information and services via computer works very well for people who know what they need; but for the individual who is overwhelmed by his or her life situation and has no idea where to turn, information without some guidance in how to use it is not very helpful. Individuals who have no experience with the human-services delivery system are unlikely to know what to look for or how to search for a list of alternatives and select an appropriate service provider. I&R specialists are more than mere conduits to the information. A trained I&R specialist can listen to the situation, assess the individual's needs, and facilitate the selection of suitable resources to meet those needs. People often need help to translate their problem into solution options. Person-to-person contact with a trained I&R specialist is vital for those who need it. Technology should never replace the support of the I&R specialist but enhance it.

An analysis of 14,645 calls for services for seniors at Akron, Ohio's Senior Information Line in 1996 revealed 65% of calls were from seniors, 25% from caregivers, and 10% from others. Of the callers 74% were female, 76% were white, and 63% reported low income. Handling a senior I&R call generally takes longer (averaging 10 to 15 minutes) than handling generic I&R calls (5 to 10 minutes). Senior calls take longer because seniors often have multiple needs and don't know what types of assistance are available, they operate at a slower pace, and they often need the I&R specialist to advocate for them and make calls on their behalf.

As the information hub of a senior center, the I&R program needs to ensure that there is a wide variety of choices for accessing the resource data. Access may be provided through a number of mechanisms including person-to-person contact, resource libraries, guest speakers, electronic directories, kiosks, or direct on-line contact. Senior centers need to develop a well-coordinated and publicized continuum of access points that enables people to find the information they need in the way that is most convenient for them. The continuum must be balanced to represent all degrees of need. For example, an individual in a crisis situation may need a case manager while computer savvy seniors can be left to their own devices with a kiosk. Those individuals who can function independently should be encouraged to access the information on their own, freeing the I&R staff to provide additional support to those who need the consultation services of a trained professional. By helping seniors understand the human-services delivery system, senior centers empower them to search for information and make choices independently as needs arise. The I&R process reinforces the individual's capacity for self-reliance.

A study of five diverse agencies that offer I&R services in Detroit was conducted to determine whether there was a common set of outcomes for the I&R services provided. The study's findings suggest that there are two types of I&R: regular and enhanced. Regular I&R clarifies needs, identifies resources, provides referrals, and educates the caller about what to expect when contacting the referral. Enhanced I&R services take additional action on the caller's behalf, which may include advocating for the caller, providing emergency assistance and crisis intervention, linking to a service, and follow-up.

Four common initial outcomes of I&R services were identified: Callers' understanding of their needs was increased; their understanding of their options was increased; callers became more educated about accessing needed services; and they were connected to resources that would meet the identified need.

The intermediate outcome of I&R services is that the customer is empowered to use these new skills and knowledge to connect successfully with the referral. The long-term outcome of a successful referral is obtaining the needed resources and resolving the problem. Enhanced I&R added to these outcomes.

Effective communication is the key to a successful I&R contact. As the older population grows increasingly diverse, differences in language, customs, culture, and information needs will present communication challenges for the I&R specialist. The I&R specialist needs to be sensitive to cultural attitudes that make it difficult for people in some cultures to share information about themselves or seek help. Information in languages other than English, multilingual staff, or translation services to communicate effectively may be necessary. Outreach activities improve access and heighten visibility of the I&R program.

To improve the visibility of the I&R program, it can be publicized by a variety of methods to reach targeted populations:

- personal contact
- speaking engagements
- community meetings
- booths at community events, organizations, and businesses
- public service announcements
- paid advertisements
- radio and television

- feature articles
- community and corporate newsletters
- displays and bulletin boards
- telephone directories
- Internet Web pages
- printed materials such as brochures, posters, and business cards
- billboards and banners
- placards on public transportation
- mailings
- promotional items such as magnets

THE STRUCTURE OF I&R

To operate effectively, I&R programs in senior centers need adequate space, equipment, staff, training, and resources to ensure that staff can effectively perform their duties. Financing should be sufficient to enable the I&R staff to provide adequate service and maintain the standards for professional information and referral. An annual evaluation to measure the effectiveness of I&R services must be conducted.

Because of the vast number of service providers in each community, information needs to be gathered and maintained at the local level. In most areas, unfortunately, numerous organizations maintain their own databases of human-services resources. Some are comprehensive for their own geographic areas; others, such as senior centers, specialize in resources for specific populations. There is likely to be significant overlap and duplication of effort. Maintaining updated information is difficult, labor-intensive, costly, and time-consuming. To best meet the information needs of the community, hub agencies are needed to develop a central database of human-services resources and to keep it updated. If multiple databases are absolutely necessary, they should be coordinated through a central resource to avoid duplication of effort. Senior centers would benefit from the development of a central database of human services that all can share, resource files that could serve as a foundation, and staff with the requisite information-management skills.

In order for information to be meaningful and of use to the individual, it must be organized and presented in a consistent and logical manner. The AIRS/INFO LINE Taxonomy of Human Services is a common classification system that structures and organizes human-services information for I&R programs. By using a common language that bridges the gap between disciplines, it also meets the needs of professionals who are working collaboratively on behalf of participants. The I&R program can use its indexing and organizational skills to help computer users save time when searching for services by providing them access to preselected Web sites.

In July 2001, the Federal Communications Commission granted the abbreviated dialing code 211 for community information and referral nationwide. The Coalition—a group of nonprofit organizations made up of the Alliance of Information and Referral Systems, the United Way of America, United Way 211 of Atlanta, Georgia, the United Way of Connecticut, the Florida Alliance of Information and Referral Services, and the Texas I&R Network—had petitioned the FCC to designate 211 as a single point of access to multiple social service organizations. Based on the successful experience of communities that have already implemented 211, the Coalition believes that letting people access their community's social services by a short, simple, universal number will increase the number of people helped by service organizations.

The key reasons for designating 211 include the following:

- 211 eliminates confusion and complicated searches through phone books.
- 211 serves people not covered by 911 and 311.
- 211 serves vulnerable people not otherwise helped. Some people in crisis are not able to search for phone numbers at all. These people may be illiterate, incapacitated by crisis (such as natural disaster), travelers who don't know where to turn, elderly, or non-English speaking.
- 211 is efficient. Setting aside 211 gives people one number to call when they are in crisis so that they won't have to dial agency after agency searching for appropriate help.
- 211 can help deliver services more efficiently by using centralized data in the community.
- 211 will raise the visibility of I&R.
- 211 builds on an existing infrastructure and the joint experience of the almost 1,000 AIRS members and 1,400 United Way locations across the country.

THE SENTINEL PROJECT

Abuse of elders takes many forms, and the I&R specialist needs to have a clear understanding of the local protective service system, state statutes regarding elder abuse, reporting requirements, and the risk factors that may contribute to making elders vulnerable. It is estimated that for every identified case of abuse or neglect, at least five go undisclosed. To address hidden abuse or neglect, the National Center on Elder Abuse introduced the Sentinel Project, a national initiative to help hidden victims of abuse. Because I&R is the gateway to community services, I&R specialists are in a unique position to act as sentinels to identify and assist older persons who are at risk. To better serve them, specialists and adult protective services need to understand each other and work together. The two systems can link through cross-training, protocols for reporting abuse or neglect, and interagency meetings to promote greater understanding.

ON-LINE SUPPORT GROUPS

A major Internet resource that I&R programs can tap is the growing number and variety of on-line self-help support groups. Self-help groups have traditionally met people's needs for information, education, support, and empowerment, and their therapeutic potential has been recognized in recent studies. An estimated 25 million Americans (18% of the population) have participated in a support group at some time in their lives. Now, groups that do not exist in the community are becoming available on the Internet. The barriers that prevent the formation of, or access to, local support groups include the rarity of many illnesses or conditions, severe physical or mental disabilities that restrict travel and access, lack of transportation; the remoteness of some locales, and time constraints. Continued need for health information to manage and improve individuals' health has contributed to the growth of support groups both on- and off-line. As the cost of computers has declined, more people are using the Internet to share their concerns and provide practical information and emotional support to others.

Computer-based support networks provide mutual support through listservs or e-mail discussion groups and Web sites that provide interactive message boards and real-time chat programs. On-line self-help groups can help people with a broader range of illnesses, disabilities, or problems. Although they lack some of the advantages of the personal contact found in face-to-face groups, they do provide for the exchange of information and support and are available 24 hours a day. Of more than 1,000 self-help support groups known to the Self-Help Clearinghouse, upwards of 90% are available through Internet Web sites or an e-mail address.

SUGGESTED ACTIVITIES

INFORMATIONAL PROGRAM TOPICS

- financial planning
- end-of-life care
- retirement planning
- estate planning
- women and wealth
- investing
- legal services
- long-term-care options
- housing options

I&R SERVICES

- caregiver resource center
- resource library with brochures, applications, and other information
- kiosks with preselected Web sites
- resource directory, accessible on-line or printed
- eldercare workplace seminars
- benefit fair
- assistance completing benefit applications
- VITA income tax assistance
- insurance counseling
- agency presentations
- speaking engagements
- assistive devices demonstrations
- forum to meet the candidates (pre-election)

BIBLIOGRAPHY

Administration on Aging. (2001). *Information and assistance services for the elderly.* [On-line]. Available: http://www.aoa.gov/may98/ia.html

Alliance of Information and Referral Systems. (2001, April). Creating a certification program for I&R specialists in the field of aging. *Alliance of Information and Referral Systems Newsletter.*

Alliance of Information and Referral Systems. (1995). *Out of the shadows. Information and referral bringing people and services together.* Joliet, IL: Author.

Alliance of Information and Referral Systems. (2000). *Standards for professional information and referral.* Joliet, IL: Author.

Downs, C. (2001, March). Gateway sentinels: Protectors of the elderly. *Information and Referral Reporter.* National Aging I&R Support Center.

Hutchinson, B. (1994). Bridging the gap: Enhancing communication with older adults. *Information and Referral. The Journal of the Alliance of Information and Referral Systems, 16,* 79–94.

Hwalek, M., Bruni, M., Barbas, S., Lyle, P., Pitchford, C., Quarterman, C., & Rodriquez-Kitkowski, L. (1998). Measuring the outcomes of information and referral services. *Information and Referral. The Journal of the Alliance of Information and Referral Systems, 20,* 31–44.

National Council on the Aging. (2001). *Ten benefits that millions of seniors are missing out on.* Washington, DC: Author.

Pennsylvania Association for Information and Referral. *Information and referral: The linking service.* Mansfield, PA: Author.

Pierson, S., & Mozina, M. (1997). Senior info line—A specialized I&R service targeted at the elderly. *Information and Referral. The Journal of the Alliance of Information and Referral Systems, 19,* 1–10.

Sales, G. (2000). I&R leadership in the information age. *Information and Referral. The Journal of the Alliance of Information and Referral Systems, 22.*

Sales, G. (2001). The role of information and referral in the national information infrastructure. An AIRS position paper. Seattle, WA: Alliance of Information and Referral Systems, pp. 139–157.

211.org. (2001). FCC approves 211 for information and referral. [On-line]. Available: www.211.org

White, B. J., & Madara, E. J. (2000). Online mutual support groups: identifying and tapping new I&R resources. *Information and Referral. The Journal of the Alliance of Information and Referral Systems, 22,* 63–82.

RESOURCES

Alliance of Information and Referral Systems (AIRS)

PO Box 31668
Seattle, WA 98103
206-632-2477
www.airs.org

The Alliance of Information and Referral Systems improve access to services for all people through the mechanism of information and referral. AIRS meets this goal through its publications, international training conferences, local I&R associations, and I&R clearinghouse. AIRS' publications include:

- *Standards for Professional Information and Referral*
- *AIRS Newsletter*
- *Information and Referral: The Journal of the Alliance of Information and Referral Systems*
- *Directory of I & R Services in the U.S. and Canada*
- *A Taxonomy of Human Services: A Conceptual Framework with Standard-ized Terminology and Definition for the Field*
- *Creating a 211 Service*, a comprehensive guide to developing a 211 Information and Referral Service

American Self-Help Clearinghouse
100 Hanover Ave., Suite 202
Cedar Knolls, NJ 07927
973-625-3037
http://www.mentalhelp.net/selfhelp/
Publications include *Self-Help Sourcebook* and the national self-help group database, www.selfhelpgroups.org. This searchable database includes information on over 700 self-help support groups, ideas for starting groups, and opportunities to link with others to develop needed new national or international groups.

BenefitsCheck*Up*
http://www.benefitscheckup.org
BenefitsCheck*Up* is a free, online service that identifies federal and state assistance programs for older Americans. BenefitsCheck*Up* is a service of the National Council on the Aging.

FirstGov
c/o GSA
750 17th Street, NW, Suite 200
Washington, DC 20006
www.firstgov.gov
FirstGov™ is an official United States Government Web site, a single online portal with information from all 27 million federal agency Web pages.

Info Line
PO Box 4307
El Monte, CA 91734
818-350-1841
Info Line co-published *A Taxonomy of Human Services* with AIRS.

National Association of Area Agencies on Aging
1112 - 16th Street NW, Suite 100
Washington, DC 20036
202-296-8130 (nationwide AAA listings)
800-677-1116 (national Eldercare locator)
http://www.n4a.org/
The National Association of Area Agencies on Aging (N4A) is the umbrella organization for the 655 area agencies on aging (AAAs) and more than 230 Title VI Native American aging programs in the U.S. Through its presence in Washington, D.C., N4A advocates on behalf of the local aging agencies to ensure that needed resources and support services are available to older Americans.

The National Aging Information Center (NAIC)
Administration on Aging
330 Independence Avenue SW, Room 4656
Washington, DC 20201
202-619-7501
http://www.aoa.gov/naic/
The National Aging Information Center serves as a central source of information on aging for older people, their families, and those who work for or on behalf of older persons. NAIC resources include program and policy-related materials for consumers and practitioners as well as demographic and other statistical data on the health, economic, and social conditions of older Americans.

National Aging I&R Support Center (NIRSC)
National Association of State Units on Aging
1225 I Street, NW, Suite 725
Washington, DC 20005
202-898-2578
http://www.narusa.org
The National Association of State Units on Aging (NASUA) is a national non-profit membership organization comprised of the 57 state and

territorial government agencies on aging. The Administration on Aging provides funding for the National Information and Referral Support Center at NASUA, which is operated in partnership with the N4A and the Alliance of Information and Referral Systems. The National Aging I&R Support Center provides technical assistance, consultation, and training to State and Area Agencies on Aging and local I&R providers funded under the Older Americans Act. NIRSC maintains a database of annotated bibliographic listings of training and technical assistance materials and a skills bank of individuals willing to share their I&R expertise. NIRSC operates an Information and Referral Conference on the AGE-NET electronic bulletin board and conducts the annual National Aging I&R Symposium. Publications include *National Standards for Older Americans Act Information and Referral Services; Assessment Guide for Older Americans Act Information and Referral Services;* and *How to Link Elders to Services: A Training Manual for Staff Providing Information and Referral Services to Older Americans.* NIRSC provides training, technical assistance, aging I&R specialist certification program, and publishes the *Information and Referral Reporter* newsletter.

National Center on Elder Abuse
1225 I Street, NW, Suite 725
Washington, DC 20005
202-898-2586
http://www.elderabusecenter.org
The National Center on Elder Abuse (NCEA) consists of a partnership of six agencies: the National Association of State Units on Aging (NASUA), the American Bar Association Commission on Legal Problems of the Elderly (ABA), the Clearinghouse on Abuse and Neglect of the Elderly (CANE), the Goldman Institute on Aging's San Francisco Consortium for Elder Abuse Prevention (GIOA), the National Association of Adult Protective Services Administrators (NAAPSA), and the National Committee for the Prevention of Elder Abuse (NCPEA).

Resource Directory for Older People
National Institute on Aging
Public Information Office
Building 31; Room 5C27
31 Center Drive, MSC 2292
Bethesda, MD 20892-2292
301-496-1752

http://www.nih.gov/nia/related/aoaresrc/resource.htm
The *Resource Directory for Older People*, a cooperative effort of the National Institute on Aging (NIA) and the Administration on Aging (AoA), is intended to serve a wide audience including health and legal professionals, social service providers, librarians, and researchers, as well as older people and their families. The directory lists Federal agencies, AoA-supported resource centers, professional societies, private groups, and volunteer programs.

2-1-1.org
United Way of Connecticut Infoline
1344 Silas Deane Highway
Rocky Hill, CT 06067
860-571-7500
http://www.211.org
2-1-1 is the national abbreviated dialing code for free access to health and human services information and referral. The site is maintained by the United Way of Connecticut.

CHAPTER SIXTEEN

Grandparenting Issues

LOUISE

It's Thursday, a little after noon. Looking out of my office window I see Louise making her way to Vintage with a small child in tow for the weekly support-group meeting for parenting grandparents. Louise walks the two blocks to Vintage each week, because she has learned it's not only okay, but also important to do something for herself. Once inside the room, the entire time is devoted to the grandparent. Child care is provided in a separate room away from the support-group meeting. On this particular day the group begins by dimming the lights and listening to a relaxation tape, as they put their problems and concerns from the past week "on the back burner." A massage therapist has stopped by and she quietly moves from one grandparent to another offering shoulder massages. There are a lot of "ahs" and sighs as they begin to relax.

The lights come on and the grandparents begin to work on a craft project, again something for themselves. Once a month they'll make something and today it is a large mug for tea or coffee. As they work, they begin to talk about the past 7 days.

The facilitator is there to assist them, but a lot of the support they get is from one another. Today they are worrying about their finances, and the facilitator asks if perhaps a resource can be found in the community to help the group work on budgeting. They all agree, and the facilitator will make arrangements to find someone in the coming weeks. With the craft project completed, it's time for refreshments, and the grandchildren are brought back to join them. As the group ends there are lots of hugs, and you can hear them saying, "See you next week" or "Call me someday."

At 65, Louise will tell you this is not what she expected to be doing at this age. A widow, Louise has been the adoptive mother of her niece's three children since they were preschoolers. They are now 14, 16, and 17.

Additionally, she cares for two grandsons, ages 4 and 6, who are with her "off and on."

Louise has been through all the stages with her kids and is thankful for the support she gets at Vintage. She was one of the first parenting grandparents to come to Vintage when we started the program about 6 years ago. She says it is good to listen to other people in a similar situation and to share experiences, often helping one another.

Anger management has been a real issue for Louise. By listening to others and using different methods to discipline her children, she now no longer feels the need to "curse at the kids or whack them." She looks forward to coming each week, and says the group has "helped her a lot." The stresses and burdens felt by parenting grandparents are often unique to them. In the support group they find others like themselves, and as they work through issues together, find a more positive way to raise their grandchildren while finding time for themselves.

Between 75% and 80% of people 65 years and older are grandparents. Grandchildren are an important part of their lives and many take the opportunity to nurture active relationships with their grandchildren. The majority of grandparents regularly see their grandchildren or travel to visit with them. When they can't see them, they keep in touch by talking on the phone or by e-mail or by sending a card or letter.

Increased life expectancy presents more opportunity for grandparents to know their grandchildren not only as infants and young children, but as adolescents, young adults, and parents. It also makes it more common for grandchildren to have four living grandparents throughout their childhood. As parents continue to find themselves constrained by busy lifestyles, the grandparent-grandchild relationship will continue to grow in importance. As these relationships develop and evolve, so will the needs of the grandparent, providing programming and service opportunities for senior centers.

AARP conducted a grandparenting survey that explored many facets of the grandparent-grandchild relationship including communications, grandparent roles, activities, spending patterns, relationships, and values. This national survey of 823 grandparents aged 50 and older found that 82% of grandparents had seen a grandchild in the previous month, 7 in 10 had shared a meal with a grandchild, half had watched a television comedy or had their grandchild spend the night, and about 4 in 10 shopped for clothes, took part in exercise or sports, watched educational television, attended a religious service, or watched a video together. Half say they frequently play the role of friend or companion for a grandchild. A number of factors affect the relationship especially the grandparent's age, health, and the geographic distance between grandparent and grandchild.

An increasing number of grandparents are finding their later years different from what they expected. Many older Americans approaching or in retirement suddenly find themselves caring for and raising their grandchildren. Frequently this responsibility occurs because of a sudden unfortunate event or set of circumstances involving the natural parents. This may require special coping skills for handling family crises that involve three generations—them, their children, and the grandchildren. Unfortunately, the development of programs and policies to address the special needs of grandparents and their grandchildren has not kept pace.

A grandparent stepping in to raise grandchildren or other relatives is not a new development. What is new is the growth in this phenomenon. According to the U.S. Census in 1970, 2.2 million, or 3.2% of American children, lived in a household maintained by a grandparent. By 1997, this number had risen to 3.9 million, or 5.5%, representing a 76% increase. Substantial increases occurred among all types of households maintained by grandparents, regardless of the presence or absence of the grandchildren's parents, but were the greatest among children with only one parent in the household. Though nearly half of the grandparent households with a grandchild include the child's mother, about 1 million families in the United States are made up of grandparents who are raising their grandchildren without one of the children's parents. Since 1990, the greatest growth occurred in the number of grandchildren residing with their grandparents only, with neither parent present. Grandparents who serve as surrogate parents represent all socioeconomic and ethnic groups. The majority of grandparents raising their grandchildren are younger than 65. Almost half of grandparent caregivers are between the ages of 50 and 64, and 19% are 65-plus.

Grandparenting styles and experiences vary according to ethnic background. In the United States, Black, Asian American, Italian American, and Hispanic Americans are more likely to be involved in the lives of their grandchildren than members of other groups. Black grandmothers historically have played a more important role in child rearing and maintaining extended family stability than White grandmothers have. Black children are more likely (13%) to live with a grandparent than White children (3.9%) or Hispanic children (5.7%). Most families headed by grandparents live in or near cities and have less than a high-school education, and more such families live in the South than in all other areas of the United States combined.

Research suggests that split-generation households are formed when parents are no longer able to take care of their children because of physical or mental illness, incarceration, substance abuse, parental abuse or neglect, severe economic problems, or because the grandparent did not want the grandchild to go to a foster home. Grandparents have formal or informal custody of their grandchildren in a minority of grandparent-led households. More often, grandchildren and parents live with grandparents in three-generation families, usually because of problems that parents encounter living independently, such as separation or divorce, unemployment, or economic need. In both situations, these families appear to form as a result of parents' economic and other needs, not because of a preference for living in an extended-family household. Better job opportunities, availability of public assistance, lower housing prices, and higher parental income reduce the chances that parents and grandchildren live with grandparents. Three-generation households are more common if the mother was a teenager, unmarried, or had a medical disability at the time she gave birth.

Though grandparents often have raised their grandchildren in times of family crisis, the proportion of families in crisis situations is growing. Approximately 10% of grandparents head a grandparent-grandchild household at any one time. The number of grandparents and grandchildren who have ever lived together at some point in their lives is higher, because many grandchildren live with grandparents for a relatively short time. A grandparent maintains the household in three fourths of families that have both grandparents and grandchildren. In the remaining one fourth, parents maintain homes in which grandparents and grandchildren live together. Of the nearly 4 million children living with their grandparents, 2.5 million live in three-generation households; nearly 1.5 million live in split-generation households. The frequency of three-generation households is much higher for younger children than for older children. Split-generation households are about equally common for all ages and are equally common in center cities and in rural areas. Grandparents in split-generation households, however, are older, less likely to be working, and more likely to have health or disability problems than grandparents in three-generation households.

Grandparent caregivers can be divided into three types. Custodial grandparents have legal custody of their grandchildren. Typically, severe problems existed in the child's nuclear family. The second type is grandparent caregivers who provide daily care for their grandchildren, but do not have legal custody. The child's parent may or may not live in the home. These grandparents focus on providing an economically and emotionally stable environment for the child and often on helping the parent. The third type is grandparents who provide day care. These grandparents tend to be least affected by their caretaking role because the children return home at the end of the day.

Grandparents may resume a parenting role for a variety of reasons, most of which revolve around problems related to the child's parent. The reasons grandparents raise their grandchildren are varied, but all result in a great deal of responsibility for the grandparent who takes on the task. Of the grandparents maintaining households for their grandchildren, the majority are grandmothers. Among all family types, grandmothers who maintain households alone are much more likely than grandparents in other family types to face economic hardship. Grandmothers in grandmother-only households are less likely to have graduated from high school, are less likely to be employed or to have been employed full time or full year, are more likely to be Black and rent their homes, and are more likely to be poor when compared to other grandmothers.

Studies indicate that children who live in grandparents' homes do not fare as well economically as those who live in their parents' homes. Grandchildren residing in grandmother-only families are much more likely than grandchildren in any other family type to be in poverty. Grandmothers in grandmother-only families are also more disadvantaged because no spouse or parents of the grandchildren are the household to help shoulder the burden of providing care and financial support.

Many grandparents in this situation suffer from economic difficulties. Because many older people are already living on a low income, taking on the care of a grandchild may put their economic future in jeopardy. Some grandparents are forced to make job-related sacrifices, while others who were comfortably retired quickly deplete their funds when they take on the responsibility of a grandchild.

Grandparent caregivers face a myriad of challenges in nearly all aspects of their lives when they assume the role of parent. They are prone to psychological and emotional strain as well as feelings of helplessness and isolation. Even those who find great satisfaction in raising their grandchildren often feel disappointment, anger, resentment, blame, guilt, and serious concern about family finances. (Parents may grieve the loss of their estranged child even if they recognize that the decision to remove the child from their care is in the child's best interests.)

Health is an issue for some grandparents. Studies have found significant health problems among grandchildren who are being raised by their grandparents and among the grandparents themselves. Grandparents who are raising grandchildren appear to be in poorer health than their counterparts and some studies have noted high rates of depression, poor self-rated health, and multiple chronic health problems. Grandparent caregivers often neglect their own physical and emotional health because they give priority to the needs of their grandchildren.

Irrespective of their health, though, is the issue of stamina. Many grandparents report feeling both emotionally and physically drained. They may fear they will be unable to meet the demands of parenting as a result of their fatigue and possible health problems. Older grandparents also worry about what will happen to their grandchildren if something happens to them.

The circumstances that bring a child into a grandparent's care can result in various difficulties in child rearing. For instance, children who were prenatally exposed to drugs or who have suffered from abuse or neglect may suffer from physical or emotional problems that may make it difficult to provide care for them. In many cases, behavioral problems can also become an issue. Other children may make fun of them because their "parents" are so old, or question their real parents' whereabouts, which may cause some resentment toward the grandparent by the grandchild.

Taking on a parental role affects an individual's lifestyle and his or her relationships with family and friends. Grandparents who raise their grandchildren are continuing their parenting role at a time when they normally would relinquish it. Many grandparents report a loss of time for themselves. Once their children leave home, many older adults replace their role and responsibilities as a parent with an expanded social network. Raising a grandchild often isolates grandparents from this network. The responsibilities of caregiving often prevent grandparents from participating in activities, while friends who are free from parental responsibilities may not wish to include young children in their activities.

Grandparents may also become isolated from other members of the family who may resent the role that they have taken on. Grandparenting and parenting roles traditionally differ widely in the kinds and levels of responsibility involved. Grandparents cannot be grandparents to the child who is under their parenting care, and this may cause role confusion in the family. Additionally, these grandparents must deal with the trauma that precipitated their role as caregiver. For instance, if the child's parent has died, the grandparent must cope not only with his or her own grief, but also with the grief of their grandchild. An adult child's problems with drugs or alcohol, abuse or neglect, or teenage pregnancy requires grandparents to cope with the loss of their hopes and expectations for their own son or daughter.

There are benefits to the grandparent-caregiver role as well. A majority report experiencing a greater purpose for living. Providing care to their grandchildren helps some caregivers to feel young and active. Other rewards include a chance to raise a child differently, to nurture family relationships, to indulge their grandchildren, continue family histories, to feel valued in their caregiving role, and to receive love and companionship from their grandchild. Many grandparents enjoy the opportunity to break norms regarding age-appropriate behavior through play with their grandchildren. Caregiving relationships can strengthen the ability of extended families to give one another the support they need.

Grandparents who are raising grandchildren encounter problems that may require them to seek legal authority in order to make decisions on behalf of their grandchildren. They may need legal authority to get their grandchildren medical care, enroll them in school, and to enable them to receive immunizations and vaccinations, public assistance, and supportive services. Grandparents can find themselves in need of respite services, affordable housing, and access to medical care.

State and area agencies on aging across the country have instituted programs and services to assist grandparent caregivers. Many have published information guides and have established resource centers to assist grandparent caregivers to identify and access available services. Other important interventions offered include respite services and support groups. Some grandparent caregivers need help with legal and financial matters or they may need to know more about schools and day care. Others need help dealing with the emotional ups and downs of parenting the second time around. Short-term respite care for young and school-age children often tops the wish list of grandparent caregivers.

Senior centers can use many strategies to support grandparents who are raising and educating their grandchildren and help them identify and access services. Such services may help reduce the isolation that is commonly cited as a major problem for grandparents who are raising their grandchildren. Grandparents often need resource information and may not be aware of the services available to help their grandchild academically or to help the child deal with emotional and psychological problems. By partnering with an organization that provides services to children and families or with local schools, senior centers can help grandparents with the grandparenting role. In 1994 Vintage partnered with Parental Stress Center, a kinship program, to provide support to parenting grandparents through the Grandparents as Parents (GAP) program. A support group meets weekly at Vintage. The group is cofacilitated with staff from Vintage and the Parental Stress Center.

Grandparent caregivers often need financial assistance to house, feed, and clothe their grandchild or grandchildren, and they need to know where to go to for help. They might also need health insurance, information about schools, and quality child care. Grandparents who are raising grandchildren with special needs require information about special education and community support services.

Grandparent caregivers often face legal issues such as custody, adoption, guardianship, and foster care. They need help understanding, identifying, and negotiating the legal and social service system, including mediation services, legal services and resources, and social service and family service agencies.

Both grandparent caregivers and grandchildren often deal with various mental health issues such as grief, anger, confusion, resentment, and depression. Grandparent support groups provide an opportunity to meet others who share similar experiences, knowledge, strengths, and hopes and provide a place to belong and a network of support. Support groups provide a combination of activities, including discussion of common problems; emotional support; education for members through guest speakers who talk about health, insurance, legal, financial, educational, or psychological and emotional issues; and assistance with solutions to specific problems.

Ask grandparents what they need then find ways to fulfill these needs either directly or by referral to available services and supports. To identify grandparents who are raising their grandchildren, ask school officials or agencies that are working with older adults, families, or children to refer grandparents who are raising children to you. Promote the program through posters, flyers, press releases, ads, announcements, or letters to the editor in newspapers, church and synagogue bulletins, local TV, and radio. If possible, provide volunteers to care for the grandchildren or have a support group for them during the meeting.

SUGGESTED ACTIVITIES

- information and education on child development, parenting, and resources for grandparents caregivers
- telephone hot lines and warm lines
- programs on stress reduction
- short-term respite services (child care co-located with other services or provided by a parent or cooperative)
- one-on-one or group counseling for grandparents and grandchildren
- support groups and grandparenting classes for grandparents who are raising a second family
- advocacy on accessing public and private assistance and programs
- toy, clothing, and equipment exchange or lending service
- opportunities to educate the public and lobby for increased services

BIBLIOGRAPHY

Administration on Aging. (2001). *Aging Internet information notes: Grandparents raising grandchildren.* Washington, DC: Author. [On-line]. Available: www.aoa.dhhs.gov/NAIC/Notes/grandparents-grandchildren.html

American Association of Retired Persons. (1999, November). *AARP grandparenting survey.* Washington, DC: Author.

American Association of Retired Persons. (1992). *Mature America in the 1990s. A special report from Modern Maturity magazine and the Roper organization.* Washington, DC: Author.

Barber, C. E. (1994, October). *Grandparents: Styles and satisfactions.* No. 10.239. Consumer Series. Fort Collins, CO: Colorado State University Cooperative Extension. Colorado State University. [On-line]. Available: www.colostate.edu/Depts/CoopExt/PUBS/CONSUMER/10239.pdf

Casper, L. M., & Bryson, K. R. (1998, March). *Co-resident grandparents and their grandchildren: Grandparent maintained families.* Working Paper No. 26. Population Division, U.S. Bureau of the Census: Washington, DC. Available: www.census.gov/population/www/documentation/twps0026/twps0026.html

Grandparents as parents: A primer for schools. (2001). ERIC Digest. [On-line]. Available: www.ed.gov/databases/ERIC_Digests/ed401044.html

Kleiner, H. S., Hertzog, J., & Targ, D. (1998, January). *Grandparents acting as parents: Background information for educators.* Purdue Cooperative Extension Service.

Pebley, A. R., & Rudkin, L. L. (1999). Grandparents caring for grandchildren: What do we know? *Journal of Family Issues, 20*(2), 218–242.

RAND. (1999, September). *Grandparent care and welfare: Assessing the impact of public policy on split and three generation families.*

Rothenberg, D. (1996). Grandparents as parents: A primer for schools. *ERIC Digest, ED401044*, 1996-10-00.

U.S. Administration on Aging. (2000). *Grandparents raising grandchildren*. [On-line]. Available: www.aoa.gov/factsheets/grandparents.html

U.S. Census Bureau. (2001). *Grandparents and grandchildren*. [On-line]. Available: www.census.gov/population/www/socdemo/grandparents.html

U.S. Census Bureau. (1999, July 1). Nearly 5.5 million children live with grandparents. *Census Bureau Reports*. [On-line]. Available:www.census.gov/Press-Release/www/1999/cb99-115.html

U.S. House of Representatives. (1992). *Grandparents: New roles and responsibilities.* Select Committee on Aging Comm. Pub. No. 102-876.

U.S. Senate. (1992). *Grandparents as parents: Raising a second generation.* Special Committee on Aging. Serial No. 102-24.

RESOURCES

AARP Grandparent Information Center

601 E Street, NW

Washington, DC 20049

202-434-2296

http://www.aarp.org/confacts/programs/gic.html

AARP—Grandparent Information Center provides an extensive range of services including a listing of local support groups, newsletters, and useful publications.

The Brookdale Foundation Group

126 East 56th Street

New York, NY 10022

212-308-7355

http://www.ewol.com/brookdale

The Brookdale Relatives As Parents Program (RAPP) provides seed grants to support local and state agencies serving grandparents and other kin who have become the primary caretakers of their grandchildren.

Cox, Carole B. *Empowering grandparents raising grandchildren: A training manual for group leaders.* (2000). New York: Springer Publishing Co.

Dannison, Linda. *Second Time Around—Grandparents Raising Grandchildren: A Curriculum Guide for Group Leaders* The curriculum focuses on issues, including increasing grandparent well-being, effective discipline techniques, normal child/adolescent development, and legal issues. Grand-Parents Rights Organization, Dept. of Family and Consumer Sciences, Michigan University. (616) 387-3704.

Eastern Michigan University
Institute for the Study of Children, Families and Communities
203 Boone Hall
Ypsilanti, MI 48197
734-487-0372
http://www.iscfc.emich.edu/
The Institute for the Study of Children, Families and Communities explores contemporary issues and enriches family and community life through the application of scholarly research and practical expertise.

- Kinship training materials were developed to use with casework staff and kinship caregivers. They include curricula for staff and for caregivers, focusing on the needs of kinship caregivers for support, information, and a forum in which to express their views and share their stories. http://www.iscfc.emich.edu/kinship.cfm

Generations United
122 C Street, NW, Suite 820
Washington, DC 20001
202-638-1263
http://www.gu.org
Generations United focuses on promoting intergenerational strategies, programs, and policies.

University of Wisconsin-Extension
432 N. Lake Street
Madison, WI 53706-1498
608-262-3980
http://www.uwex.edu/ces/gprg/gprg.html
The University of Wisconsin-Extension maintains a Web site for grandparents raising grandchildren, professionals, legislators and policymakers, graduate students and videoconference planners to share information, find answers to questions, and learn about resources.

CHAPTER SEVENTEEN

Developmental Disabilities

GEORGE

As I sit here thinking about the first time I saw George, I suspect it was when I noticed a rather overweight man with a very full head of hair slouched in one of the white plastic chairs in the atrium. He appeared to be sound asleep and my first thought was that it would not take much for him to simply slip off the chair and have a very rude awakening when he hit the floor. He still occasionally falls asleep, but not nearly as often. George is 68 years old and resides in an assisted-living facility. He has mild mental retardation, a seizure disorder, and experiences some difficulty with coordination.

George has always been a very sociable person, attending many of the activities here at the center. He also is the official "waterer" of office plants and has become a welcome sight to staff when he appears with his watering can to keep our plants alive.

You might say George has made a successful transition to a senior center, but it wasn't until a year ago when he joined the walking group here at Vintage that he came to realize his own potential. At first he joined the short-distance walking group, many of whom have three-prong canes or walkers. This group walks inside to avoid the pitfalls of uneven sidewalks; however, within 6 months George was walking with both groups. The long distance group walks outside, weather permitting. They cover a distance of 3.1 miles twice a week. The other day I was walking through the dining room where the short-distance group was gathering when I noticed George already up and walking at a remarkable clip around the perimeter of the room.

All of the wellness classes are taught by a wellness coordinator, and the success of George and others in the class is due in large part to her ability to encourage and motivate people to get involved and stay involved. Prizes are given for walking so many miles. The initial course was to "walk" from Pittsburgh to Atlantic City. Once several walkers have accomplished this feat a huge casino party was held in their honor.

Many participants have walked farther then George, but none have accomplished as much. Once, a man who slept for lack of anything better to do, he is now taking part in exercise classes and is proud of the 30 pounds he has lost. Even more important is his feeling of well-being and increased self-esteem. In addition to the exercise classes, George spends hours in the art studio trying his hand at abstract art. He has become such a prolific artist that a one-man show is being planned to display his work.

Wellness is such a vital part of successful aging and by his example George has displayed what we all know to be true—it is never too late to develop a healthy lifestyle. George also has exemplified that success in one area will lead to success in other areas. When I asked him about the walking group he said, "For me it is a good thing."

A developmental disability is defined as a severe chronic disability that is attributable to a physical or mental impairment manifested before age 22, which is likely to continue indefinitely; results in substantial functional limitations in at least three areas (self-care, receptive and expressive language, learning, mobility, self-direction, capacity for independent living, and economic self-sufficiency); and reflects the person's need for a combination of services that are lifelong or of extended duration. Developmental disabilities may include mental retardation, cerebral palsy, autism, blindness, deafness, and other neurological conditions that result in the impairment of general intellectual functioning or adaptive behavior similar to that of a person with mental retardation.

Persons with developmental disabilities include persons with and without mental retardation. The definition of mental retardation includes significant subaverage general intellectual functioning (an IQ below 70 to 75) and related deficits in two or more adaptive skill areas. Adaptive skill areas are those daily living skills needed to live, work, and play in the community (communication, home living, community use, health and safety, leisure, self-care, social skills, self-direction, functional academics, and work). The impact on the individual can be minimal to severe. A variety of interventions, enrichments, training, special assistance, or supports can compensate for deficits in intellectual functioning. Low levels of adaptive behavior are related to institutionalization and lack of opportunities for normal life experiences and activities. Older persons with developmental disabilities are not as likely to have had the opportunity to work, attend school, or live independently in the community as their younger counterparts do today.

The American Association on Mental Retardation defines leisure as available free choice time and activities that are not related to work or other obligatory forms of activity and which are expected to promote feelings of pleasure, affiliation, happiness, spontaneity, fantasy or imagination, fulfillment, creativity, self-expression, and self-development. Leisure is essential for lifelong development and personal well-being. Leisure experiences include play behavior, recreation activities, diversion and amusement, art and creative activities, adventure challenges activities, sports and games, travel and vacations, and holiday celebrations. Leisure skills include choosing and self-initiating interests, using and enjoying home and community leisure and recreational activities alone and with others, playing socially with others, taking turns, terminating or refusing leisure or recreational activities, extending one's duration of participation, and expanding one's repertoire of interests, awareness, and skills. People with mental retardation will develop leisure skills and a leisure repertoire if provided with meaningful and structured leisure education opportunities, as well as a supportive environment.

DEMAND FOR SERVICES

The aging of our society has directly influenced the demand for developmental disability services. There is widespread uncertainty about the actual numbers of older persons with a developmental disability as many have lived with their families at home and have not interacted with the developmental disability or aging systems. In the United States, there are an estimated 526,000 adults aged 60 years and older with a developmental disability, and their numbers are expected to double by 2030 when the baby-boom generation will be in their 60s. It is estimated that the majority of persons with a developmental disability, 60% reside with family caregivers. Twenty-five percent of family caregivers are aged 60 or older. The informal system of residential care provided by families served 5 times the number served by the formal residential care system. As these caregivers age beyond their caregiving capacities, demand for services will continue to grow.

Although the prevalence of mental retardation is higher among minority group families, these families are often less likely to receive formal services for their relative with mental retardation. Less accessibility and availability of services in their communities, more positive attitudes toward family responsibility, greater availability of extended family supports, suspicion of formal structures, and cultural beliefs are some of the reasons for this difference.

Another factor that influences the demand for services is the increased life span of individuals with developmental disabilities. For example, the mean age at death for persons with mental retardation increased from 19 years in the 1930s to 66 years in the 1990s. With continued improvements in their health status, individuals with mental retardation can expect to have a life span of 70 years, equal to that of the general population. The life expectancy and age-related medical conditions of adults with mental retardation are similar to that of the general population unless they have severe levels of cognitive impairment, Down's syndrome, cerebral palsy, or multiple disabilities.

With increased longevity, it is likely that persons with developmental disabilities will live into their own retirement and outlive their family caregivers. This has stimulated a growing need for more services and supports. Persons with developmental disabilities are now surviving beyond the relevance of traditional skills-development and job programs and are experiencing retirement, a new arena for the developmental disability network. Individuals with developmental disabilities are more likely to experience restricted social roles and more limited social networks than people without disabilities, and thus may have fewer opportunities to benefit from the retirement experiences that are open to those without disabilities. Poor social networks reduce the likelihood of survival into old age.

A significant portion of individuals with lifelong developmental disabilities will experience age-related decline both biologically and functionally at a much earlier age than the general aging population. Adults with mental retardation have higher obesity and cholesterol levels, low levels of cardiovascular endurance, and poor strength levels, and they exercise less than the general population. In addition to the negative effects on health, the high levels of obesity and low levels of physical inactivity can create barriers to the performance of daily activities, including leisure activities. Older adults with developmental disabilities are often disadvantaged when attempting to access or secure social and health services. This is especially true of women with mental retardation, as they are less likely to receive Pap smears, breast exams, or mammograms than the general population, and many more are overweight compared to men with mental retardation. Inadequate health care and the lack of physical fitness are a major threat to independence and increase the likelihood that they will incur other disabling conditions as they age.

The aging of caregivers and the increasing numbers of older adults with developmental disabilities are stretching state service-delivery systems well beyond their capacity to meet current and projected demands for residential, vocational, and family support services for individuals with developmental disabilities. Large and growing waiting lists are very common in the states today. Demographic trends suggest that waiting lists will continue to grow unless a concerted effort is mounted to address them. Improved coordination between the aging and the developmental-disability service system is needed.

At the same time, there has been a major shift in approaches that support older adults with developmental disabilities and their families, including greater inclusion in the community, more person-centered choices that address quality of life, and supports provided in the natural context in which people live, work, and play.

Older adults with developmental disabilities have many of the same interests and age-related concerns as other older adults. However, they typically have had less experience and fewer opportunities in making choices and limited knowledge of potential options. Some prefer to continue participation in work or vocational activities. As many of these adults are unemployed, underemployed, or participate in day or sheltered programs with little or no pay, the prospect of retirement may take on a different meaning than it does for persons who have been employed most of their adult life and who may have retirement income beyond Social Security or SSI.

Older persons with developmental disabilities are entitled to the same array of services that are available to the general aging population, including the right to gain access to nonsegregated senior center services. They do have special needs that may not be addressed through current service-system structures but that can be met at the senior center:

- exercise and other health-promoting activities for health maintenance
- health education programs and health information materials to increase understanding of personal health and how to obtain health care
- access to services that provide maintenance and development of skills

- nutritional meals and nutrition counseling
- leisure time and recreational activities appropriate to disability and aging impairments
- peer socialization opportunities
- community exposure and involvement

INCLUSION

Positive environments foster the growth, development, and well-being of the individual. For individuals with developmental disabilities, positive environments include settings with their age peers that are appropriate for their needs and interests. The extent to which individuals with developmental disabilities experience successful aging results from the interaction of their capabilities, their environment, health, functioning, and support systems. Senior centers provide a natural context to enable older adults with a developmental disability to experience successful aging.

Community integration means being part of one's community, having the same opportunities to use public services as one's peers, and using these opportunities to live an ordinary life. Segregated programs dramatically lessen the chances for contact between people with and without disabilities. Inclusion in the senior center means being involved with and an intimate part of the senior center scene and being part of the same experiences as other persons of one's age. Senior centers provide a rich and varied choice of environments for meeting others, developing friendships, and being able to recreate, socialize, and learn new things. Friendships provide companionship for community activities and someone with whom to enjoy new experiences. The continuity of relationships over the years is an important source of security, comfort, and self-worth. Senior centers provide the opportunity to integrate, include, and enrich the quality of life for older persons with developmental disabilities. Because of the diversity of participants and senior centers, no one integration approach will work for all senior centers or for all older adults with a developmental disability.

Support for inclusion comes from many sources. Awareness of the increasing number of aging persons with intellectual disabilities led the World Health Organization, the International Association for the Scientific Study of Intellectual Disabilities, and Inclusion International to propose health and social inclusion promotion activities that would foster sound health and improve quality of life for all older people, including those with intellectual disabilities. The term *intellectual disabilities* includes mental retardation and related developmental disabilities and encompasses any set of conditions—resulting from genetic, neurological, nutritional, social, traumatic, or other factors occurring prior to birth, at birth, or during childhood up to the age of brain maturity—that affect intellectual development.

The proposal recommended that older people with intellectual disabilities have equal entitlement to medical treatment for both physical and mental disorders and good quality social provision as their peers within the society of which they are members. The fundamental principle underlying this resolution is the inclusion of older persons with intellectual disabilities in both health and social services and the wider life of the community in which they live, consistent with the progress towards inclusion that is being made for all people with intellectual disabilities across the life span.

These groups recommended that aging-supportive social and health policies focus on promoting productive or successful aging and developing infrastructures for healthy aging that can be accessed by older people with intellectual disabilities so that natural inclusion can be facilitated. Older people with intellectual disabilities may have significant physical health needs, reflecting the social and economic circumstances that have shaped their daily lives. Lifestyle choices and inadequate personal skills may have a major impact on their health and well-being. Sensory and mobility impairments, morbid obesity, poor oral hygiene, sexual behavior, and other lifestyle or personal attributes can also contribute to poor health.

Older people with intellectual disabilities need access to health services that include health promotion and support services that will guarantee the greatest possible health quality of life as they age. Service design and structures that will optimize the inclusion of people with intellectual disabilities in mainline health and social services are encouraged.

Health education programs that will compensate for risks associated with poor health habits need to be developed, especially improved nutrition and dietary habits. Targeting lifestyle may result in substantial gains in longevity, quality of life, and functional capability. Health education and preventative intervention programs should be available to older people with intellectual disabilities and to their families to the same extent they are for the wider population. All health education programs should include people with intellectual disabilities. Health education information should be designed to be intellectually accessible to older people with intellectual disabilities and their families. They need appropriate and ongoing education regarding healthy living practices in areas such as nutrition, exercise, oral hygiene, safety practices, and the avoidance of high risk behaviors such as tobacco use and substance abuse.

The United Nation's social agenda for older people states that policies and actions aimed at benefiting them must afford opportunities for older people to satisfy their need for personal fulfillment, which can be realized through the achievement of personal goals and aspirations and the realization of potential. Older people can find personal satisfaction through voluntary service to the community; continued growth through formal and informal learning; self-expression through the arts, participation in community organizations and organizations for older people, religious activities, recreation, travel; and participation in the political process as informed citizens.

The UN International Plan of Action on Aging encourages lifelong education through informal, community-based, and recreation-orientated programs for aging people. Recently, the importance of education and leisure in the lives of older people with intellectual disabilities has been recognized. The plan draws attention particularly to greater participation in leisure activities and creative use of time and recommends the development of programs of learning and leisure for older people with intellectual disabilities in inclusive community settings, in contrast to segregated activities. The plan suggests promoting programs that actively encourage and support integrated and active learning and leisure engagement with appropriate support for both older people with intellectual disabilities and those providing these services. Programs providing leisure for the general aging population should be inclusive for older individuals with intellectual disabilities.

The key issues identified in the reports are as follows:

1. There is generally a lack of organized public or private sector systems that are designed to address the needs of persons with intellectual disabilities.

2. Public attitudes need to be modified to create positive and valued status for persons with intellectual disabilities and to improve public support for specialty services that are designed to aid adults with intellectual disabilities.

3. There is a need for supportive services, health surveillance and provision, and family assistance for person with intellectual disabilities.

4. Women with intellectual disabilities often find themselves a disadvantaged class and little is done universally to address their specific health and social needs.

5. Health practitioners generally fail to recognize special problems experienced by persons with lifelong disabilities who are aging.

6. There are many misconceptions about intellectual disabilities and aging: that people with intellectual disabilities are mentally ill and do not survive to old age; that disabilities are the result of some wrongful behavior on the part of parents; that adults with intellectual disabilities can only be cared for in institutions and are incapable of learning everyday skills, of being educated, or of working.

Further support for the right to leisure activities comes from the National Therapeutic Recreation Society. Their philosophical position statement encompasses three broad values:

1. Right to leisure—including leisure as part of a healthy lifestyle.
2. Self-determination—wherein the individual can express unique abilities, predilections, and preferences that are encompassed with leisure experiences.
3. Quality of life—that leisure should be fun, enjoyable, and satisfying. Quality of life also includes prevention of illness and promotion of health and functional abilities through leisure.

The traditional barriers of transportation, environmental access, attitudes, financial resources, and staff preparation present challenges to inclusive programming. Other challenges include

- Concerns for liability, client autonomy, and confidentiality limit information-sharing.
- Territorial issues that cause service fragmentation and limit coordination.
- Older persons with significantly more challenging disabilities and increasingly intense health and human service needs are living in the community.
- Older people with developmental disabilities may be unaware of community and leisure resources, lack activity-specific and social

skills, and their wants, interests, and skills may not be adequately identified.

- Some people with developmental disabilities may lack friendships, which are 75% of leisure experiences.
- Persons with disabilities often have limited discretionary income.
- Senior center staff may be unaccustomed to older people with developmental disabilities and have limited information and exposure to their needs and limitations.

SUCCESSFUL MODELS OF INTEGRATION

Neither the aging nor disability systems have been fully prepared for this demand. Historically, older persons with lifelong disabilities have either been cared for by their family caregivers or have spent many years institutionalized. In the past they did not survive to old age and they have not interacted with community service systems. As a result, professionals in aging and developmental disabilities have little experience working with one another and working with older people with developmental disabilities. For collaboration to occur, there needs to be both statewide and local focus for collaboration.

Senior centers expand the options and choices available to older adults with developmental disabilities to ensure that their retirement will be an enjoyable experience. As the most common community resource available to older adults, senior centers provide the most prevalent community integration model. However, most senior centers do not have the staff or budgets to integrate older adults with developmental disabilities into the senior center. Senior centers can benefit from staff sharing, budgetary assistance, and other cost-sharing efforts. As partners, senior center and developmental-disability service providers can benefit from grants and contracts to provide integration.

The Center Care program at Vintage was developed in response to the need to serve older adults with developmental and other disabilities in the senior center. Older adults with mental retardation were retiring from sheltered employment programs and needed a place to go for socialization and recreation. The goal of the program was to help older adults with disabilities integrate into senior center activities. A full-time staff person, the Center Care coordinator, oriented new participants, facilitated integration, provided training, and acted as the liaison to disability agencies. Funding and other resources for the program came from a variety of sources including the mental health and mental retardation network, a local agency serving older blind persons, and the United Way. Over time, the Center Care program expanded to include older adults who have a mental illness and it is now called Senior Supports.

Many models of integration exist, but all help prepare the older person who has a developmental disability to retire successfully. The goals of senior center models of integration include providing age-appropriate, integrated social and recreational opportunities and leisure education; increased social interaction skills; and the development of a personal awareness of leisure. Modeling and mentoring can help the person learn how to do the things associated with retirement. Helping someone adapt to the senior center can work better than expecting that person to know how to use the senior center naturally. Many integration models pair the older person who has a developmental disability with a friend or coach to assist with the transition and to teach retirement skills. This can be a family member, friend, volunteer, paid companion, or designated staff person. They aid by example and by direction. Securing adequate staffing via paid staff or volunteers is necessary for success.

There are some barriers that senior centers face in attempting integration: staff who are not trained to work with people who have developmental disabilities and who may have negative attitudes about integration; senior center staff do not generally provide personal care or special assistance; senior center participants are not used to mainstreaming; funding; the fear that too many developmentally disabled participants will stop the "regular" participants from coming; and individuals who are not prepared to act appropriately in the social situations presented by the senior center. Acceptance is also affected by the appearance and behavior of the senior who has a developmental disability. When efforts are made to bring together people with and without disabilities, the people without disabilities are often treated as volunteers who are responsible to the teacher or coordinator rather than as peers.

A consultant at one senior center made recommendations to help alleviate some potential barriers including adjusting the dress of the older person who has a developmental disability to suit the senior center; and teaching social rules such as table manners, appropriate greetings, and locking the doors when using the bathroom.

Some of the lessons learned from successful models of integration include the following.

For the Older Person with a Developmental Disability

- Pair with a coach, role model, mentor, escort, or staff trainer.
- Prepare the individual on how to behave.
- Teach social skills and train individuals on the "hidden rules" of the senior center.
- Allow the person to adapt at his or her own pace.
- Develop the program around each participant's interests and needs.
- Focus on strengths by building upon skills rather than focusing on deficits.
- Use others to help promote social entry.
- Begin with small groups of one or two individuals in community activities.

For the Senior Center

- Overcoming barriers is an ongoing process.
- Gain support from local office for aging and developmental-disability networks.
- The cooperation of administration and staff is crucial.
- Develop an inclusion philosophy and communicate it with enthusiasm to all staff.
- Institute community education and awareness programs for staff, community, and participants.
- Provide cross-training for staff; improve the expertise of senior center and disability staff relative to issues of aging with developmental disabilities.
- Orient developmental-disability staff to the senior center.
- Use a variety of agencies to meet each participant's needs.
- Provide ongoing, comprehensive case management once integrated into the senior center.
- Conduct activities consistent with the concept of normalization.
- Involve senior center participants.
- Emphasize the reciprocal benefits of integration.

The Partners Project, funded by the Administration on Aging, demonstrated that cooperation between the aging and disabilities systems is helped when three basic ingredients are present:

1. Some formal means of collaboration for ongoing communication between the systems
2. Outreach strategies to older adults who have developmental disabilities and their family caregivers, such as a resource fair; focus groups of clergy, health care providers, and others, to identify families that have an older adult with a developmental disability; and telephone outreach
3. Methods of building the capacities of agency staff, caregivers, and older adults with disabilities to identify and use appropriate resources that maximize the community functioning of these older adults

Successful senior-center integration ventures involved a key person to get the effort going, low-cost efforts, a strong interest in use of the senior center as an integration site, and receptivity by the senior center staff and participants.

SITE EVALUATION CRITERIA

Individual interests and talents should be matched with activities and places within the community, including senior centers. Individuals needs to know their options, how to access them, and how to behave once there. Senior center sites can be evaluated using the following criteria:

- Does the senior center culture and programs match the person's interests, skill, culture, personal habits, personality, and age?
- Does the senior center environment afford the participant the opportunity to form bonds with fellow participants?
- Does the individual have personal qualities and skills that can be enhanced at the senior center?
- Does the individual have the social skills to function independently in the senior center?
- Does the individual have the functional and adaptive behavior that would allow him or her to blend normally within the social context of the senior center?
- Does the senior center have the staff and their commitment to make integration successful?

Once a match is found, time needs to be spent supporting and encouraging relationships with others. Negative preconceptions can be reduced when senior center participants see and experience people with disabilities as good friends and active participants. This can be accomplished by positioning people with disabilities in roles, activities, and settings that suggest status and competence.

EVALUATION

Despite initial fears about introducing adults with a developmental disability into senior centers, integration experiences have proven to be highly successful and beneficial to all involved. The following criteria were developed to help determine how successful integration is for individuals:

- Have they developed relationships with others?
- Are they recognized and acknowledged by others?
- Do they communicate with others?
- Do they feel safe and comfortable in the environment?
- Are they accepted and respected by others?
- Do they have a physical presence? Are they part of the fabric of life at the senior center?
- Have they taken on any responsibilities?
- Do they make contributions to organized activities and benefit from the contributions of others?
- Are they invited by others to join in, volunteer, and participate in activities?
- Are they missed when they are absent, and do they miss others when they are absent?

BIBLIOGRAPHY

American Association on Mental Retardation. Leisure as an adaptive skill area. *AAMR Leisure and Recreation Division Newsletter, 5*(2), 2–4. Washington, DC: Author.

American Association on Mental Retardation. (1992). *Mental retardation: Definition, classification, and systems of supports.* Washington, DC: Author.

Ansello, E. F., Coogle, C., & Wood, J. *Partners: Building inter-system cooperation in aging with developmental disabilities.* Richmond, VA: Virginia Center on Aging, Virginia Commonwealth University.

Braddock, D., Hemp, R., Parish, S., & Rizzolo, M. (July 2000). *The state of the states in developmental disabilities.* Chicago: Department of Disability and Human Development, University of Illinois at Chicago.

Carter, M. J. (1995). *Brief encounters: Community connections in TR.* Morgantown, WV: Presentation at West Virginia Therapeutic Recreation Association Conference.

Evenhuis, H., Henderson, C. M., Beange, H., Lennox, N., Chicoine, B., & Working Group. (2000). *Healthy aging—Adults with intellectual disabilities: Physical health issues.* Geneva, Switzerland: World Health Organization.

Fujijura, G. (1998). Demography of family households. *American Journal on Mental Retardation, 103,* 225–235.

Harlan, J., Todd, J., & Holtz, P. (1997). *A guide to building community membership for older adults with disabilities.* Bloomington, Indiana: Center for Aging Persons with Developmental Disabilities, Institute for the Study of Developmental Disabilities, Indiana University.

Heller, T., & Factor, A. (1999). *Older adults with mental retardation and their aging family caregivers.* Chicago: Rehabilitation Research and Training Center on Aging with Developmental Disabilities, Institute on Disability and Human Development, University of Illinois at Chicago.

Heller, T. *Aging with mental retardation: Emerging models for promoting health, independence and quality of life.* Chicago: Article supported in part by funding from the Rehabilitation Research and Training Center on Aging with Mental Retardation, University of Illinois at Chicago, through the U.S. Department of Education, National Institute on Disability and Rehabilitation, Grant No. H133B980046.

Hogg, J., Lucchino, R., Wang, K., Janicki, M. P., & Working Group. (2000). *Healthy aging—Adults with intellectual disabilities: Aging and social policy.* Geneva, Switzerland: World Health Organization.

Janicki, M. P., & Keefe, R. M. (1992). *Integration experiences casebook. Program ideas in aging and developmental disabilities.* New York: New York State Office of Mental Retardation and Developmental Disabilities.

Janicki, M. P., & Breitenbach, N. (2000). *Aging and intellectual disabilities—Improving longevity and promoting healthy aging: Summative report.* Geneva, Switzerland: World Health Organization.

Janicki, M. P., & Breitenbach, N. (2000). *Healthy aging—Adults with intellectual disabilities: Summative report.* Geneva, Switzerland: World Health Organization.

Lutfiyya, Z. M. (1997, September). *The importance of friendships between people with and without mental retardation.* The Arc's Q&A on Friendships. [On-line]. Available: thearc.org/faqs/friend.html

National Therapeutic Recreation Society. (1996). *National therapeutic recreation society philosophical position statement.* Ashburn, VA: Author. [On-line]. Available: www.nrpa.org/branches/ntrs/philos.htm

Rimmer, J. H. (1997, November). Aging, mental retardation and physical fitness. *Aging with mental retardation.* Arlington, TX: The ARC of the United States.

Snyder, A., Dom, H., Biegel, D., & Beisgen, B. (1986). *Service coordination for the blind and visually impaired elderly.* Pittsburgh, PA: Vintage, Inc. and Pittsburgh Blind Association.

RESOURCES

Administration for Children and Families
Administration on Developmental Disabilities
U.S. Department of Health and Human Services
HHH 300-F, 370 L'Enfant Promenade, SW
Washington, DC 20447
202-690-6590
http://www.acf.dhhs.gov
The Administration for Children and Families (ACF), within the Department of Health and Human Services is responsible for federal programs that promote the economic and social well-being of families, children, individuals, and communities.

American Association on Mental Retardation (AAMR)
444 North Capitol Street, NW, Suite 846
Washington, DC 20001-1512
202-387-1968 or 800-424-3688
http://www.aamr.org
American Association on Mental Retardation is the oldest and largest interdisciplinary organization of professionals concerned about mental retardation and related disabilities.

The Arc of the United States
1010 Wayne Ave., Suite 650
Silver Spring, MD 20910
301-565-3842
http://thearc.org/
The national organization of and for people with mental retardation and related developmental disabilities and their families.

National Rehabilitation Information Center (NARIC)
1010 Wayne Avenue, Suite 800
Silver Spring, MD 20910
800-346-2742 or 301/562-2400
http://www.naric.com
The National Rehabilitation Information Center collects and disseminates the results of federally funded research projects. NARIC is funded by the National Institute on Disability and Rehabilitation Research to serve anyone, professional or lay person, who is interested in disability and rehabilitation.

Rehabilitation Research and Training Center on Aging with Mental Retardation
Department of Disability and Human Development
The University of Illinois at Chicago
1640 West Roosevelt Road
Chicago, IL 60608-6904
800-996-8845
www.uic.edu/orgs/rrtcamr/index.html.
The Rehabilitation Research and Training Center on Aging with Mental Retardation's mission is to promote the independence, productivity, community inclusion, full citizenship and self-determination of older adults with mental retardation through a coordinated program of research, training, technical assistance and dissemination activities.

National Therapeutic Recreation Society
22377 Belmont Ridge Road
Ashburn, VA 20148
703-858-0784
http://www.nrpa.org/
The National Therapeutic Recreation Society mission is to advance parks, recreation, and environmental conservation efforts that enhance the quality of life for all people.

CHAPTER EIGHTEEN

Sensory Impairments

MARIO

Ask any staff member to open his or her desk drawer and 9 chances out of 10 you will find a ceramic item made by Mario. A peek into my desk reveals several items he has made, including an eyeglass case and a pin designed with grapes and grape leaves. The grapes are a takeoff on the Vintage logo, Mario's second home for over a decade. A veteran of World War II, a husband, a father, and a grandfather, Mario lost his sight suddenly due to complications from diabetes. For a proud active man, this loss was unbearable. Left with only dime-sized blurred vision, Mario worked to relearn daily tasks at Pittsburgh Blind Association (PBA). Thoughts of suicide frequently were on his mind and his wife, Rita, was desperate to help him. Rita worked nearby at that time and she knew Vintage was a place where older adults went to take part in activities. Somehow she convinced Mario to give Vintage a try. PBA worked with the Vintage staff, teaching them to guide a sightless person around the center and providing additional information on supporting other participants with low vision.

Kay, the ceramic teacher, took Mario under her wing and patiently worked with him to take a ball of clay and mold it into his own creation such as: merry-go-rounds, cars, baby buggies, Nativity scenes and an array of smaller items. Before long we noticed a coffee pot in the studio, with Mario brewing a pot for his fellow artists. He frequently also made pizelles for everyone.

Ceramics at Vintage opened up a whole new arena for Mario. Over the years he has served on the House Council, took numerous day trips with his friends, assisted with Columbus Day activities, and dressed up as our in-house Santa Claus each December. The hidden talents we find in so many of the people who come to Vintage never ceases to amaze those of us who work here. We are aware of how fortunate we are to have a wonderful volunteer like Kay, who was in the right spot at the right time to help Mario discover one of his many talents. Mario's success at Vintage spurred the agency to create a program for other impaired seniors in tandem with PBA. This program has expanded over the years to include seniors not only with physical limitations but also those with a mental health or mental retardation diagnosis.

A year and a half ago, Mario died of complications from diabetes and his friends at Vintage mourned his passing. We all have fond memories of this man who discovered new things about himself, and in return gave so much to this agency.

Many older adults experience sensory impairments that interfere with their ability to function independently and their involvement in activities that add quality to life. These impairments include visual (blindness, severe visual impairment, and low vision); hearing (partial or total loss); and speech (expressive and receptive aphasia). Sensory perceptual processes are the fundamental links that connect us with the external and internal environment.

VISUAL IMPAIRMENTS

The term *visual impairment* covers a wide range and variety of vision, from blindness and lack of usable sight to low vision, which cannot be corrected to normal vision with standard eyeglasses or contact lenses, to moderate visual impairment and an inability to read the fine print in a daily newspaper.

More than half of the new cases of blindness each year involves a person aged 65 or older. One in six—or 5 million—Americans aged 65 and older are blind or severely visually impaired, and this population is expected to more than double by the year 2030. Most persons who are older and blind are newly blind, have some remaining vision, and experience other physiological, psychological, and social problems.

The proportion of adults reporting some form of visual impairment increases dramatically with age, from 5% in the under-20 age group, to 17% for those 65 years and older. Twenty-six percent of adults aged 75 years and older report a vision impairment.

Although self-reported vision impairment cuts across all social and economic strata, specific groups of Americans are at greater risk. In 1992, among individuals with visual impairments, approximately 80%

were White, 18% were Black, and 2% were from other races. Blacks make up only 12% of the general population of the United States, and thus are overrepresented among individuals with visual impairments. In general, vision impairment is more prevalent among those people who have fewer social and economic resources, compared to those who report no vision impairment. Persons with vision impairments are more likely to be women, poor, unmarried, living alone, non-White, not a high-school graduate, in fair or poor general health, and lack health insurance.

Blindness and severe visual impairments are conditions whose handicapping effects vary with the individual, depending on the degree of remaining useful sight, the person's ability to use residual sight effectively, and the presence of other impairments. The onset of blindness may be met with depression, loneliness, fear, anxiety, anger, and helplessness. Mobility and daily living skills (telling time, meal preparation, handling money) and the ability to communicate through reading and writing may be lost or impaired. In general, the psychosocial needs of blind older persons focus on regaining as much independence as feasible and regaining status and self-esteem.

The majority of middle-aged and older Americans have limited knowledge of the relationship between vision loss and aging. The oldest, poorest, and least educated respondents to the Lighthouse National Survey on Vision Loss were the most likely to be ill informed, believing that all older people become visually impaired as a part of the normal aging process. People with vision impairments and their family members were also more likely to be misinformed.

Individuals should be encouraged to have their impairment assessed. Many older persons fail to seek help for vision loss because of a misconception that vision loss is a natural result of aging. Low-vision aids and vision services that can help improve vision are often underutilized. In healthy aging eyes, changes in vision can be corrected by eyeglasses or contact lenses. People with low vision experience one or more of three types of vision problems:

1. Overall blurred vision that can be caused by cataracts, scars on the cornea, or diabetic retinopathy
2. Loss of central or center vision, frequently caused by macular degeneration
3. Loss of peripheral or side vision, most commonly caused by glaucoma or stroke

When older persons experience vision loss, they need to receive appropriate and timely eye medical care. A low-vision specialist can determine the extent of any remaining vision and prescribe special optical devices that can make the best use of the vision by magnifying, filtering, or increasing the usable field of vision. Low-vision services and devices and vision rehabilitation services can help people with visual impairments continue to live in their own homes and communities. If the vision loss cannot be completely corrected and interferes with the individual's ability to do everyday tasks, vision-related rehabilitation services can help maintain or restore function and assist individuals in regaining self-sufficiency and maintaining their quality of life.

Rehabilitation services are provided by specially trained vision-related rehabilitation professionals, such as low-vision specialists, orientation and mobility instructors, and rehabilitation teachers. Vision-related rehabilitation services include

- low-vision examinations and devices
- individual counseling to help with adjustment to vision loss
- support groups
- training in adaptive techniques to assist with home and personal management skills (meal preparation, personal care techniques, managing money, labeling medications); communication skills (large print, computers with screen magnification, tape recorders, Braille, writing guides, telephones, and timepieces); and mobility skills (learning to orient oneself in familiar and unfamiliar environments, to ask for assistance from others when appropriate, and to move about using a long white cane)

Knowledge about the availability of local vision-rehabilitation services is seriously lacking, creating a huge gap between the need for services and access to services. More than one third (35%) of middle-aged and older Americans do not know if there are local public or private agencies in their community that provide services for people with vision impairments. This is especially true among older persons and those with severe vision impairments.

All evidence points to the underutilization of both vision rehabilitation services and adaptive devices by people with impaired vision. Yet when used, these interventions and devices are considered very important in improving quality of life. Although very few adults use adaptive devices, those who do consider them an important part of their daily lives.

The use of vision rehabilitation services is even less prevalent than the use of optical and adaptive devices. When asked why they have not used these services, a sizable number report being unfamiliar with their availability. Among people with general health-care insurance, a significant percentage do not have coverage for even basic eye-care services while the majority lack, or are unaware of, coverage for vision rehabilitation services or devices.

The majority of people with vision problems adapt very well or somewhat well to their vision loss. Yet substantial numbers report significant consequences on the quality of their everyday lives. Half of all people with impaired vision report that their vision problem interferes to some degree with what they want to do in their daily lives. The inability to read standard-sized print, books, newspapers, and other material poses the most severe barrier in connection with their vision loss. Thirty-eight percent report at least some interference with their leisure activities because of their vision problem. Isolation and lack of socialization are major problems for individuals who are blind or visually impaired, and needs assessments have identified the need for social and recreational opportunities, including avocational training to learn new skills or adapt old ones. Loneliness is a very serious or somewhat serious problem for 31% of people with severe vision impairments.

The large majority of middle-aged and older Americans fear blindness more than other physical impairments. Only mental or emotional illness is feared more. The Lighthouse survey respondents generally expressed positive attitudes towards people with vision impairments and their capabilities. However, when confronted with an individual with a visual impairment, nonimpaired middle-aged and older Americans expressed mixed reactions and attitudes towards vision loss. Many reported feeling awkward or embarrassed because they do not know how to behave with people who are visually impaired.

HEARING IMPAIRMENTS

The population of those who are deaf or hard of hearing is estimated at approximately 28 million persons, or 10% of the total U.S. population. Older individuals were more likely than any other age group to have hearing problems serious enough to affect the quality of communication and interpersonal relationships—one third of the population 65 and older and half of adults aged 85 and older. In fact, impaired hearing affects more older adults than any other chronic condition. Hearing impairment impacts safety, quality of life, and the ability to live independently.

The term *hearing impairment* refers to any degree of loss in the ability to discern loudness or pitch outside the range for normal. *Deaf* refers to a condition where hearing is impaired to a profound degree. Hearing loss that occurs with increasing age is known as *presbycusis*, wherein hearing loss is permanent, affects both ears equally, is greater for high-pitched sounds, is more common and severe for men, and gradually worsens with age. Often it is difficult to know how much hearing loss is due to aging and how much is attributed to other factors. Prolonged exposure to noise, injury, medications, disease, and heredity are all factors that affect hearing and some of these factors can be reversed. Examination and test results from a qualified professional provide the basis for determining the best treatment for a hearing impairment.

Many older people with hearing impairments are not receiving appropriate treatment or using potentially beneficial devices. Some do not seek treatment because they are not aware of their hearing loss or because they believe nothing can be done to treat or compensate for it. Others do not want to call attention to their loss. There is also a general lack of education and of awareness of the value of hearing and its impact on a positive lifestyle. Unlike the eyeglass industry, which has succeeded in convincing its public that good vision is an important component to a quality life, hearing professionals have not been as successful.

A variety of approaches such as the use of hearing aids, other rehabilitation devices, or aural rehabilitation services can be used to compensate for hearing impairment. Aural rehabilitation services, including counseling, speech-reading, and auditory training, can help older persons with hearing impairments reduce anxiety, facilitate better use of residual hearing, and achieve more realistic expectations regarding remediation of hearing loss. These approaches can improve the ability to communicate even when the underlying problem cannot be cured. Some individuals may benefit from speech-reading (lipreading), which allows a person to receive visual cues from lip movements as well as facial expressions, body posture, hand gestures, and the environment. Auditory training may include hearing-aid orientation, but also may be designed to help a person who is hearing-impaired identify and handle specific communication problems. Speech-reading and auditory training can significantly reduce the handicapping effects of hearing loss or impairment in later life. If needed, counseling may help individuals understand their abilities and limitations in a way that maintains a positive self-image.

Hearing loss is potentially the most serious of all sensory impairments. The list of problems associated with hearing loss include fatigue, irritability, embarrassment, tension, stress, anxiety, depression, negativism, avoidance of social activities, withdrawal from personal relationships, rejection, threat to personal safety, loneliness, dissatisfaction with life, and unhappiness at work. Hearing loss is often progressive following a gradual onset and may not be recognized for some time. Negative social attitudes about growing old and becoming hard of hearing causes some older people to deny their hearing loss. Hearing loss may significantly impair the ability to successfully cope with, or adapt to, other age-related losses. When hearing impairment occurs at a later age, the loss is particularly difficult to contend with. After a lifelong ability to communicate, the barriers imposed by hearing loss may seem insurmountable. Unlike vision loss, it is not easily recognized by others, and it rarely prompts empathy and understanding.

Hearing loss is often unbalanced. For example, a person may hear low tones but not be able to hear high tones well. In conversation, such a person won't be able to hear complete words clearly and must piece the communication together, which can lead to misunderstandings. Asking someone to speak louder often doesn't resolve the problem because it is a tone deficiency. With added amplification, all tones are amplified, which prevents comprehension. Although the hearing-impaired person can hear many sounds, the ability is lost to hear those tones that allow comprehension of the spoken word. It is this inability to get the full message that adds stress and exhausts people who are hard of hearing to the point that they want to avoid social situations.

After numerous such occasions, the person's self-image is damaged. A hearing test and an explanation of the effects of the loss may alleviate some of these negative feelings. Many assistive devices are available to help the person who is hard of hearing to communicate, and knowing about these devices can make a big difference. It is also important that people learn to be more assertive about their communication needs, asking others to repeat what was said when they don't understand and asking for help when needed.

People tend to avoid situations where they know they cannot function, which easily leads to isolation. Certain acoustic conditions may lend themselves to good comprehension and enjoyment, but in other situations, persons who are hard of hearing may be able to hear but understand only parts of the conversation or comprehend little or nothing. Because it is often impossible to know ahead of time how well they will be able to hear, some choose to stay at home, even though they may desperately wish to participate. Those who do participate may experience frustration and disappointment.

People with normal hearing can be spoken to and understand what was said in the presence of other sounds. Many older people with hearing impairment have a decreased ability to tune out background noises and thus have more difficulty hearing in a noisy setting. People who are hard of hearing often have difficulty hearing others when performing simple tasks, and they must stop in order to concentrate on what is being said. They must focus so much on trying to understand the conversation that their awareness of the discussion suffers and memory is impaired. Older adults who respond without actually hearing what was said may risk being labeled cognitively impaired instead of hearing-impaired.

Senior centers can play an important role in educating seniors and their families about vision and hearing loss and rehabilitation services and assisting them in accessing services. Senior centers can also sponsor self-help groups, which have been effective in promoting awareness of sensory impairments and the needs of sensory-impaired people.

INCLUDING PEOPLE WITH SENSORY IMPAIRMENTS IN THE SENIOR CENTER

People who are visually or hearing-impaired have a great range of interests and want to participate in the gamut of daily activities. Senior centers should plan appropriate interventions and support measures to maintain and strengthen social interactions. Simple changes can help older adults who have a sensory impairment to enjoy a higher quality of life. They may need training in various adaptive techniques in order to do so.

For many older Americans, membership and participation in a senior center is a lifeline to the community. Like other older Americans, older people who are sensory impaired also want to be full and active participants. The following are suggestions to help senior centers include people who are sensory-impaired in the senior center:

• Contact local agencies that serve the visually or hearing-impaired, either the state rehabilitation agency or a local private rehabilitation agency. They can provide information about the special needs and capabilities of older sensory-impaired persons.

• Have a rehabilitation professional from a local agency come to the senior center and provide in-service training for staff members on how to include sensory-impaired people in programs and activities.

• Arrange for training about sensory impairment for senior center members with normal hearing and vision. This can make them feel more comfortable with their sensory-impaired counterparts and help them get involved.

• Be welcoming. When a sensory-impaired person joins the senior center, have a staff member or another senior chat with the newcomer and find out his or her interests. Establish a buddy system for orientation to the center and its programs.

• When people who are sensory-impaired are introduced to the senior center, they should be given an orientation tour of the building or facility so they become aware of structural features, landmarks they can use to orient themselves, and potential hazards.

• Respect the abilities of sensory-impaired members. Many sensory-impaired seniors will want to be more than just participants and may also want to assume leadership roles within the center. Such roles may include initiating a new center activity about which they have expertise, becoming a member of a planning committee, or joining the board of directors.

• Older people who are sensory-impaired should be treated with dignity and courtesy. Their level of independence and capabilities, as well as their needs for assistance, should be respected.

• Older people who are sensory-impaired should have all aspects of the program explained and described to them.

• Older people who are sensory-impaired should be encouraged to move around the senior center unaided, to take part in a full plan of activities, and to do everything as independently as possible.

• Older people who are sensory-impaired should be encouraged to participate in outings and trips, and where assistance is needed, a buddy system or other assistance should be provided.

• The local rehabilitation agency can provide advice about how to adapt crafts programs, dance classes, choral groups, and other activities so that members who are sensory-impaired can participate.

• Provide verbal instruction in addition to visual demonstration to help seniors who are visually impaired to be successful at crafts, dance, and other activities.

• Where written materials are needed, such as the lines in a play or the words to the music, consult the local vision rehabilitation agency about how to get these materials in large print, Braille, or on audiocassette.

• Written announcements that apply to everyone should be provided to people who are blind or visually impaired in accessible media in large print, Braille, or on audiocassette; whenever possible, these announcements will be read by staff members to older persons whose sight is impaired.

• Suggest or provide low-vision devices such as magnifiers, needle threaders, large-print reading materials, large-print cards and games, and high-contrast computers to maximize sight.

• The environmental needs of older people who are sensory-impaired, such as appropriate lighting and the safe arrangement of furniture to minimize obstacles, should be taken into consideration.

• People who are blind or visually impaired should be informed in advance about changes in the environment, such as the rearrangement of furniture, so that they can reorient themselves.

Senior center staff may not be educated in sensory impairments and are probably not familiar with agencies that serve those who are sensory-impaired. This is probably also true for older adults with a sensory impairment and for their caregivers, if they have one. Individuals with sensory impairments may not be identified or the degree of impairment may not be known. Vision loss is often gradual and not perceived until severe or complete loss of function occurs. Senior center staff should be trained on aging and sensory impairments, low vision and accessing resources, avoidance of overprotection and an emphasis on promoting independent functioning, terminology, the impact of sensory impairments on the individual, sensitivity training, mobility instruction techniques, use of adaptive devices, and communication skills.

A report prepared by Vintage and Pittsburgh Blind Association under a contract with the Pennsylvania Department of Aging identified the need to increase social and educational opportunities to blind and visually impaired older persons who were underserved by the aging network. As a result of the report, Vintage developed a program to reach out to blind and visually impaired older adults. Integrating older people with sensory impairments into the senior center can make a big difference in the overall quality of the senior center program and in the quality of life for older persons who are sensory-impaired. Establishing relationships with agencies that serve those who are sensory-impaired can help ensure that older adults with sensory impairments are integrated into the senior center and participate in a supportive environment. Consultants such as occupational therapists, orientation and mobility instructors, and rehabilitation counselors can work with and advise staff, conduct staff training, assess the senior-center site for accessibility, and develop and evaluate the treatment plan for individuals who use the center. A mobility instructor can orient seniors who are visually impaired to the senior center, and peer counselors can be used to provide support in using the center.

A comfortable and functional environment for individuals who are sensory-impaired should be part of universal design for older people, benefiting all older individuals. Making facilities and programs and activities safe and accessible for older participants who are sensory impaired does not necessarily require a great deal of time, energy, or money. It is a matter of knowing the basics and planning for easy access to the senior center.

ENVIRONMENTAL MODIFICATIONS

LIGHTING

- Provide plenty of floor lamps and table lamps in recreation and reading areas.
- Replace burned-out light bulbs regularly.
- Place mirrors so that lighting doesn't reflect off them and create glare.
- Use adjustable blinds, sheer curtains, or draperies for window coverings, because they allow for the adjustment of natural light.
- Keep a few chairs near windows for reading or doing crafts in natural light.
- Use nonglare surfaces that do not reflect light.

FURNITURE

- Arrange furniture in small groupings so that people can converse easily.

- Make sure there is adequate lighting near furniture.
- Avoid upholstery and floor covering with patterns. Stripes and checks can create confusion for people who are visually impaired.

ENVIRONMENTAL

- Maintain a clutter-free environment. Place furnishings strategically to reduce the likelihood of falls and collisions and to encourage conversation.
- Replace worn carpeting and floor covering.
- Tape down or remove area rugs.
- Remove electrical cords from pathways, or tape them down for safety.
- Use nonskid, nonglare products to clean and polish floors.
- Keep desk chairs and table chairs pushed in.
- Move large pieces of furniture out of main traffic areas.
- Make sure that lighting is uniform throughout.
- Place drinking fountains and fire extinguishers along one wall only throughout hallways to allow individuals who are visually impaired to trail the other wall without encountering obstacles.
- Make certain that stairway railings extend beyond the top and bottom steps.
- Mark landings in a highly contrasting color.
- Provide acoustical control to decrease noise or increase amplification.
- Use specialized alarm systems.

COLOR CONTRAST

- Place light objects against a dark background.
- Install doorknobs that contrast in color with doors.
- Paint the woodwork of the door frame a contrasting color.
- Mark the edges of all steps and ramps with paint or tape of a highly contrasting color.

PROGRAMMATIC

- Use talking tapes to report on daily and weekly activities and events.
- Staff should be trained and receptive to working with individuals with sensory impairments.

- Use captioned programs on the TV.
- Provide escort services for trips.
- Provide programs that focus on multiple senses, forms of communication, and expression.

SIGNS

- Place all signs at eye level, with large lettering according to specifications outlined in the Americans With Disabilities Act (ADA).
- Provide Braille signage according to ADA specifications.
- When making signs by hand, use a heavy black felt-tip pen on a white, off-white, or light yellow, nonglossy background.

PRINTING

- Large-print type should be used, preferably 18-point, but at a minimum 16-point.
- Select fonts with easily recognizable characters, such as standard roman, sans serif, or arial. Use boldface type because the thickness of the letters make the print more legible. Avoid decorative fonts, italics, and all capital letters.
- Spacing between letters should be wide because text with letters very close together is difficult to read for many people who are visually impaired, particularly those who have central visual field defects such as macular degeneration.
- The use of different-colored lettering for headings and emphasis is difficult to read for many people with low vision. When used, dark blues and greens are most effective.
- Contrast is one of the most critical factors in enhancing visual functioning, for printed materials as well as in environmental design. Text should be printed with the best possible contrast. For many older people, light lettering—white or light yellow—on a dark background, usually black, is easier to read than black lettering on a white or light yellow background.
- Avoid using glossy finish paper as it creates glare.
- The recommended spacing between lines of text is 1.5 rather than single-spaced. Many people who are visually impaired have difficulty finding the beginning of the next line when single-spacing is used.

TELEPHONES

- Provide some telephones with large-print keypads or dials.
- Provide telephone amplifiers that increase the level of sound.
- Provide assistive devices such as TDD (Telecommunication Device for the Deaf).

These basic environmental design and safety tips can go a long way toward making a comfortable and accessible environment for older persons who are sensory impaired and for everyone else who uses the facility and services. Increasingly, these elements must be incorporated into universal design. Orientation and mobility instructors can assess the senior center, point out obstacles, and make suggestions for adaptations to improve accessibility to the senior center and to activities.

FACILITATING COMMUNICATION WITH PERSONS WITH SENSORY IMPAIRMENTS

Guidelines have been developed to facilitate communication and interaction with people who are sensory-impaired.

COMMUNICATING WITH A PERSON WHO IS BLIND OR VISUALLY IMPAIRED

- Announce that you are in the room and say who you are and what you are doing.
- If you are entering a room with someone who is visually impaired, describe the room layout, other people who are in the room, and what is happening.
- Tell the person if you are leaving. Let the person know if others will remain in the room or if he or she will be alone.
- Stand where you can be seen or let the person know where you are. Try to avoid talking from behind the person.
- Speak distinctly to the person. Do not raise your voice unless the person has a hearing impairment.
- Talk directly to the person, not through an intermediary.
- When you speak, let the person know whom you are addressing.
- Explain what you are doing as you are doing it.

- Always answer questions and be specific or descriptive in your responses.
- Leave things in the same place you found them. Do not move furniture or other articles without informing the person who is visually impaired.
- Allow the person to take your arm for guidance.
- Do not take care of tasks for the person that he or she would normally do, such as change television channels, cut meat, salt and pepper food. First ask if the individual needs help, then offer to assist.
- Ask how you may help: increasing the light, reading the menu, describing where things are, or in some other way.
- Call out the person's name before touching. Touching lets a person know that you are listening. Allow the person to touch you.
- Treat the person like a sighted person as much as possible.
- Use the words "see" and "look" normally.
- Legal blindness is not necessarily total blindness. Use large movements, gestures, and contrasting colors.

COMMUNICATING WITH A PERSON WHO IS HEARING IMPAIRED OR DEAF

- Wait until you are directly in front of the person, have that individual's attention, and you are close enough to the person before you begin speaking.
- Be sure that the individual sees you approach, otherwise your presence may startle the person.
- Face the person who is hard of hearing directly and be on the same level with him or her whenever possible. Never speak directly into an individual's ear.
- Avoid eating, chewing, or smoking while talking; your speech will be more difficult to understand.
- Keep your hands away from your face when talking.
- Recognize that people who are hard of hearing hear and understand less well when they are tired or ill.
- Reduce or eliminate background noise as much as possible when carrying on conversations.
- Speak in a normal fashion without shouting. See that the light is not shining in the eyes of the person who is hearing-impaired. Avoid overarticulating.

- If the person has difficulty understanding something, find a different way of saying it rather than repeating the same words over and over.
- Be concise; use simple, short sentences to make your conversation easier to understand.
- Write messages if necessary.
- Allow ample time to converse with a person who is hearing-impaired. Being in a rush will compound everyone's stress and create barriers to a meaningful conversation.
- Use a pictogram grid or other device with illustrations to facilitate communication.
- Utilize as many other methods of communication as possible to convey your message (i.e., body language, pictograms).
- Enhance speech through facial expressions, gestures, and visual aids.
- Give a person who is hearing-impaired time to respond to the message, and allow longer pauses between your sentences.

COMMUNICATING WITH A PERSON WITH APHASIA

Aphasia is a total or partial loss of the power to use or understand words. It is often the result of a stroke or other brain damage. People with expressive aphasia are able to understand what is said; persons with receptive aphasia cannot. Some individuals may have both expressive and receptive aphasia. Expressive aphasia is like having a word on the tip of your tongue and not being able to call it forth. The following are some suggestions for communicating with individuals who have aphasia:

- Be patient and allow plenty of time to communicate with a person with aphasia.
- Be honest with the individual. Let them know if you do not understand what they are telling you.
- Ask the person how best to communicate.
- Allow the person with aphasia to try to complete their thoughts. Avoid being too quick to guess what the person is trying to express.
- Encourage the person to write the word he or she is trying to express and read it aloud.
- Use gestures or point to objects if it is helpful in supplying words or adding meaning.

- Use a pictogram if needed to fill in answers to requests such as "I need" or "I want." The individual can point to the appropriate picture.

SUGGESTED ACTIVITIES

- Self-help support groups
- Hearing and vision screening programs
- Educational programs on sensory impairments and adaptive aids
- Rehabilitation services, in partnership with rehabilitation organizations
- Resource-fair, featuring agencies that serve those who are sensory-impaired and adaptive aids
- Sensitivity training for staff and participants

BIBLIOGRAPHY

Administration on Aging, National Aging Information Center. (2001). *Aging Internet information notes: Hearing loss and older adults.* Washington, DC: Author. [Online]. Available: www.agingstats.gov./NAIC/Notes/hearingloss.html

American Foundation for the Blind. (1998, August 1). *A Bill of Rights for older Americans who are blind or visually impaired.* New York: Author.

American Foundation for the Blind. (1998, December). *Communicating comfortably with a person who is visually impaired.* New York: Author.

American Foundation for the Blind. (2000, September). *Creating a comfortable environment for older individuals who are visually impaired.* New York: Author.

American Foundation for the Blind. (1998, October). *Integrating older persons who are visually impaired into a senior center.* New York: Author.

American Foundation for the Blind. (2000, September). *Low vision and older persons.* New York: Author.

American Foundation for the Blind. (1999, January). *Special services to help older persons experiencing vision loss.* New York: Author.

Barber, C. E. (1996). *Age-related changes in hearing.* Colorado: Colorado State University Cooperative Extension.

Hard of Hearing Advocates. (1999). *Emotional factors of HOH.* Framingham, MA: Author.

Holt, J., Hotto, S., & Cole, K. (1994). *Demographic aspects of hearing impairment: Questions and answers.* Center for Assessment and Demographic Studies. Washington, DC: Gallaudet University.

Kelly, M. (1995, November–December). Consequences of visual impairment on leisure activities of the elderly. *Geriatric Nursing, 16*(6).

Lighthouse International. (1994). *The Lighthouse National Survey on Vision Loss: The experience, attitudes and knowledge of middle-aged and older Americans.* Executive summary. Louis Harris and Associates, Inc. Arlene R. Gordon Research Institute. New York: Author.

Snyder, A., Dom, H., Biegel, D., & Beisgen, B. (1986). *Service coordination for the blind visually impaired elderly.* Pittsburgh, PA: Vintage and Pittsburgh Blind Association.

U.S. Congress, Office of Technology Assessment. (1986). *Hearing impairments and elderly people—A background paper.* Washington, DC: U.S. Government Printing Office.

RESOURCES

American Foundation for the Blind (AFB)
11 Penn Plaza, Suite 300
New York, NY 10001
800-232-5463
http://www.afb.org/
The American Foundation for the Blind is a leading national resource for people who are blind or visually impaired, the organizations that serve them, and the general public.

American Speech-Language-Hearing Association (ASHA)
10801 Rockville Pike
Rockville, MD 20852
800-498-2071 or 301-897-5700
http://www.asha.org
The American Speech-Language Hearing Association is the professional, scientific, and credentialing association for audiologists, speech-language pathologists, and speech, language, and hearing scientists. ASHA's mission is to ensure that all people with speech, language, and hearing disorders have access to quality services to help them communicate more effectively.

Hard of Hearing Advocates (HOHA)
245 Prospect Street
Framingham MA 01701
508-875-8662
http://www.hohadvocates.org
Hard of Hearing Advocates helps hard of hearing (HOH) people by creating and implementing programs/solutions where HOH people have undue problems.

Lighthouse International
111 East 59th Street
New York, NY 10022-1202
212-821-9200 or 800-829-0500
http://www.lighthouse.org
Lighthouse International is a leading resource worldwide on vision impairment and vision rehabilitation.

National Institute on Deafness and other Communication Disorders
National Institute of Health
31 Center Drive, MSC 2320
Bethesda, MD 20892-2320
http://www.nidcd.nih.gov/
The National Institute on Deafness and Other Communication Disorders (NIDCD) is one of the Institutes that comprise the National Institutes of Health (NIH). NIDCD conducts and supports research in the normal and disordered processes of hearing, balance, smell, taste, voice, speech, and language.

National Federation of the Blind
1800 Johnson Street
Baltimore, MD 21230
410-659-9314
http://www.nfb.org
The National Federation of the Blind (NFB) provides public education about blindness, information and referral services, literature and publications, adaptive equipment, advocacy services, development and evaluation of technology, and support for blind persons and their families.

National Eye Institute Information Center
National Institutes of Health
3 Center Drive, Building 31
Bethesda, MD 20892
301-496-2234
http://www.nei.nih.gov
The National Eye Institute of the National Institutes of Health, conducts and supports research that helps prevent and treat eye diseases and other disorders of vision.

National Library Service for the Blind and Physically Handicapped
The Library of Congress

1291 Taylor Street N.W.
Washington, DC 20542
202-707-5100
http://www.lcweb.loc.gov/nls
Through a national network of cooperating libraries, National Library Service for the Blind and Physically Handicapped administers a free library program of braille and audio materials.

CHAPTER NINETEEN

Mental Health

GLADYS

The last time I saw her, she was sitting outside the offices of The Western Pennsylvania Hospital Vintage Community Care for Seniors, after seeing the physician. She was waiting for her Access ride, which provides transportation for older adults in Allegheny County. It occurred to me then that Gladys had spent a lot of time waiting for others.

Hers is a long story, beginning about six years ago when I first met her at Vintage. You could always recognize Gladys as she made her way around the building. A small, stooped African American woman, she always wore a heavy coat all day in the winter and a lighter coat in the summer. She used a walker to help her walk and to carry the several plastic bags that held all the supplies she needed for crocheting. She would hook her bags over the handles of the walker, a trick that many seniors use to get around independently. You could not only see Gladys, but you could also hear the thud-stop, thud-stop rhythm of her walker as she went to lunch or to a classroom.

As far as we could tell, Gladys had two loves: her son and her crocheting. Often she would stop me in the hall to show me a new pattern for a project she was about to begin. Vintage has at least two groups that do needlework and it was some time before I realized that Gladys did not seem to join the women in a classroom in the morning, but rather did her work alone or with a friend in the hall. Following lunch she would go to a classroom and continue her craft, until some point late in the day when her son, a man in his 60s, would arrive in a battered van to pick her up. Gladys always told us her son was a singer, just waiting for his big break to record with some famous artist. In the meantime, he sang at local churches and did home repairs.

As time went by, it became apparent to staff that Gladys was experiencing some problems with incontinence. Several nurses spoke to her with little or no success; Gladys would always deny any problem. It was when some of the other women began to ignore her that our wellness coordinator spoke with both Gladys and her son. Gladys apologized, telling us that her son was remodeling their bathroom and soon all would be well. She did agree to use incontinence products, but never seemed to have the money to purchase an adequate supply. She would accept what we gave her. It was also about this time that she agreed to see the doctor and received some prescriptions, but never got them filled.

In December of 2000, Gladys was at her usual post in the hall when someone told me that the odor there was very bad and someone needed to do something. I collected some clean, dry clothing from the country store and got an incontinence product from adult day care. Approaching Gladys I whispered to her that I had some supplies for her and suggested we go to the ladies' room. Her son was sitting beside her, as he had begun coming to Vintage recently and would join his mother for lunch. On this particular day he said nothing. As we made our way slowly down the hall, she once again apologized, saying that she was in "this condition" because they had spent the night in the car. I knew that the low temperature the previous night had been 7°. After Gladys was taken care of in the ladies' room, the decision was made by the staff to report her situation to Protective Service. Protective Service is not one of the services Vintage provides, but we do partner with another agency in our area that does provide this service, which assures the welfare and safety of older adults. Once interviewed by Protective Service they determined that Gladys was of sound mind and had both the right and ability to make her own decisions. Protective Service workers will tell you that it is not uncommon to see how people choose to live. It is their responsibility as an agency to determine if the client is capable of making sound judgments, even if those judgments do not meet the standards we set for ourselves. Gladys and her son said they had adequate housing and soon would be moving into their newly remodeled home. They left Vintage and disappeared. Participants told us they had seen the son at church, but Gladys was not with him. Knowing that Protective Services had done all they could, Vintage made the decision to file a missing person's report to the police. Gladys was finally located living with a friend in a nearby community. She was sleeping on the sofa in the living room.

Shortly thereafter we learned that Gladys's son had had a massive heart attack and died instantly while doing some home repair work. A staff member attended the funeral, which was held in the church that Gladys had always attended. After the funeral, Gladys began calling Vintage participants, asking if she could please come and live with them. She said she would be "just fine on the sofa for a few days." It was clear that Protective Services needed to be involved again and at this point they brought her to see a doctor. Eventually, with several agencies and a hospital involved, housing was found for Gladys in a personal-care home. We know now that she is clean, she will be warm on a cold winter night, and she is getting adequate food.

On the day that I last saw her outside the physician's office, she was dressed in a clean black-and-white outfit and sat clutching her purse. When I offered my condolences on her son's death, she opened her purse and took out a small plastic photo album. She showed me several pictures of her son and when she finished she looked up at me with tears in her eyes and said, "You know if only he hadn't died, I know he would have gotten the break he had been waiting for to make a recording."

Mental stress and mental disorders take a significant toll on the health and productive functioning of older adults. A substantial proportion of the population aged 55 and older, 20%, experience specific mental disorders that are not part of normal aging. Four of the 10 leading causes of disability in the U.S. are mental disorders—major depression, bipolar disorder, schizophrenia, and obsessive-compulsive disorder. Many people suffer from more than one disorder at a given time. Far more attention has been paid to the physical than to the mental and emotional losses of aging. Yet findings indicate that the correlation between physiological and psychological variables increases with age. Older adults face many problems that could be beneficially treated with psychological interventions. These problems include stress, bereavement, alcohol and drug abuse, serious or chronic mental disorders (such as anxiety and depression), and psychological components of physical diseases.

The mental disorders that affect older people are often undiagnosed and untreated, contributing to high rates of suicide among older people. There is a high level of misdiagnosis of depressive disorders among older people. Depression and anxiety disorders impose risks to physical health and to recovery from serious medical conditions. Depression can have a serious negative impact on social, emotional, and physical health. Improved assessment and treatment of mental disorders of older persons could have a significant impact on their quality of life and on the economic costs associated with their health care. Success rates for the treatment of mental illness are as high or higher than for most physical illnesses. A potential barrier to seeking help for mental disorders may involve the older adult's viewing and presenting psychological symptoms as a normal part of aging. It is important that older adults, their caregivers, and senior center staff be able to distinguish between normal and abnormal aging processes.

Although there has been an increasing recognition of the mental-health needs of older people, it has been difficult getting services to older people due to a combination of factors:

- The stigma associated with mental illness, especially among older people, discourages treatment and is an excuse for inaction.
- Inadequate understanding by older people and the professionals who serve them of the realities of aging and mental illness.
- The feeling of powerlessness, a symptom of depression, discourages treatment.
- Inadequate insurance coverage.
- Insufficient resources to fund and staff the services needed.
- Fragmentation and duplication of services by aging and mental-health service providers whose responsibilities for older adults may overlap.
- The lack of alternative service modalities for reaching those who are unlikely to seek traditional mental-health services.

Approximately 2% of the population over age 54—about 1 million persons—has a chronic mental illness other than dementia. Over the next 30 years, their number will double as the baby boomers reach old age. This generation of persons with chronic mental illness have spent considerably less time in mental institutions than earlier generations and consequently will need to negotiate health and social service systems that may not be prepared to deal with them.

Historically, older persons have been underserved by the mental-health system and little attention has been paid to elders who have a lifelong history of psychiatric disability. The growth of the older population of adults who are seriously and persistently mentally ill who live in the community is a new phenomenon. In the recent past, when older people with a serious mental disorder were discharged from a psychiatric facility, they frequently went to a nursing home.

Older persons with schizophrenia comprise the majority of those with serious and persistent mental illness. There is little research available on older persons with schizophrenia, and there are few age-appropriate clinical, rehabilitative, or residential programs for older patients with chronic mental illness. Critical gaps exist in the understanding of the nature and treatment of schizophrenia in older persons. There is evidence that these deficiencies are even more pronounced in minority areas.

The prevalence rate of aging persons with schizophrenia is about 1%, and about 85% are living in the community. There has been a dramatic decline in the number of persons with schizophrenia living in mental institutions. In tandem with the decline in the number of inpatients is an increase in the number of older outpatients, which increases the pressure for community programs to provide services to older persons.

Despite the presence of significant symptoms, older persons with chronic mental illness generally receive little support from the mental-health system beyond medication, and there have been few changes to accommodate older persons with serious and persistent mental illness. Older adults account for only 6% of the caseload of community mental-health centers, and only 2% of the caseload of mental-health private practice. However, they do appear to be overrepresented in inpatient mental-health populations, as over half of public mental-hospital beds are occupied by adults over 65. More than half of these people receive no psychiatric care prior to their admission, making the admission their first contact with the mental-health system.

Because about two thirds of patients in mental hospitals are discharged to their families, caregivers' needs also need attention. More older relatives are caring for middle-aged persons with chronic mental illness. Caregiving for those who are chronic mentally ill is complex, and caregivers are burdened around issues of responsibility (e.g., who will care for the patient when the caregiver becomes incapacitated or dies), as well as the behavioral concomitants of the illness.

Several reasons for underserving the older population have been identified. First, older adults do not generally seek mental-health services, as they tend to utilize their primary physician for most mental-health-related care. Second, members of the older generation values their independence and ability to resolve personal problems on their own. Third, as mental-health treatment is often considered to be for those with severe impairment, it tends to carry a negative stigma among older adults. Additionally, some mental-health professionals have demonstrated a bias against working with older individuals.

Many older adults experience loss with aging—loss of social status and self-esteem, loss of physical capacities, and the deaths of friends and loved ones. But in the face of loss, many older people have the capacity to develop new adaptive strategies and move in a positive direction, either on their own, with informal support from family and friends, or with formal support from mental-health professionals.

Older people who are at risk of developing mental-health problems may include those who experience one or more of the following:

- advanced age
- bereavement and other losses
- change in health status
- disruption in family structure or function
- functional disability
- lack of adequate financial support
- minority status
- recent discharge from a hospital or institution
- relocation
- retirement
- stressful living conditions such as isolation or crime
- substance abuse

Vintage served many older adults with mental-health needs who were not known or were not actively involved with the mental-health system. Older people who have, or are at risk of developing, mental disorders should be considered a priority population with special needs. Preventive and rehabilitative services that are responsive to the needs and preferences of older people are needed to identify ways to prevent adverse reactions and to promote positive responses to loss in later life. Senior center programs can help identify older persons with mental-health needs and identify the barriers that prevent them from getting the care they need. Behavioral care must be available and accessible.

Even those who are physically frail can manage their overall health if their mental functioning is adequate. But if mental functioning is impaired—through altered mood that can undermine motivation, or psychosis that reduces capacity to negotiate reality, or memory impairment that compromises the execution of necessary tasks—then the individual's health and safety is at significantly increased risk.

Loneliness can be brought on by the absence of a needed relationship or group of relationships and lack of meaningful contact with others. Studies find loneliness to be associated with depression, frequency of doctor's office visits, risky sexual behavior in gay men, and the likelihood of nursing home admission. Loneliness among older adults, as a whole, has been found to be in the range of 27% to 35% or more, and as high as 50% for those aged 90 and older. Given the prevalence of loneliness and the frequency of its adverse effects on health in later life, loneliness among the aging population needs to be addressed as a mental-health issue.

Some of the key public education areas to be addressed include warning signs, coping strategies, the stigma of mental illness among older persons, education for family caregivers, and availability of services. Senior center staff also need training in mental disorder identification, referral skills, and available resources. The availability of an on-site counselor-social worker at Vintage Senior Center enabled older persons with mental-health needs to be identified and their needs addressed in a nonthreatening environment. The counselor made referrals and worked with physicians and mental-health providers to coordinate services, led support groups and provided individual counseling. Support for this position was found through the United Way and private sources. It is important that both the aging and mental health systems work together to coordinate services, and having a designated staff person to do this facilitates the provision of services to persons in need. Unfortunately, very few senior centers have on-site counselors or social workers.

DEMENTIA

Dementia is a mental disorder characterized by the loss of the ability to think, reason, and remember. It is not a normal part of the aging process, and it is caused by some underlying condition affecting the brain. Eventually, the symptoms associated with dementia become severe enough to interfere with work performance, social activities, and daily functioning. Symptoms of dementia vary, but all dementias involve some impairment of memory, thinking, reasoning, and language. Personality changes and abnormal behavior may also occur as dementia progresses.

Many different conditions can cause dementia. Alzheimer's disease accounts for more than half of all cases of dementia, but as many as 50 other conditions may cause dementia. Alzheimer's disease is a progressive degenerative disease of the brain that affects as many as 4 million Americans. The risk increases greatly with age. Symptoms vary from person to person, but generally include forgetfulness, confusion, disorientation, and a decline in cognitive abilities, such as thinking and understanding. The disease progresses to affect behavior, language, reasoning, reading, and writing. Behavioral symptoms include agitation, anxiety, delusions, depression, hallucinations, insomnia, and wandering.

As individual progress through the disease, their needs change, as do the needs of their caregivers. In the early stages of the disease, individuals with Alzheimer's disease and their families may not know what to expect or understand the changes taking place. Many families don't know about available services. Informed individuals and caregivers experience less anxiety and are better able to cope with stressful situations. Professional counseling and support groups can help the individual and their family deal with their emotions and stress.

A diagnosis of Alzheimer's disease is made through the process of elimination. Early diagnosis is important as many treatable conditions can cause dementia, including depression, alcohol use, thyroid disease, heart disease, stroke, malnutrition, dehydration, reaction to medication, head injury, and eye and ear problems. There is no cure for Alzheimer's disease but expert medical care and support can enhance the individual's quality of life.

Another common form of dementia is vascular dementia. This condition results either from narrowing and blockage of the arteries that supply blood to the brain or by strokes that cause an interruption of blood flow within the brain. As many as 30% to 40% of people with Parkinson's disease, a progressive, degenerative disease of the nervous system, will develop dementia during the later course of the disease.

Lewy body disease, Huntington's disease, Creutzfeldt-Jakob disease, and Pick's disease are other causes of dementia. Delirium, a state of temporary but acute mental confusion, is common in older people who have lung or heart disease, long-term infections, poor nutrition, medication interactions, or hormone disorders. Depression is often mistaken for dementia in older adults. When depression is severe, poor concentration and a limited attention span may develop. When dementia and depression occur together, the intellectual deterioration can be more extreme. Depression, alone or in combination with dementia, is treatable.

Inevitably, some senior center members will exhibit symptoms of dementia and senior center staff will have to intervene, particularly when the individual lives alone. It can be very difficult getting the person to a doctor to receive a proper diagnosis. People with dementia may try to remain independent but require supervision. They may no longer be able to attend the senior center independently because of their confusion and disorientation. Other senior center members may try to protect them. Adult day services co-located with the senior center can provide the individual who has dementia with an opportunity to maintain a social network and level of activity similar to what they experienced at the senior center.

DEPRESSION

Major depressive disorder is the leading cause of disability in the United States. More individuals with mental illness experience depression than any other illness, with nearly 10 million Americans of all ages, socioeconomic classes, races, and cultures being affected. For those over 65 years of age, 10% to 15% are affected by depression. Depression is a potentially fatal disease due to suicide, accidents due to impaired concentration, and increased risk of substance abuse, yet fewer than one third of those with depression will receive proper medical care. Without proper treatment, 80% will experience a recurrence within 3 years.

Depression affects mood, thought, body, and behavior. For some, it occurs in one or more relatively severe episodes, known as major depression. Others have chronic, less severe symptoms of depression known as dysthymia. Still others have bipolar disorder, where episodes of terrible lows alternate with excessive highs. Depressive disorders often co-occur with anxiety disorders and substance abuse.

Feeling sad or blue is a natural part of life but depression is not. For the most part, a person who is blue can continue to carry on with regular activities. Feeling sad is generally transient and the person will eventually return to their normal mood state. Clinically depressed persons suffer from symptoms that interfere with their ability to function in every day life. When clinically depressed, the affected older person may experience feelings of diminished self-esteem or even lose the will to live. As these symptoms develop, the older person may stay in bed, remain undressed in the morning, and show little interest in their own well-being and in doing things that in the past brought them pleasure. Appetite and sleep may be affected and lethargy may set in. There may be suicidal thoughts. If left undiagnosed and untreated, depression may last months or even years, lead to disability, aggravate symptoms of other illnesses, lead to premature death, or result in suicide. Depression is a medical illness that should be diagnosed and treated by trained professionals.

Recognizing depression in older individuals is not always easy. One of the biggest obstacles to getting help for depression can be a person's attitude. Many people think that depression will go away by itself, or that they're too old to get help, or that getting help is a sign of character weakness. Additionally, those who are depressed may fear being labeled mentally ill. The attitude of society reinforces fears and adds barriers to accessing care. It often is difficult for a depressed older person to describe how he or she is feeling. Sometimes the person's family and friends think that the person will just snap out of it, but unfortunately, a person suffering from depression does not just get over it. Another complicating factor is that many older people, disabled by or at risk for mental disorders, find it difficult to afford and obtain needed medical and related health care services.

When properly diagnosed and treated, however, most people recover from depression. In all populations, 80% of those experiencing even severe depression return to normal life with treatment. Good coping skills, a social support network, early detection, and medication and psychotherapy have been proven to be very helpful in minimizing depression in older persons. Psychotherapy assists the person with depression in recognizing and changing depressive thoughts.

The most common symptoms of late-life depression are

- persistent sadness
- diminished interest or withdrawal from regular social activities
- slowed thinking or response
- lack of energy or interest in things that were once enjoyable
- excessive worry about finances or health
- frequent tearfulness
- feelings of worthlessness or helplessness
- significant weight change
- pacing and fidgeting
- changes in sleep patterns (inability to sleep or excessive sleep)
- difficulty concentrating or making decisions
- staring off into space (or at the television) for prolonged periods of time

Depression often runs in families. Children of depressed parents have a higher risk of being depressed themselves. People with low self-esteem or who are very dependent on others seem to be vulnerable to depression. The death of a loved one, divorce, moving to a new place, money problems, or any sort of loss can contribute to depression. People without relatives or friends to help may have even more difficulty coping with stress. Sadness and grief are normal responses to loss, but if they linger or are severe, professional help should be sought.

Research has established a strong connection between physical and mental health. Chronic or serious illness is the most common cause of depression in older persons and depression will often worsen the symptoms of other illnesses. Long-term or sudden illnesses can bring on or aggravate depression. Some medicines cause depressive symptoms as side effects. For example, medical disorders may contribute biologically to depression, as with an underactive thyroid. People who are medically ill may become depressed as a psychological reaction to the prognosis, pain, and incapacity caused by the illness or its treatment, as in cancer. It is also possible that depression and a general medical disorder occurring together may be unrelated. Fatigue, high or low mood, sedation, and difficulty with memory or concentration can be depressive symptoms but can also occur as side effects of medication.

Weight loss, sleep disturbance, and low energy occur in depression and also in diabetes, cardiovascular disease, vitamin or mineral imbalances, and endocrine disorders. Symptoms of apathy, poor concentration, and memory loss are found in depression and in Parkinson's and Alzheimer's diseases. Depressive symptoms may also include achiness or fatigue, which are present in many other conditions. In addition, some illnesses may hide the symptoms of depression. For this reason the older adult may not report the depressive symptoms to a doctor, family or friends.

Mental disorders can lead to or exacerbate other physical conditions by decreasing the ability of older adults to care for themselves, by impairing their capacity to rally social support, or by impairing physiological functions. Clinical depression symptoms have been estimated to occur in as many as one third of persons with any medical condition, and the rates in some specific conditions may be even higher. Research suggests that recognition and treatment of co-occurring depression may improve the outcome of the medical condition, enhance quality of life, and reduce the degree of pain and disability experienced by the medical patient. Untreated depression worsens the prognosis for patients with cancer, heart disease, stroke, AIDS, Parkinson's disease, and most other major illnesses.

Treatment of depression can improve a patient's overall quality of life in several ways. It may enhance the ability to follow the treatment regimen for a co-occurring medical condition, decreasing complications and improving the eventual outcome. In addition, effective management of depression can lessen the degree to which the patient is irritable, demanding, or experiences overall problems in functioning, any of which may contribute to slower or more difficult recovery and greater stress and disability from the medical condition. Finally, controlling the depression will often improve the cognitive symptoms that are a part of some illnesses.

Depression can be confused with or masked by other problems in addition to physical illness, particularly dementia. Pseudodementia is used to describe depression in older people that often occurs following major life losses. Because its symptoms can mimic dementia (e.g., withdrawal, confusion, and memory loss), it is important to distinguish the two through a professional assessment.

Depression also occurs more frequently in persons with other psychiatric disorders, especially anxiety disorders. In such cases, detection of depression can result in more effective treatment and a better outcome for the patient. Substance abuse disorders (including alcohol and prescription drugs) frequently coexist with depression. Substance use must be discontinued in order to clarify the diagnosis and maximize the effectiveness of psychiatric interventions. Additional treatment is necessary if the depression remains after the substance use and withdrawal effects have ended.

The loss of a spouse is common in late life and bereavement is a natural response to the death of a loved one. The symptoms of bereavement—crying and sorrow, anxiety and agitation, insomnia, and loss of appetite—do not constitute a mental disorder. However, they still warrant clinical attention because as a highly stressful event, bereavement increases the probability of and may cause or exacerbate mental and somatic disorders and it is a well-established risk factor for depression. At least 10% to 20% of widows and widowers develop clinically significant depression during the first year of bereavement. Widowed men are at a greatly increased risk for death in the period immediately following their wives' deaths. Without treatment, such depressions tend to persist, become chronic, and lead to further disability and impairments in general health. Despite cultural attitudes that older persons can handle bereavement by themselves or with support from family and friends, it is imperative that those who are unable to cope be encouraged to access mental-health services. Bereavement is not a mental disorder but, if unattended, can have serious mental-health and other health consequences. Preventive interventions, including participation in self-help groups, have been shown to prevent depression among widows and widowers.

For some older persons the holidays can be an especially difficult time. The stress associated with holidays may stir feelings of loss or separation. Older adults may feel more acutely the passing of time and the absence of family and friends who have died or moved away. Traditional reunions and rituals that were observed in the past may no longer be possible and the holiday season may seem meaningless in their absence. Though it is normal to feel subdued, reflective, and even sad in the face of these losses, some older adults may experience a more serious case of depression. The factors contributing to holiday blues or depression in older persons include financial limitations, loss of independence, being alone or separated from family, failing eyesight that lessens the ability to write or read holiday correspondence, and loss of mobility or the inability to get to religious services or holiday celebrations.

SUBSTANCE ABUSE

Substance abuse, particularly of alcohol and prescription drugs, is one of the fastest growing health problems facing the country, affecting as many as 17% of older adults. Yet even as the number of older adults suffering from these disorders climbs, the situation remains underestimated, underidentified, underdiagnosed, and undertreated. Health care providers tend to overlook substance abuse and misuse among older people, mistaking the symptoms for those of dementia, depression, or other problems common to older adults. Age-associated changes in pharmacokinetics and physiology may alter drug tolerance in older adults. Compared to a younger adult, a similar amount of alcohol consumed by an older individual may lead to increased intoxication due to decreased tolerance to alcohol.

In addition, older adults are more likely to hide their substance abuse and less likely to seek professional help. Problems of identification may be compounded because older adults often live alone, which makes detection of problems more difficult. Many relatives of older individuals with substance abuse disorders, particularly their adult children, are ashamed of the problem and choose not to address it. The result is thousands of older adults who need treatment and do not receive it.

Another assumption that inhibits identification is the belief that older adults do not respond to treatment, a misperception contradicted by studies showing that older adults are more likely to complete treatment and have outcomes that are as good or better than those of younger patients. Ageism also contributes to the problem and to the silence. Younger adults often unconsciously assign different quality-of-life standards to older adults. There is an unspoken but pervasive assumption that it's not worth treating older adults for substance abuse disorders. Behavior that is considered a problem in younger adults does not inspire the same urgency for care among older adults. Along with the impression that alcohol or substance abuse problems cannot be successfully treated in older adults, there is the assumption that treatment for this population is a waste of health care resources.

Older adults who self-medicate with alcohol or prescription drugs are more likely to characterize themselves as lonely and to report lower life satisfaction. Alcoholism is more prevalent among older African Americans, Hispanic men, and men in general. Older women with alcohol problems are more likely to be a widow, to have had a problem-drinking spouse, to have experienced depression, and to have been injured in falls. Alcohol may elevate the older adults' already high risk for injury. Depressive disorders are more common among older persons than among younger people and tend to co-occur with alcohol misuse. Among persons older than 65, those with alcoholism are approximately 3 times more likely to exhibit a major depressive disorder than are those without alcoholism. Among persons older than 65, moderate and heavy drinkers are 16 times more likely than nondrinkers to die of suicide, which is commonly associated with depressive disorders.

In general, older people consume less alcohol and have fewer alcohol-related problems than younger persons, yet alcohol abuse and dependence are likely to increase as baby boomers reach older age, with heavier drinking habits than current cohorts of older adults. Persons born after World War II may show a higher prevalence of alcohol problems than persons born in the 1920s, when alcohol use was stigmatized. Alcohol use was also less common in the 1930s through the 1950s than it has been since the 1960s. Younger birth cohorts in the twentieth century tend to have increasingly higher rates of alcohol consumption and alcoholism. Because there is a clear relationship between early alcohol problems and the development of alcohol problems in later life, drinking among older adults is likely to become an even greater problem in the near future. The prevalence of alcohol problems in old age is expected to increase, especially among women, for birth cohorts entering their 60s in the 1990s and beyond.

Cross-sectional data suggest that there is a low prevalence of illicit drug use among the current older population. However, longitudinal data from the National Survey on Drug Abuse suggest that there could be in excess of 1 million more individuals using illicit drugs among baby boomers than previous generations. In the 1970s, as many as one fourth of baby boomers reported using an illicit drug in the past month. As they aged, the prevalence of baby boomers' using illicit drugs declined sharply until they reached their early 30s and illicit drug use leveled out at about 5%. This compares to a prevalence rate of approximately 3.8% among age-comparable individuals from the previous generation. In general, substance abuse decreases over a person's life span, but as increasing proportions of younger substance abusers are surviving into late life, the number of older drug abusers in our population is expected to increase and will impact the need for, and use of, treatment programs and other resources.

Ideally, every older adult should be screened for alcohol and prescription drug abuse as part of their regular physical examination. In the interim, self-administered and self-scored mass screenings can be a part of a larger presentation on the topic of alcohol's effects on older adults. Self-administered and machine-scored computerized screens can be conducted at senior centers with access to computers. However, many senior centers, health care, and social service providers are unaware that effective, validated instruments are available for screening older adults or they are intimidated by the prospect of using them. Many screens, moreover, take only a few minutes to administer, and require little or no specialized training to score and interpret.

Research has shown that 10% to 30% of nondependent problem drinkers reduce their drinking to moderate levels following a brief intervention by a physician or other clinician. A brief intervention is one or more counseling sessions, which may include motivation-for-change strategies, patient education, assessment and direct feedback, contracting and goal setting, behavioral modification techniques, and the use of written materials such as self-help manuals. Brief intervention techniques can be conducted by trained clinicians, health care workers, psychologists, social workers, and professional counselors.

SUICIDE

Suicide is the eighth leading cause of death in the U.S., and persons over 65 years have the highest rate of suicide. Comprising only 13% of the U.S. population, individuals aged 65 and older accounted for 19% of all suicide deaths in 1997. The highest rate is for White men aged 85 and older: 64.9 deaths per 100,000 persons in 1997, about 6 times higher than the national U.S. rate of 10.6 per 100,000. For some older persons, suicide is seen as a way to maintain control over the dying process. More men than women complete suicide but more women than men attempt suicide. It is estimated there are about 10 attempted suicides to one completion.

The risk factors for suicide frequently occur in combination. Almost all people who kill themselves have a mental or substance abuse disorder or both, and the majority have depressive illness. Social factors such as broken relationships, death of a loved one, or disputes with family members may contribute to depression. Other risk factors include fire-arms in the home (over half of all suicides are committed with guns), substance abuse, prior suicide attempts, and exposure to the suicidal behavior of others. Adverse life events in combination with other risk factors such as mental or substance-abuse disorders and impulsivity may lead to suicide. The strongest risk factors for attempted suicide are depression, alcohol abuse, cocaine use, and separation or divorce.

Studies indicate that the most promising way to prevent suicide and suicidal behavior is through the early recognition and treatment of depression and other psychiatric illnesses. There are two categories of suicide prevention. First are general preventive measures designed to address suicide and suicidal behaviors in the context of broader issues such as mental health, helping older adults cope with loss and depression, and recognition and treatment of substance abuse disorders. The second is crisis intervention. Because there are signs that a suicidal person may exhibit, senior center staff must be able to identify persons in need. Access to crisis centers, hot lines, peer support groups, and other sources of help will assist in suicide prevention.

SENIOR SUPPORT SERVICES

It is important to promote mental health and minimize the negative outcome of mental-health problems by providing mental-health services and supports in the community that extend beyond traditional, formal treatment settings. One model of a community support program is Senior Support Services at Vintage, a pilot project for providing comprehensive senior center services to older adults who have a mental health and/or mental retardation disability. Vintage collaborated with Allegheny East Mental Health/Mental Retardation to develop the program to focus on the physical, mental, and social wellness of the participants. The program was designed to address the significant service gap between the number of older adults with a mental health or mental retardation diagnosis and the number utilizing direct services, by developing age-appropriate support and treatment. Supportive services include staff support to access and participate in program options and specialized services such as assistance and training with daily living skills. Mental-health clinical services and supports, including psychiatric rehabilitation, are available through group and individual sessions at Vintage.

Through support networks, self-help groups, education, and other means, older people, families, and communities are assuming an increasingly important role in treating and preventing mental health problems and disorders among older persons.

SUGGESTED ACTIVITIES

- self-help support groups on mental health topics such as grief, loss, Alzheimer's disease and depression
- mental health supports and services on-site in partnership with mental-health providers
- resource fair with agencies providing mental-health supports
- educational programs on normal aging, warning signs of depression, Alzheimer's disease, substance abuse, and others
- mental fitness exercises
- screening programs on depression and memory loss

BIBLIOGRAPHY

Administration on Aging. (2001). Alcoholism and aging. *Aging Internet information notes.* Washington DC: Author. [On-line]. Available: www.aoa.dhhs.gov/naic/notes/alcoholabuse.html

Allegheny County Health Department. (1998, April). Alzheimer's disease. *Health Beat.* Pittsburgh, PA: Author.

Allegheny County Health Department. (1999, July/August). Suicides. *Health Beat.* Pittsburgh, PA: Author.

National Institute of Mental Health, Office of Communications and Public Liaison. (1999). *Awareness and treatment can improve overall health and reduce suffering.* Bethesda, MD: Author.

Bane, S. D. (1996). *Mental health and aging.* Kansas City, MO: National Resource Center for Rural Elderly, Center on Aging Studies, University of Missouri-Kansas City, MO.

Blow, F. C. (2001). Substance abuse among older adults. *Treatment Improvement Protocol (TIP) Series 26.* Washington, DC: U.S. Department of Health and Human Services.

Cohen, C., Cohen, G., Blank, K., Gaitz, C., Katz, I., Leuchter, A., Maletta, G., Meyers, B., Sakauye, K., & Shamoian, C. (2000, February). Schizophrenia and older adults. An overview: Directions for research and policy. *American Journal of Geriatric Psychiatry, 8,* 19–28.

Cohen, G. (2000, August). The future of being old in America. A mental health perspective. *American Journal of Geriatric Psychiatry, 8,* 185–187.

Cohen, G. (2000, November). Loneliness in later life. *American Journal of Geriatric Psychiatry, 8,* 273–275.

Gitlitz, R., & Gibbs, D. (1999). *Aging with a psychiatric disability.* Brooklyn, NY: G& G Geriatric and Disability Care Management, Inc.

Jewish Healthcare Foundation. (2001, March). Moving toward the ideal in mental health services. *Branches.* Pittsburgh, PA: Author.

Joint Committee on the Mental Health of Older People for the Pennsylvania Department of Aging and the Pennsylvania Department of Public Welfare/Office of Mental Health. (1994). *Joint policy statement on the mental health of older people.* Harrisburg, PA: Author.

Mayo Foundation for Medical Education and Research. (2000, December 18). *Dementia and memory loss.* Rochester, MN: Author.

National Clearinghouse for Alcohol and Drug Information. (1995, Spring). *Making prevention work.* Rockville, MD: Author. NCADI Inventory Number MPW002. [On-line]. Available: www.health.org/govpubs/mpw002/index.htm

National Institute on Alcohol Abuse and Alcoholism. (1998, April). *Alcohol alert.* No. 40. Bethesda, MD: Author.

National Institute of Mental Health. (1999). *Older adults: Depression and suicide facts.* Washington, DC: Author.

National Institute of Mental Health. (1999). *Suicide facts.* Washington, DC: Author.

National Institute of Mental Health, Office of Communications and Public Liaison. (1999). *The unrecognized link: Depression co-occurring with medical conditions.* Bethesda, MD: Author.

Patterson, T., Lacro, J., & Jeste, D. (1999, April). Abuse and misuse of medications in the elderly. *Psychiatric Times, 16*(4). [On-line]. Available: www.psychiatrictimes. com/p990454.html

RESOURCES

Alzheimer's Association
919 North Michigan Avenue, Suite 1000

Chicago, IL 60611-1676
312-335-8700
800-272-3900
http://www.alz.org
The Alzheimer's Association, a national network of chapters, is the largest national voluntary health organization committed to finding a cure for Alzheimer's and helping those affected by the disease.

Alzheimer's Disease Education and Referral Center (ADEAR)
PO Box 8250
Silver Spring, MD 20907-8250
301-495-3311
800-438-4380
www.alzheimers.org
The Alzheimer's Disease Education and Referral Center and Web site provide information about Alzheimer's disease and related disorders. The ADEAR Center is a service of the National Institute on Aging.

The American Association for Geriatric Psychiatry
7910 Woodmont Avenue, Suite 1050
Bethesda, MD 20814-3004
301-654-7850
www.aagpgpa.org
The American Association for Geriatric Psychiatry is a national association representing and serving its members and the field of geriatric psychiatry. It is dedicated to promoting the mental health and well being of older people and improving the care of those with late-life mental disorders.

American Psychological Association
Division of Adult Development and Aging
750 First Street, NE
Washington, DC 20002-4242
202-336-5500 or 800-374-2721
www.apa.org
The American Psychological Association is a scientific and professional organization that represents psychology in the United States.

National Alliance for the Mentally Ill
Colonial Place Three

2107 Wilson Blvd., Suite 300
Arlington, VA 22201-3042
703-524-7600 or 800-950-NAMI
http://www.nami.org
NAMI's efforts focus on support to persons with serious brain disorders
and to their families; advocacy for nondiscriminatory and equitable
federal, state, and private-sector policies; research into the causes, symptoms and treatments for brain disorders; and education to eliminate
the pervasive stigma surrounding severe mental illness.

National Depressive and Manic Depressive Association
730 N. Franklin, Suite 501
Chicago, IL 60601
312-642-0049 or 800-826-3632
http://www.ndmda.org
The National Depressive and Manic-Depressive Association educates
patients, families, professionals, and the public concerning the nature
of depressive and manic-depressive illness as treatable medical diseases;
fosters self-help for patients and families; works to eliminate discrimination and stigma and improve access to care; and to advocate for research.

National Foundation for Depressive Illness, Inc.
PO Box 2257
New York, NY 10016
212-268-4260 or 800-239-1265
http://www.depression.org.
The National Foundation for Depressive Illness educates the public
about depressive illness, its consequences, and its treatability.

National Institute on Alcohol Abuse and Alcoholism (NIAAA)
6000 Executive Boulevard—Willco Building
Bethesda, MD 20892-7003
http://www.niaaa.nih.gov/
The National Institute on Alcohol Abuse and Alcoholism supports and
conducts biomedical and behavioral research on the causes, consequences, treatment, and prevention of alcoholism and alcohol-related problems.

National Institute of Mental Health (NIMH)
6001 Executive Boulevard, Rm. 8184, MSC 9663

Bethesda, MD 20892-9663
301-443-4513
http://www.nimh.nih.gov
The National Institute of Mental Health is part of the National Institutes
of Health.

National Mental Health Association (NMHA)
1021 Prince Street
Alexandria, VA 22314-2971
703-684-7722 or 800-969-6642
http://www.nmha.org
The National Mental Health Association is the country's oldest and
largest nonprofit organization addressing all aspects of mental health
and mental illness. NMHA works to improve the mental health of all
Americans through advocacy, education, research and service.

National Resource Center for Rural Elderly
Center on Aging Studies
University of Missouri-Kansas City
5215 Rockhill Road
Kansas City, MO 64110
816-235-1747
http://iml.umkc.edu/casww/
The National Resource Center for Rural Elderly is a national focal point
for programs and services for rural elders. The Center focuses on mental
health and health care coordination services. The Center provides technical assistance and focused in-service training, conducts short-term
research; and identifies Best Practice Programs. Publications include:

- *Mental Health and Aging: Textbook*
- *Mental Health and Aging: Instructor's Manual*
- Mental Health and Aging: Bibliography
- Mental Health and Aging: Programs that Work

Substance Abuse and Mental Health Services Administration (SAMHSA)
U.S. Department of Health and Human Services
Center for Substance Abuse Prevention (CSAP)
Rockwall II, 5600 Fishers Lane
Rockville, MD 20857

301-443-0365
http://www.samhsa.gov/
National Clearinghouse for Alcohol and Drug Information: http://
www.health.org/

CHAPTER TWENTY

Caregiving

PAULA AND EMILY

The first time I met Paula was when she interviewed for a position at Vintage. My first impression, and one that remains to this day, is that she has a genuine love of life. Nothing pleases her more than to sing a song, decorate a room, plan a party, take a trip, or help a friend. Paula rarely, if ever, says no to anyone or anything. The oldest of three children, Paula mentioned during the interview that her mother was showing signs of dementia and had also been diagnosed with lymphoma. The family planned to move their mother, Emily, from her apartment in Virginia to a younger sister's home in New Jersey. Paula and her brother would take turns having their mother visit them. The first time Emily came to spend time with Paula and her husband, plans were made to help her mom feel comfortable and safe. Paula spoke to the Vintage staff who cares for clients with dementia to learn as much as possible to help Emily adjust to a new situation. Drawers were labeled so items of clothing could easily be found and a routine was quickly established. Paula also arranged for Emily to attend Vintage's adult day care.

Paula became the primary caregiver the following year when Emily moved in with her permanently. As with everything Paula undertakes, this too was met with enthusiasm. Emily was included in all the family activities, and Paula would frequently take her mom shopping at a local mall to purchase a special blouse or sweater. Emily began attending the adult day care five days a week and always had a friendly greeting for the staff.

The first time Paula hired a sitter so that she and her husband could go out to dinner and a movie was very difficult. Once again she sought the counsel of Vintage staff who work with caregivers and who are able to offer suggestions and support. It is never easy to be the designated primary caregiver, a situation that differs with each family and with the disease of the loved one. For Paula, each decision she has made for her mother has been hard. Paula always weighs what is in the best interest of her mother, as opposed to her own needs or the needs of her husband. A woman of strong faith, she knows assisted living will soon be necessary for her mother. Until that time, Paula continues on her course of providing loving care to the person we have all come to know as Emily.

If you were to ask Paula about this journey with her mother, this is what she would tell you after thoughtful consideration:

This was not a test. This was not some awful joke being played on us by a cruel, insensitive God. My God is not like that. This was by far the hardest journey my mom and I have ever taken, and the ride goes on. This journey has been a series of good-byes for my mom and me. My mom was always the quintessential lady, raising us girls to always be polite, sit with our legs crossed, carry a hanky, say thank you, etc. Good-bye.

Her dementia has changed that part of her, substituting rudeness where once there was sweetness, and inconsiderate of the feelings of others where once there was genuine caring. Good-bye.

Mama never swore (at least in front of us or in public) and we were severely reprimanded if we even thought about it. Now, I cringe when she swears at the aides and nurses who are trying to help and care for her and even at me. Good-bye.

We used to love to shop—she always loved clothes and she was always interested in her appearance. Dementia has taken that away too and she clings to one particular shirt (for comfort, I suppose) or one ugly pair of shoes and doesn't understand the importance of bathing. Good-bye.

There always was a smile and a certain light in her eyes when she saw her kids or our kids. The smile when I visit her is still there, but the light of recognition is gone. She knows me just as Paula, a nice lady who visits and brings fresh flowers each week, not Paula her oldest daughter. Good-bye.

That's the thing about some journeys—you always plan to return and find things as you left them. These good-byes are permanent and adding up every day. Mom and I can't go back, and the ride is getting more difficult as the days go by. She must be so confused and sad . . . I know I am.

HARRY

Every morning he arrived at Vintage long before the doors were opened. It didn't bother him that he had to stand and wait. Dressed in a jacket, jeans, sneakers, and a baseball cap, Harry enjoyed being at the door to greet the staff as we arrived at work. If any of us had even the smallest of packages he was immediately offering to help us. For five years, our staff knew we had a willing set of hands. Helping others was a trademark of Harry. Carrying a tray for someone in the dining room or getting coffee for a volunteer at the registration desk, he was always there to assist in a quiet unassuming manner.

So what do we know of this man? We know that as a young man he lived with his mother and twin brother. Illiterate, he worked most of his life in a bowling alley. A recovering alcoholic, Harry had been sober for 12 years when he came to Vintage. If he hadn't become terminally ill, we probably never would have really known him. We'd see him playing chess with a friend, enjoying a fish sandwich in the café, or occasionally hanging out in the billiards room. For the most part, Harry came to Vintage for the familiar faces and the social activities.

Illness changed everything. When Harry was diagnosed with cancer, we became his family. Staff took on the responsibility of being caregivers by taking him to doctor's appointments, sitting in waiting rooms during surgery, and being there when he was returned to his hospital room. This may not seem too unusual in the day of the transported family, but with Harry it was anything but usual. We don't know why Harry was suspicious of hospitals and doctors but he surely was. He discharged so many physicians and hospitals that we lost count.

As Harry's condition worsened, he chose to refuse treatment. A proud man, he valued his freedom and admitted once that like Frank Sinatra, he "wanted to do it his way." Near the end of his life he was willing to accept a hospice program. They, along with Vintage and his many friends of all faiths and races, allowed him to make his own decisions, affording this proud man an opportunity to die with dignity.

Following his death, Vintage made all the arrangements for his funeral, including a memorial service held at Vintage, which was attended by well over 100 people. Once he said to me, "I don't know what I would do if I couldn't come to Vintage." His many friends who mourned his death equally rewarded his feelings about Vintage. Although he was a man without a family in the traditional sense, Harry was rich with people who truly cared about him.

As many as 12.8 million Americans of all ages need assistance from others to carry out everyday activities. It is projected that by the year 2040 the population of older persons who are severely disabled and need help with personal activities of daily living (bathing, eating, dressing, and toileting), with instrumental activities of daily living (cooking, cleaning, laundry, transportation), with transfer or mobility, or who require skilled care will increase by 90%.

The National Family Caregiver Support Program (NFCSP) was developed by the Administration on Aging of the U.S. Department of Health and Human Services. It was modeled after successful long-term care programs in California, New Jersey, Pennsylvania, and other states, and after listening to the needs expressed by hundreds of family caregivers in discussions held across the country. The program calls for all states, working in partnership with area agencies on aging and local community-service providers, to have five basic services for family caregivers:

- information to caregivers about available services
- assistance to caregivers in gaining access to services
- individual counseling, organization of support groups, and caregiver training to caregivers to assist the caregivers in making decisions and solving problems relating to their caregiving roles
- respite care to enable caregivers to be temporarily relieved from their caregiving responsibilities
- supplemental services, on a limited basis, to complement the care provided by caregivers

A caregiver is anyone who provides unpaid assistance to another adult who is ill, disabled, or needs some help. Caregiving usually starts for a health-related reason, from either a crisis or a chronic condition that worsens. Caregiving for family members is very common. A recent study by the National Alliance for Caregiving and AARP (NAC/AARP) found that in about 1 in 4 households, a person over the age of 18 had provided care to someone aged 50 or more at some point during the previous year. The number of informal caregivers in the U.S. is estimated to be 20 million to 25 million. These informal caregivers (family members or friends of the care receiver) provide approximately 80% of the care to those who are chronically ill in the U.S. About two thirds of caregivers help aging parents or others over the age of 65, but the remainder care for nonelderly persons such as children, spouses, or other relatives and friends. The proportion of Americans age 60-plus with at least one parent alive has risen dramatically from 7% in 1900 to 44% in 2000.

Approximately 7 million caregivers provide or manage care long-distance (living at least an hour away). The number providing long-distance care is expected to double in 15 years. A survey on long-distance caregiving by the National Council on the Aging suggests a growing market for private businesses and the voluntary sector. Long-distance care is a large and growing concern to baby boomers. The average age of the caregivers interviewed was 46, and nearly half of them were boomers. The survey indicates that approximately 3.3 million boomers are providing long-distance care. Senior centers should look for opportunities to respond to this emerging market and find better ways of helping the caregiver and care receiver.

Caregivers include spouses, adult children, and other relatives and friends. Of the older persons receiving paid and unpaid assistance, 95% have family and friends involved in their care. Studies have shown that the degree of caregiver involvement has remained fairly constant for more than a decade, despite increased geographic separation, greater numbers of women in the workplace, and other changes in family life.

In most families, one person assumes the role of primary caregiver because they live closest geographically, are closer to the parent emotionally, and/or are the kind of person who takes charge of the situation. While the role of the primary caregiver is probably the most time consuming and stressful, all those involved face similar issues.

The NAC/AARP study found the average age of care receivers was 77 years and almost 1 in 4 are over the age of 85. The average age of caregivers was 46; 24% of these were 50 to 64 years of age and 12% were 65 and older. Caregivers providing the most intensive care were much more likely to be at least 65 years old than any other caregiver. Caregivers taking care of parents are more likely to be older themselves as the proportion of Americans aged 60 with at least one parent alive has risen dramatically this century, from 7% in 1900 to 44% in 2000. The typical caregiver is a married woman in her mid-40s, providing an average of 18 hours of caregiving per week, working full-time, lives near the care recipient, and has an annual household income of approximately $35,000. Thirty-one percent of caregivers take care of two or more people, and the majority of caregivers (64%) are employed. A study by Metlife found the average length of time spent on caregiving was about 8 years, with about one third of the respondents providing care for 10 or more years; the NAC/AARP study found the average duration of caregiving to be 4.5 years. Almost all respondents reported helping the care recipient with some expenses, most frequently with food, transportation, or medications.

Although each caregiving situation is different, caregivers are likely to experience stress from their caregiving responsibilities for a loved one. Caring for an aging relative is frequently a multiyear commitment, with huge investments in time, money, and emotions. Caring for an older person with disabilities can be physically demanding, particularly for older caregivers. One third of all caregivers describe their own health as fair to poor, and some caregivers fear the people they are caring for will outlive them. Many individuals become depressed or anxious and others report physical ailments associated with the stress of caregiving. Twenty-five percent of care receivers are either bedridden or use wheelchairs, and their needing to be lifted and carried can result in muscle strain and back pain for the caregiver.

Surveys show that most caregivers do have help. However, getting help and using it productively involves people skills. Though family members are not the only ones who can assist, working with other family members constructively can be challenging. The primary caregiver needs help to overcome barriers to cooperation and to create the supportive network they and the care receiver need.

CARING FOR A PERSON WITH A COGNITIVE IMPAIRMENT

An estimated 16% to 23% of families across the U.S. may be caring for an adult with a cognitive impairment, including Alzheimer's disease, Parkinson's disease, stroke, head injury, or AIDS dementia. The projected dramatic increase in the size of the older population will result in a corresponding increase in the number of older adults with cognitive impairments. Cognitively impaired persons typically require special care, including supervision (often 24-hour), specialized communication techniques, management of difficult behaviors, incontinence, and help with activities of daily living (ADLs), for example, bathing, eating, transferring from bed to a chair or wheelchair, toileting, and other personal care.

Caring for a person with a cognitive impairment is particularly hard work and these caregivers need help, including physical and emotional support, education and training, financial assistance, and respite care. These caregivers spend more time in the daily tasks of caregiving, provide more help with the activities of daily living, and they provide the most difficult type of care. They are twice as likely to be dealing with feeding and incontinence, one of the most challenging caregiving tasks. Older caregivers are more likely to be living with the person needing care, providing more than 40 hours of direct care each week, providing the most intensive care, and providing care for more than 5 years. As a result, they are more likely to report physical strain, high levels of emotional stress, family conflict, and financial pressures. Yet the majority of these caregivers have never received any training to help the care receiver with the activities of daily living.

INFORMAL CARE

In general, formal services are used by relatively few caregivers and care recipients. National data indicate that only about 9% of caregivers and 5% of care receivers receive all their care from formal, community-based providers. The vast majority of long-term care is provided informally and privately at no public cost. Informal caregivers provide assistance with daily activities, including eating, bathing, and dressing, or shopping, transportation, and taking medications. This form of care is generally unpaid and may help avoid or delay institutional placement of the individual or the need for more formal, or paid, caregiving services. Families are more inclined to provide services directly than to purchase them for the care receiver. Female caregivers typically provide assistance with personal care, housekeeping tasks, and meals, while male caregivers provide assistance with home repairs, transportation, and financial management.

Older people prefer to remain in their own homes if they need care. Difficulty bathing, eating, and toileting are the activities that most clearly signal declines in an older person's ability to live independently. Coresidence is more likely for dementia caregivers, especially at the later stages of disease. When the caregiver and care receiver live together, there is usually greater caregiving involvement and less use of formal services. Research shows there was a 16% reduction in co-residence over the 10-year period from 1987 to 1997, probably because of the growth of support services, such as home health care, that enable care receivers to remain in their own homes.

The NAC/AARP survey identified and described the experiences of caregiving. According to the survey, 79% of caregivers provided assistance with transportation, 77% with grocery shopping, 74% with housework, 60% with meal preparation, 56% with managing finances, 54% with arranging and supervising outside services, and 37% with medications. Caregivers provide assistance with personal ADLs including assisting with transfer in/out of chairs (37%), dressing (31%), bathing (27%), toileting (26%) and feeding (19%). On average, caregivers spend 18 hours per week on caregiving, with almost one fifth of caregivers providing constant care for 40 or more hours per week. Differences in amounts and types of care are directly influenced by the type and extent of the care recipient's impairment. For example, dementia caregivers provided more hours of care, more types of care, and were more likely to help with personal ADLs than nondementia caregivers.

The study suggests that caregivers provide care without a perception that they lack the services they might need. The main reason caregivers gave for not using services and assistive devices was that they had no need for them. However, the second most frequent reason for not using a service was not being aware of it. This was particularly true for caregivers providing the most intensive caregiving. The perception or knowledge that a service is not available also contributes to its nonutilization. Fifteen percent of caregivers said they or the care receiver were too proud to use adult day care or a senior center.

The majority of caregivers are women. The average age of caregivers is influenced by the age of care recipients—the older the care recipient, the older the caregiver. Spouses are the first source of caregiving assistance, providing the most extensive and comprehensive care. Often they are the only caregiver. Children are the next source of informal care, with daughters more likely than sons to be the caregiver. Friends and neighbors are mobilized in the absence of family caregivers or as supplemental sources of assistance. However, caregiving for older persons with dementia is less frequent among extended family and friends, probably because of the greater commitment and involvement required. In general, one person tends to provide the majority of informal care and there is little sharing of care. Secondary caregivers are often few in number and provide much less care, and then on an intermittent basis.

The survey reported a higher incidence of caregiving among Asian American (32%), Black (29%), and Hispanic (27%) households than in the general population. Caregivers in these three minority groups are more likely to provide care for more than one person and more likely than White caregivers to live with the care recipient and to have help from other persons. Black caregivers are the most likely to be taking care of a relative other than an immediate family member or grandparent.

The caregiver's personal situation influences how caregivers respond to the care receiver's needs and how they interface with the formal service system. Older men and women appear to perceive their need for assistance differently. Men receive more informal care than women. Older men are more likely to receive help with personal care, housekeeping tasks, and meals, activities that may require more time than the assistance with transportation, shopping, and home repairs, which were more frequently received by women. In addition, while men receive more care, on average they are likely to get that help from only one person, usually their spouse. Older women, on the other hand, have larger numbers of caregivers, typically two to four.

Differences in types and related amounts of assistance received are also influenced by traditional gender- and social-role stereotypes. Older people continue to do those tasks of daily living with which they feel familiar and for which they have skills. They receive help in those areas with which they are unfamiliar or less skilled. Caregivers' expectations of the recipient may also differ according to the older person's gender and therefore be an additional determinant of the kind of care provided.

An older person's living arrangement is a predictor of the level of care received. Older people who are living with a spouse or others were likely to receive substantially more care than those who lived alone, while those living alone are more likely to use paid formal help. Studies have found that those who were not married, lived alone, and lived in public housing were less likely to have informal caregivers available for assistance and therefore were more likely to rely on formal services for assistance. Living alone has consistently emerged in studies as a major predictor of institutionalization of older individuals. Despite the frequency of chronic and long-term illnesses or conditions requiring care, very few care receivers live in a nursing home or assisted-living facility. One fifth live in the same household as their caregiver, more than 50% live alone, and the rest live with another family member or friend.

THE EFFECTS OF CAREGIVING

The personal, social, and health impacts of caregiving are well documented. One in five caregivers in the National Alliance for Caregiving and Alzheimer's Association study said the biggest difficulties they face in providing care are the demands on their time or not being able to do what they want. Constraints or restrictions of caregiving on time for leisure, social, and personal activities have been consistently reported. Overall, the majority of caregivers reported less time for other family members and giving up vacations, leisure time, or hobbies. Other difficulties include watching or worrying about the care receiver's deterioration; the care receiver's attitude; and location, distance, or inconvenience. These impacts are greater for dementia caregivers.

The majority of caregivers are working full- or part-time. Between 1987 and 1997, the percentage of working caregivers rose from 55% to 64%, an increase of 9%. It is expected that this trend will continue and there will be more caregivers in the work force in the future, including long-distance caregivers. Working caregivers juggle the competing demands of caring for a chronically ill or disabled parent, raising a family, and managing a career. Work is a financial necessity and a source of satisfaction for many, yet the responsibilities of caregiving and doing well on the job often conflict. People who want to do both well can be caught in the middle. The Metlife research revealed that caregiving responsibilities seriously affected the productivity of caregivers, particularly because of altered work schedules, increases in absenteeism, early retirement, turnover, and decreases in on-the-job effectiveness. Working caregivers sacrifice leisure time, incur significant losses in career development, salary, and retirement income and often suffer stress-related illnesses. Eventually, some 12% quit their jobs to provide care full-time. Yet few companies have employer-sponsored programs or eldercare services for employee caregivers (only 23% of companies with 100 or more employees). For all of these reasons, finding practical ways to cope and get help are especially important for caregivers.

Caregivers often report their health to be worse than do noncaregivers. Depression among nondementia caregivers was twice that of the general population. Prevalence rates of depression among dementia caregivers have been as high as 43% to 46%. Though rates of depression across studies of dementia caregivers vary, the consistent finding is that dementia care is psychologically distressing.

The care of older adults who are disabled can be burdensome, but caregiving stress is not universal. It is important not to generalize the needs of dementia caregivers to nondementia caregivers. The needs of both groups of caregivers should be distinguished in order to accurately identify how best to assist caregivers in each group because their stressors and needs may differ.

Many caregivers report no or minimal negative effects of their helping role, and caregiving is described in positive terms. The biggest rewards of caregiving are knowing that the care receiver is well cared for, personal satisfaction in knowing one is doing a good deed or giving back or fulfilling family obligations, the care receiver's appreciation or happiness, seeing the care receiver's health improve, and spending time together. Neither the disability status nor the amount and type of care provided are related to caregiver burden. Problem behaviors, such as the wandering associated with dementia, have been consistently related to greater caregiver burden and role overload. These caregivers are also more likely to be depressed. Caregiver well-being is enhanced by a sense of mastery, the quality of the relationship with the care receiver, and feeling supported in the role.

Several studies reported that caregivers used the following methods of coping: prayer (74%), talking with friends or relatives (66%), exercise (38%), and hobbies (36%); 16% sought professional help or counseling. Most caregivers use multiple coping mechanisms, and the number of coping mechanisms increases as the level of care increases.

Studies have found that people do not plan for how and when they will assume a caregiving role—it just happens to them. Not only do most adults fail to plan for how they will provide care for their parents or other relatives, most caregivers also do not plan for changes in caregiving needs or for their own future health, financial, and long-term-care needs. A common coping strategy is to "take one day at a time." This works as long as the situation is stable or changes gradually. A major acute health event that suddenly increases the need for care may find the caregiver unprepared and require formal intervention. Yet most people will not seek out information until they need it. General information sessions about community services are frequently not well attended. One strategy is to engage a caregiver in planning shortly after experiencing such an event, when they are more likely to be receptive to new information and formal assistance. A vast majority of caregivers have thought about their own long-term-care needs as a result of their caregiving experience.

The Survey of Family Caregivers in New York City is important for its implications regarding the need for training and support for lay caregivers. The survey found that nearly 60% of New Yorkers who provide unpaid personal care for a relative or friend who is seriously ill, disabled, or older said that professionals did not give them the training necessary to perform caregiving tasks related to the activities of daily living (bathing, toileting, transferring, etc.). The caregivers reported significant lapses in training to perform medical tasks like changing bandages on wounds, using medical equipment, and managing medications. Improper techniques, such as for lifting, can injure a caregiver and put the care receiver at risk as well. The United Hospital Fund and Visiting Nurse Service, cosponsors of the survey, recommended that caregivers be better prepared to deal with the technical aspects of in-home care and the emotional issues that accompany in-home caregiving. Caregivers need education in the care tasks they are assuming, adequate home health care, and emotional support.

Support and counseling have been shown to be successful in prolonging the time that caregivers provided care at home, particularly during the early to middle stages of dementia. Support should focus on the factors that contribute to overload and on an attempt to intervene in a way that prevents stress rather than simply relieving it. Support services should address issues of evaluating the older person's needs, coming to terms with the needs of the recipient versus the caregiver's ability and willingness to provide care, and developing strategies to prevent overload, by training caregivers in technical skills or in obtaining emotional support before they actually need it. The challenge is to identify caregivers and intervene before they become caregivers or perceive the need for outside intervention. Given that restrictions on personal and leisure time are the most frequently reported caregiving impact, primary caregivers need help to identify other informal and formal sources of care to provide respite. It is also important not to assume that older members of minority groups don't need as much help because they have larger caregiving networks.

Most caregivers are women, but male spousal caregivers are highly involved and want to care for their wives. However, they may need skill training or supportive services (especially personal care) in order to do so, particularly if the care recipient requires extensive and personal care. Male caregivers in these situations are usually older and are less likely to be prepared and skilled to provide the care needed. They might also be challenged by their own health conditions or physical disability.

Caregivers end their caregiving role when higher levels of care are required, there is a need for constant supervision, or problem behaviors are manifested. Other reasons include a sense that the benefits of caregiving do not outweigh caregiving stress, not having a good relationship with the care recipient, lack of confidence in one's ability to provide more care, and not being a close relative.

If caregivers feel overwhelmed or overloaded by their caregiving responsibilities, they are more likely to experience physical and emotional problems. The assessment of at-risk caregivers should include their feelings about their caregiving responsibilities, their ability to manage multiple demands, their confidence in their caregiving skills, their organizational, and their time-management skills.

Dementia care, particularly the manifestation of problem or disruptive behaviors, is particularly stressful. Developing interventions to specifically address these behaviors by changing the older person's behavior or by developing the caregiver's skills to manage the behaviors is needed. Suggested interventions include skills training, education, and counseling. Caregivers need help in determining the optimal mix of formal services and informal care in order to ensure the well-being of both care recipient and caregiver. Transition to a special-care environment, including assistance with appropriate timing and with negotiating a role for continued involvement of the caregiver is another important issue.

The challenges senior centers face in providing services to caregivers in the future include

- changing sociodemographics of the older population and the impact on the caregiver and care receivers;
- projected changes in active life expectancy and the compression of disability, meaning higher needs for care but perhaps for shorter periods of time at advanced ages;
- the availability and ability of families—which will be smaller and older—to care for very old and perhaps severely disabled elders; and
- the increased ethnic diversity of the population, underscoring the need for culturally sensitive and appropriate services and service delivery mechanisms.

END-OF-LIFE CARE

It is inevitable that the staff of the senior center will deal with the death of its members and their own grief and the grief of their family and friends. It is important to help all involved through the grieving process.

Planning for incapacity and other end-of-life issues and communicating their desires to their clergy or spiritual advisor, family and friends, and doctor increases the chances that the older adult's wishes will be carried out. Older adults can benefit from information that will help guide them in their decisions about what kind and how much care is wanted when they are incapacitated or death is expected, where they want to die, and whom they want to care for them. They can benefit from the opportunity to discuss the ethical, moral, and religious implications of their decisions. In some cases, those older adults with no family members turn to their "family" at the senior center for guidance.

Although caring for loved ones and friends as they die clearly requires expert medical attention, families and friends also need to advocate for their loved one to ensure that expert care is provided and that the dying person is not allowed to suffer in pain or with other unaddressed symptoms. Many older adults need to learn how to advocate for the person they are caring for.

Educational programs and information about advance directives are important topics for older adults and family caregivers. They need help understanding living wills, health-care powers of attorney, and DNR (do not resuscitate) orders. Information about hospice services and palliative care will help the planning process.

Palliative care focuses on ways to ease pain and make life better for people who are dying and for their loved ones. Palliative care means taking care of the whole person—body, mind, spirit—heart and soul. It looks at death and dying as something natural and personal. The goal of palliative care is to provide the best quality of life until the very end of life.

Ira Byrock learned from caring for people who are dying that good dying is wellness in dying. Providing opportunities to listen to people's life stories, helping them in their reminiscences, and creating a safe place for families to say hard things are important to dying well. Dying is a part of the life of the individual and the family and the dying need to be honored for that life.

Reflecting on and reassessing life achievements promotes mental and emotional well-being and combats depression. The opportunity to reminisce can help older people tap into forgotten resources within themselves and come to terms with events and feelings they may not have had time to reflect upon and think through at the time they occurred.

A bereavement program can help people who have lost a loved one cope with their loss. American or religious customs concerning death, the grief process, relationships with friends and family, strategies, local resources, and personal goal-setting are some ideas for discussion. How to help someone through grief is another good topic.

CAREGIVER NEEDS

Denise Bown and Donna Grove Hipskind have identified four stages of caregiving, a concept that describes the path caregivers take: from (a) worrying that caregiving will become part of their lives in the next few months (anticipatory caregiver); to (b) regularly meeting the needs of their aging relatives (freshman caregiver); to (c) meeting those needs year after year (entrenched caregiver); and finally, to (d) dealing with grief and feelings of loss due to a change in the caregiving role, whether due to nursing home placement or death (caregiver in loss). Caregivers and those who help them need to learn to identify and adjust to their changing needs.

STAGE I: THE ANTICIPATORY CAREGIVER

A person anticipates becoming a caregiver in the next 12 to 18 months because of a decline in a friend or relative's health and recognition that they will need help. The caregiver may feel conflicted about the care recipient's illness or disease, as well as confused about what is part of the normal aging process and what is not. Due to inexperience, the caregiver cannot plan and prepare for an emergency because he or she can't envision what an emergency would be. The key to this stage is to help the caregiver gather information about the care recipient's health and financial status and about organizations and people who can help, for the individual might be unsure of what questions to ask and lack the experience to find the needed information.

STAGE II: THE FRESHMAN CAREGIVER

The freshman caregiver has been a caregiver for a short time and needs to involve others to help care for the care receiver. Sometimes freshman caregivers have false expectations about the situation itself or about the help they'll receive from others. The freshman caregiver might act for the care recipient and not with them, eliminating their input in important decisions. Freshman caregivers need help working with their family members to ensure they communicate the care recipient's status and the help needed.

STAGE III: THE ENTRENCHED CAREGIVER

The entrenched caregiver may feel tired, guilty, and run-down. There may be unresolved issues between the caregiver and the care recipient, making it difficult for the caregiver to be an effective. Entrenched caregivers need to know how important it is to take care of themselves and to involve those who can provide respite and emotional support so that they continue to provide care. Counseling services may be needed.

STAGE IV: THE CAREGIVER IN LOSS

The caregiver in loss may need help to make a successful transition through the grieving process from those who can help, such as a bereavement counselor or a support group.

Several national caregiving studies conducted by the National Alliance for Caregiving found that caregivers desire information, education, and resources on the financial and health aspects of caregiving. Caregivers also need and want information to help them plan for their own future needs and cited the need for a central place to go or call to find out what help is available. Respondents to the Caregiving Boom study said they found health-related information to be the most valuable, including what to expect with a particular disease, and how to care for someone with a disease. They also value information on how to provide basic care, how to deal with the stresses of caregiving, paying for long-term care, managing the use of medications, and how to balance caregiving with work and family. Information to facilitate caregiving, such as finding and evaluating in-home services, was also reported as being helpful. More respondents named a health professional as the most valuable source of information. Younger caregivers are more likely than older caregivers to say they like receiving information on the Internet.

OPPORTUNITIES FOR SENIOR CENTERS

The large number of long-distance caregivers and the cost-sharing requirements under the new Family Care Givers program of the Older Americans Act presents a unique opportunity for senior centers to develop programs that respond to the needs of the private pay market.

Caregivers often learn through trial and error the best ways to help the care receiver maintain routines for eating, hygiene, and other activities at home. Senior centers can help caregivers maximize caregiving abilities and the care receiver's independence and health by providing programs and services to meet their special needs.

PREVENTIVE HEALTH CARE

- maximizing the care receiver's independence and health
- exercise programs that help improve strength, balance, and mobility and prevent accidents
- care for the caregiver
- self-care regimens
- avoiding burnout
- stress management and coping skills

EDUCATIONAL PROGRAMS

- disease-specific information, including what to expect and caring for someone with the disease
- normal aging
- coping with Alzheimer's disease and other forms of dementia
- providing assistance with the activities of daily living (giving medications, bathing, transferring, etc.)
- maintaining a good quality of life while caregivng
- planning for caregiving
- caregiving tips
- training to improve caregiving skills
- planning for long-term care
- balancing work and caregiving
- communicating with health professionals and advocating for the care receiver
- how to hire a home-care employee
- determining whom to involve and asking others for help
- conducting a family meeting
- communicating with and involving others
- dealing with changed family relationships
- the "sandwich generation"—caring for older parents and children
- long-distance caregiving
- coping with grief and loss
- power of attorney
- advance directives and living wills
- financial and legal planning
- choosing a nursing home or other care options
- home modifications to ensure home safety
- assistive devices that can enhance the care receiver's independence and safety

- managing problem behaviors (individuals who are cognitively impaired may experience a range of behavioral problems including communication difficulties, aggressive or impulsive behaviors, memory problems, incontinence, poor judgment, and wandering)
- driving and transportation concerns

ACTIVITIES

- opportunities for the caregiver to participate in center activities
- opportunities for the care receiver to be mentally stimulated and involved in activities

INFORMATION AND REFERRAL (I&R)

Information on topics needed by caregivers such as:

- public benefits and entitlements
- respite care services
- long-term care insurance planning
- finding help; local caregiving resources and community care options
- national caregiver resource organizations
- caregiving services
- selection and evaluation criteria for services such as in-home health care
- selection and evaluation criteria for nursing homes or assisted-living residences

Senior centers can tap into the National Council on the Aging's comprehensive, 50-state, on-line service, Benefits Check Up, that enables organizations quickly and easily to let an older person or caregiver learn about benefits they are eligible for and where and how to apply.

OUTREACH PROGRAMS

- outreach to identify caregivers and their needs

CAREGIVER RESOURCE CENTER OR LIBRARY

- Internet access to caregiving resources
- books, CDs, articles, and other information on caregiving
- brochures from community service providers

COUNSELING SERVICES AND SUPPORT GROUPS

- for the caregiver to provide emotional support and caregiving tips, information on community resources from others who have learned from experience, and relief from the isolation some caregivers experience
- for the care receiver on coping with loss and impairment
- a professional counselor to help caregivers and care receivers cope with feelings of anger, frustration, guilt, loss, or competing personal, work, and family demands.

ELDERCARE

Eldercare is recognized by a growing number of employers. Senior centers that provide services to caregivers can extend these programs to employers who want to provide eldercare services. Support for employees who have caregiving responsibilities can take a variety of forms:

- information on local I&R services or resource centers
- caregiver support groups
- caregiver information fairs
- lunch-time seminars on topics such as long-distance caregiving
- telephone hot line
- articles or information in employee publications and Intranet sites

BIBLIOGRAPHY

Byock, I. (1997). *Dying well: The prospect for growth at the end of life.* New York: Riverhead Books.

American Association of Retired Persons. (2001). *Balancing work and caregiving.* Washington, DC: Author. [On-line]. Available: www.aarp.org/confacts/care give/balance.html

American Association of Retired Persons. (2001). *Planning for caregiving.* Washington, DC; Author. [On-line]. Available: www.aarp.org/confacts/caregive/planning.html

Brubaker, T. (1985). Caregiver's action plan. *Continuing Care Coordinator, 4*(6).

Family Caregiver Alliance. (1998). *Fact sheet: Caregiving.* San Francisco, CA: Author. [On-line]. Available: www.caregiver.org/factsheets/caregiving.html

Family Caregiver Alliance. (1996). *Fact sheet: Work and eldercare.* San Francisco, CA: Author. [On-line]. Available: www.caregiver.org/factsheets/work_eldercare.html

Family Caregiver Alliance. (1996). *Incidence and prevalence of the major causes of adult-onset brain impairment in the United States and California.* San Francisco, CA: Author.

Grove Hipskind, D., & Brown, D. M. (1998). *The four stages of caregiving. Unlocking the blocks: Your keys to successful caregiving.* Park Ridge, IL: Tad Publishing Co. [On-line]. Available: www.caregiving.com

Levine, C., Kuerbis, A., & Gould, D. A. (1997). *A survey of family caregivers in New York City: Findings and implications for the health care system.* New York: United Hospital Fund.

Metlife® Metropolitan Life Insurance Company, Mature Market Institute. (1999). *The Metlife juggling act study. Balancing caregiving with work and the costs involved.* New York: Author.

National Alliance for Caregiving. (1998). *The caregiving boom: Baby boomer women giving care.* Bethesda, MD: Author.

National Alliance for Caregiving. (1999). *Caring today, planning for tomorrow.* Bethesda, MD: Author.

National Alliance for Caregiving and AARP. (1997). *Family caregiving in the U.S.: Findings from a national survey.* Bethesda, MD: Author.

National Alliance for Caregiving and Alzheimer's Association. (1999). *Who cares? Families caring for persons with Alzheimer's disease.* Bethesda, MD: Author.

Ory, M. G., Hoffman, R. R., Yee, J., Tennstedt, S., & Schulz, R. (1999). Prevalence and impact of caregiving: A detailed comparison between dementia and non-dementia caregivers. *The Gerontologist, 39*(2), 177–186.

Pandya, S. M., & Coleman, B. (2000) *Caregiving: Involving others* AARP: Washington, DC.

Tennstedt, S. (1999, March 29). *Family caregiving in an aging society.* Presented at the U.S. Administration on Aging Symposium: Longevity in the New American Century. Baltimore, MD.

U.S. Congress Office of Technology Assessment. (1990). *Confused minds, burdened families.* Washington, DC: Author.

Wagner, D. (1997). *Comparative analysis of caregiver data for caregivers to the elderly 1987 and 1997.* Bethesda, MD: National Alliance for Caregiving.

Wagner, D. L. (1997). Long-distance caregiving for older adults. *Healthcare and aging.* Washington, DC: National Council on the Aging.

RESOURCES

Aging with Dignity
PO Box 1661
Tallahassee, FL 32302-1661
850-681-2010
http://www.agingwithdignity.org
Provides a simplified advance directive form that is a useful guide and is legally valid in most states.

American Association of Retired Persons (AARP)
601 E Street NW
Washington, DC 20049
202-434-2277
http://www.aarp.org
AARP is a membership organization for people 50 and over. AARP provides information and resources on consumer, legal and caregiver issues; and advocacy on legislation. AARP Widowed Persons Service programs offers one-to-one outreach, group meetings, support groups, educational meetings, guest speakers, online discussion groups, publications and training materials on bereavement, and referrals to community resources.

Careguide, Inc.
210 N. University Drive, Suite 700
Coral Springs, FL 33071
954-796-3727
http://www.careguide.com
CareGuide is a caregiving Web site. CareGuide is partnered with leading caregiving organizations, including the American Society on Aging, Assisted Living Federation of America, National Alliance for Caregiving, and National Association of Professional Geriatric Care Managers.

Family Caregiver Alliance
Family Caregiver Alliance
690 Market Street, Suite 600
San Francisco, CA 94104
415-434-3388
http://www.caregiver.org/
Family Caregiver Alliance supports and assists caregivers of brain-impaired adults through education, research, services and advocacy. FCA's Information Clearinghouse covers current medical, social, public policy and caregiving issues related to brain impairments.

Interfaith Caregivers Alliance
One West Armour Blvd.
Suite 202
Kansas City, MO 64111
816-931-5442
http://www.interfaithcaregivers.org/

Interfaith Caregivers Alliance (originally known as the National Federation of Interfaith Volunteer Caregiver) has existed to develop and support interfaith volunteer caregiving programs across America.

Last Acts
Partnership for Caring, Inc.
1620 Eye Street NW, Suite 202
Washington, DC 20006
202-296-8071
http://www.lastacts.org
Last Acts is a call-to-action campaign to improve care at the end of life. Last Act's goals are to bring death related issues out in the open and help individuals and organizations pursue better ways to care for the dying

National Alliance for Caregiving
4720 Montgomery Lane
Bethesda, MD 2084
301-718-8444
http://www.caregiving.org
The National Alliance for Caregiving has developed a template for resource guides-the *Local Resource Guide for Caregivers.*

National Association of Area Agencies on Aging
927 15th Street, NW, 6th floor
Washington, DC 20005
202-296-8130 (nationwide AAA listings)
800-677-1116 (national Eldercare locator)
http://www.n4a.org/
The National Association of Area Agencies on Aging (N4A) is the umbrella organization for the 655 area agencies on aging (AAAs) and more than 230 Title VI Native American aging programs in the U.S. Through its presence in Washington, D.C., N4A advocates on behalf of the local aging agencies to ensure that needed resources and support services are available to older Americans.

National Association of Professional Geriatric Care Managers
1604 N. Country Club Road
Tucson, AZ 85716
602-881-8008
http://www.caremanager.org/

National Association of Professional Geriatric Care Managers is a non-profit, professional organization of practitioners whose goal is the advancement of dignified care for the elderly and their families.

The National Hospice and Palliative Care Organization (NHPCO)
1700 Diagonal Road, Suite 300
Alexandria, VA 22314
703-837-1500
www.nhpco.org
NHPCO is a resource for professionals and volunteers providing service to patients and their families during end of life.

U.S. Administration on Aging
Department of Health and Human Services
200 Independence Avenue, SW
Washington, DC 20201
202-619-0724
http://www.aoa.gov
The Administration on Aging supports a nationwide, toll-free information and assistance directory called the Eldercare Locator, which can find the appropriate area agency on aging to help an individual seeking assistance for their loved ones, relatives, or friends. The Office of Public Affairs publishes *Because We Care: A Guide for People Who Care.*

Washington Business Group on Health (WBGH)
777 North Capitol Street NE, Suite 800
Washington, DC 20002
202-408-9320
http://www.wbgh.com/
The Washington Business Group on Health is a non-profit, health policy and membership organization of national and multinational employers. WBGH works to stimulate and foster corporate leadership and partnership in promoting performance-driven health care systems and competitive markets that improve the health and productivity of companies and communities.

CHAPTER TWENTY-ONE

Spirituality and Aging

DONNA

Every agency needs strong leadership and never is that more important than during the period of its inception. Many people contributed to starting Vintage, but the person I know best is Donna. The wife of a leading minister in our city at that time, Donna was quick to see the need for a place where our community's older residents could go during the day.

Donna and other church leaders joined forces with the Junior League of Pittsburgh to create such a place. After extensive searching they were fortunate to find space in the basement of a local church that allotted them 2 days a week for activities and a noon meal.

The historical details of Vintage's early days are well documented, but along with these facts certain stories have become legend. One concerns the name "Vintage" and how it came about. A group of founders (including Donna) were at a restaurant one evening discussing what they could name the place they had established. The Oaks was being discussed, for they were thinking of the oak tree as H. F. Chorley wrote in "The Brave Old Oak" "still flourishing after a hundred years are gone." One woman raised her glass of red wine and said. "Vintage—aging is like a fine wine—getting better with age." And so Vintage got its name.

Donna's contributions are well known and have been immeasurable. As Vintage grew, she was the person who hired the first executive director. She served on the board for more than 25 years, including 4 years as president. Like many board members during the early years, Donna was hands-on, helping with everything from preparing lunches to raising money. She continued to be invested in the agency until her retirement 2 years ago.

As a staff, we all felt Donna was our voice. She understood the importance of providing adequate compensation and recognition in order to keep good staff on the Vintage team. She found creative ways to do so, if not always through monetary means, then certainly with a personal thank-you. We all have notes from Donna expressing her genuine appreciation for something that we did for Vintage. She is a wonderful, fun-loving person who believes the whole world should know about Vintage.

Donna was also the spiritual leader of Vintage, and her influence in this area is present to this day. People of all faiths are welcomed, indeed encouraged, to come to Vintage. She along with the staff created an Annual Spirituality Conference, which was held each spring. Listening to Donna speak at the 20th anniversary of Vintage in 1993, it was clear that her work at Vintage had been a mission for her. Her loving, prayerful guidance of our agency in its earliest days has been a cornerstone of all we have been and all we will be.

I recently sat down with her and asked her to sum up her feeling about this "place" called Vintage that she and others had established 28 years ago and this is how she responded:

> *I always liked our mission statement "to raise the quality of life for older adults by developing and utilizing their potential." My joy in serving Vintage was to see people coming every day and bringing their untapped talents. Many had worked at what could be called unglamorous jobs all their lives and were too tired at the end of their work day to try singing in a chorus, or joining a dance team, or an art education class, but now their day had come. It was always a thrill to me to see the polished productions the various groups put together. It brought much happiness and pride into their lives. It proves the adage that when one door closes another opens. Some of our Vintagers had looked so long at the closed door that they had to be shown that another was opened to them. I have always believed that every human being has an undeniable right to develop his capabilities, so long as they do not deny the same right to others. God gave us life for happiness, and I am sure that humans will never be made lazy or indifferent by an excess of happiness. Happiness lies within each one of us. External conditions are the accidents of life. The great, enduring qualities are love and service and these are what I found at Vintage in abundance, and every bit as redemptive as whatever I did to serve my church.*

People of all ages search for meaning in their everyday activities. Expressions of spirituality through religious practice or compassion, service to others, or passing on wisdom to succeeding generations (generativity) can bring deep personal satisfaction, comfort, and peace to older adults and thus help them age more successfully.

Religion is generally recognized to be the practical expression of spirituality—the organization, rituals, and practice of one's beliefs. Religion offers a way to express spirituality with social support and a sense of belonging through religious affiliations. Religion includes specific beliefs and practices, while spirituality is much broader. Spirituality includes a system of beliefs that encompasses love, compassion, and respect for life. Spirituality is about existence; individuals' relationships with themselves, others, and the universe; and a search for meaning in life. Individuals may experience both spirituality and religion very privately within themselves (internally), and externally, through social interaction with persons and organizations.

Research has found that people do not necessarily become more religious as they age, but religion and associated activities are common among older adults. Nine out of 10 older adults rate religion as important in their lives. Many of the present cohort of older persons were religious in their youth, and a large percentage of them will retain their religious interest. Spirituality and faith development is lifelong; it does not end at any particular age or life stage. Yet senior adult ministry is the least developed of all ministries, and aging is the only major life stage that is not focused on in most churches.

Maturing adult-life stages offer special opportunities for spiritual development. Surveys indicate that a majority of older persons (76%) today regard religion as highly important in their lives. More than half of all older persons attend religious services on a weekly basis. Numerous studies have shown that even when poor health prevents public religious participation, many older persons compensate with high levels of nonorganizational religious activities such as frequent prayer, meditation, and Bible reading. In addition, when asked to describe the ways they cope with stressful events, older people most often talk about their religious faith and their prayer life.

Evidence is accumulating that religious beliefs and practices contribute to well-being in later life. Compared to nonreligious older persons, those who are religious have better functional health and higher levels of adjustment as indexed by levels of depression, suicide rates, anxiety, and alcohol abuse. Through their discovery and utilization of spiritual resources, older persons may experience their lives as meaningful even in the face of multiple, serious challenges to satisfaction with life

To cope successfully with these challenges, older adults can fortify themselves with spiritual-wellness skills. A significant correlation between religion and coping has been found, and most older persons report that religion helps them cope or adapt with losses or difficulties. In addition, there is a positive relationship between religion and physical health. Studies have related happiness, morale, and health to spirituality. In an important study affirming the interrelationship of physical and mental health, Idler and Kasl examined the relation between disability, depression, and mortality. They found that for men, religion had a buffering effect, reducing the probability that they would become depressed following disability.

Older adults may turn to spirituality and religion when they experience difficult life-changing events and personal losses, such as the loss of a spouse or child. Losses and life changes increase in later life and challenge older adults. Such losses can also threaten the strength and stability of spirituality in older adults, who may experience distress or psychological conditions in reaction to these events and losses. Just when religious support is needed most, older persons may be less able to access it due to failing health, problems with mobility, or lack of transportation.

Observations of older adults have shown increased reflection, less concern for material things, and more interest in quality and satisfaction with life as they age. There is a greater emphasis on inner experiences that facilitate expanding consciousness. Many older persons derive a sense of meaning in life through their sense of connectedness to nature. Studies suggest that life satisfaction increases simultaneously with aging as a shift takes place from the material world to the cosmic. Some older adults may have experiences that seem mystical as spirituality extends beyond the physical, material, and self, to a state called transcendence. This may occur in responses to illness or other life-changing occurrences. It is thought that transcendence appears through creative work, religious beliefs, children, identification with nature, and mystical experiences. Time to meditate, contemplate, and reflect can be healthy for older adults.

Older adults' increasing interest in self-awareness, the search for meaning and personal development has created new opportunities for education in seniors centers. The activities of Sage-ing Centers™, based on the concept of spiritual eldering, includes activities encouraging personal growth, social activism and mentoring of skills and experiences to younger generation. The Spiritual Eldering Institute® in Boulder, Colorado spearheads the spiritual eldering movement. The Institute is a multi-faith organization dedicated to the spiritual dimensions of aging and conscious living, affirming the importance of the elder years, and teaching individuals how to harvest their life's wisdom and transform it into a legacy for future generations. The Sage-ing Center movement evolved from the work of Zalman Schacter-Shalomi and Ronald S. Miller and described in *From Age-ing to Sage-ing: A Profound New Vision of Growing Older*. Schachter-Shalomi, a rabbi dreading retirement, realized that he must recontextualize aging as the anticipated fulfillment of life as opposed to an inevitable decline.

Federal and state government involvement with faith-based organizations has become more evident, but the evolution of this partnership has not been without public policy debate and judicial scrutiny. Public policy activity in the area of spirituality first occurred as part of the While House Conference on Aging in 1961. In 1972, the National Interfaith Conference on Aging was held, which led to the formation of the National Interfaith Coalition of Aging (NICA). The National Interfaith Coalition of Aging is a source of leadership to religious and spiritual communities. NICA developed a definition of spiritual well-being that would be acceptable to different faith groups, which included Jewish, Eastern Orthodox, Roman Catholic, and several Protestant denominational leaders: "the affirmation of life in a relationship with God, self, community and environment that nurtures and celebrates wholeness." Spiritual well-being offered a way of changing the focus from religious activities to spiritual satisfaction, thus avoiding the issue of separation of church and state. The 1981 White House Conference on Aging did not include a section on spirituality, reportedly to avoid violating the relationship between church and state. However, NICA passed 45 recommendation that focused on spirituality. President Bill Clinton called on religious and spiritual organizations and delegates to the 1995 White House Conference on Aging to address the religious needs of older adults and their spiritual well-being.

A survey of the participants of the White House Conference on Aging who were architects of the recommendations found that faith is critical to their quality of life. Ninety-eight percent said religion adds meaning to their lives. More than 90% said religion has changed in importance in their lives; they apply their faith more in everyday life and see it as a source of hope and the key to true fulfillment of meaning in life. Contentment in aging comes from knowing that their lives have meaning, from giving to others, and from knowing that God is with them. Half or more of the respondents said aging well means "to have purpose and a sense of worth," "to accept the changes that occur physically to me as I grow older," or "to become more reconciled with myself and my life." With regard to caring and caregiving, God and one's religious congregation were seen as important support for caregiving, and God and God's love were the strongest motivators. In terms of the gift of self, respondents saw their faith as a primary motivator for volunteerism.

Research findings indicate that older adults gain richly from their efforts when they engage in purposeful activity where they are genuinely assisting others. Their contributions bring them heightened levels of satisfaction, fulfillment, physical energy, self-worth, and well-being. They see themselves as valuable, enjoy a high sense of utility, and believe that what they are doing is worthwhile.

CULTURAL TRADITIONS AND SPIRITUALITY

Cultural and religious traditions become more important with age, especially to different ethnic populations. Religious practices often provide comfort and give people strength to cope with the stress in their lives. As various groups look for solutions to their unique problems, their healing often comes from within their own cultural and religious traditions. Although individuals within and among cultures have different philosophies and practices of spirituality, similar positive outcomes are derived. By sharing practices and traditions, participants gain a greater understanding and appreciation of other cultures and traditions.

Black women are more religious than Black men and more than all Whites. The church serves many important functions in the Black community. Studies have shown that older Blacks, especially women, attend church more frequently, participate more in church-related activities, and score higher on measures of religiosity and commitment. Women have played major roles in the organization and programs of support within their churches. Some strategies that Black women use in resolving adverse experiences include accepting reality, turning things over to a higher power, identifying life lessons, and recognizing purpose and destiny and achieving growth.

Many Blacks deal with losses, sudden changes, and abrupt endings as a way of life. Higher infant mortality, shorter life spans, greater morbidity from chronic illnesses, and increased risk for injury and death from violence can result in a chronic state of grief. To deal with losses, many Blacks rely on their strong spiritual and religious foundations for comfort. Grief that is defined, discussed, and supported can improve physical health and emotional well-being.

The Minority Recruitment Satellite (MRS) at the Alzheimer's Center of University Hospitals of Cleveland/Case Western Reserve University collaborated with the Nu Chi chapter of Chi Eta Phi Sorority and faith-based leaders in the Black community to produce the first *Matters of the Heart and Mind* grief workshop. The aim of the workshop is to help older Blacks cope with many types of losses in a safe, culturally sensitive environment that respects spiritual traditions. *Matters of the Heart and Mind* is a didactic presentation set in the context of a culturally appropriate spiritual experience. A panel comprised of ministers representing the six major faiths of Blacks in Cleveland discussed faith perspective on life after death, end-of-life care, and rituals or practices specific to each faith tradition in order to give participants of all faiths some insight into other religious traditions. The workshop ended with a healing circle led by a minister. Participants joined hands, honored lost or deceased loved ones by saying their names, and prayed a healing prayer. Each participant was given a starter plant to symbolize new life.

The workshop also includes information about how health, social, or functional problems create losses for individuals, families, and the community; how illness and death cause grief; how grieving differs from depression; and how to make practical end-of-life decisions. Information on mourning, religious customs, support and bereavement groups, and other services for individuals and families are provided. Breakout sessions cover topics such as visiting the dying and the grieving, leaving a legacy, estate, funeral and burial planning, and the legal issues surrounding death. In the evaluations, participants emphasized that they gained sensitivity to loss as experienced by Blacks across multiple faith perspectives.

STRATEGIES TO BRING SPIRITUALITY INTO OLDER ADULT LIVES

Those who design programs of all kinds for older persons are recognizing the importance of meeting spiritual needs as well as physical, psychological, recreational, and social needs. Having a conscious spiritual-wellness statement that has been carefully considered is an important step in accomplishing this goal. There are many approaches that senior centers can utilize to help older adults express their religious, spiritual, or social needs and find meaning or spirituality in their lives. Spiritual development activities and opportunities must be personal, practical, and relevant if they are to be maximally effective with older adults. Suggested strategies include the following:

- Provide professional and personal assistance to individuals who need direction and referrals to clergy, chaplains, or professionals when needs are beyond the staff's ability to help.
- Collaborate to provide pastor-in-residence programs or pastoral counseling on-site.
- Offer activities that allow for artistic expression, reminiscence, and meditation.
- Provide opportunities to connect with nature and appreciate the environment.
- Provide opportunities to share personal experiences individually or through a group. The sharing of personal experiences may be very helpful in resolving some distress that older persons may feel in their spiritual lives and serve as an outlet for emotions. It is always helpful to know that others have similar thoughts and experiences, similar losses, and ways of coping.
- Legacies given by an individual or collectively by a group are another approach to bringing meaning and spirituality into peoples' lives. The process of a life review has long been recognized to help older persons resolve past issues. These may be expressed via writing or taping memoirs, autobiographies, or life histories; reviewing and assembling personal photograph albums; developing family histories or genealogies; and taking trips to locations of spiritual significance.
- Conduct Bible-study classes.
- Conduct readings and discussion groups on topics such as searching for meaning and altruism.
- Offer workshops on topics such as the art of faithful aging and caregiving, and grief topics such as comforting the dying.
- Provide opportunities for vital involvement and the expectation that seniors are supposed to perform acts of deliberate and random kindness. Encourage the gift of time in service to others.
- Identify and provide information on resources for those wanting to expand their spiritual lives.
- Help older adults maintain an active interest in the development and growth of their personal talents and provide opportunities for them to exercise their talents.
- Help older adults see their bodies as deserving of the best care and maintenance that they can provide. Help them value their physical health and provide for their own physical self-care.

BIBLIOGRAPHY

Administration on Aging. (2001). Faith based services, spirituality, and aging. [On-line]. Available: www.aoa.gov/naic/notes/faithandaging.html

Auld, W. (2001). *Meaning and spirit for the last years.* [On-line]. Available: www.luthersem.edu/cars/Articles/articlethree.htm

Blazer, D. (1991). Spirituality and aging well. *Generations, 15*(1), 61–66.

Chatters, L. M., Levin, J. S., & Taylor, R. J. (1992). Antecedents and dimensions of religious involvement among older Black adults. *Journal of Gerontology: Social Sciences, 47,* S269–S278.

Clingan, D. F. (2001) *Aging: Gathering a spiritual perspective.* [On-line]. Available: www.luthersem.edu/cars/newsletters/1995/FRSTNEWS.HTM

Ebersole, P., & Hess, P. (1995). *Toward healthy aging: Human needs and nursing response* (5th ed.). St. Louis, MO: Mosby-Year Book, Inc.

Ellor, J. W. (1995). Special White House Conference edition. Mini Conference Resolutions. *Chronicle.* Center for Aging Religion & Spirituality. [On-line]. Available:www.luthersem.edu/cars/newsletters/frstnews.htm

Idler, E. L. (1987). Religious involvement and the health of the elderly: Some hypotheses and an initial test. *Social Forces, 66,* 226–238.

Idler, E. L., & Kasl, S. V. (1992). Religion, disability, depression, and the timing of death. *American Journal of Sociology, 97,* 1052–1079.

Johnson, R. P. (2002). Spiritual wellness and well-being. *Well Wise And Whole Monthly.* [On-line]. Available: www.senioradultministry.com/new_page_17.htm

McFadden, S. H. (2001). Religion, spirituality, and a good old age. *C.A.R.S. Newsletter.* [On-line]. Available: www.luthersem.edu/cars/Articles/articletwo.htm

Pittman, B. G., & Jackson Ledford, J. (2002). Senior centers respond to the changing educational interests of older Americans. *American Society on Aging.* [On-line]. Available: www.asaging.org/networks/learn/learnhome.cfm

Redd, D. (2001, Summer). Matters of the heart and mind: African American elders and grief. *Aging and Spirituality.* American Society on Aging.

Schacter-Shalomi, Z., & Miller, R. S. (1997). *From age-ing to sage-ing: A profound new vision of growing older.* New York: Warner Books.

Senior Adult Ministry. (2001). The state of senior adult ministry in the church today. *Well Wise And Whole Monthly.* [On-line]. Available: www.senioradultministry.com/new_page_18.htm

U.S. Administration on Aging, National Aging Information Center. (2001). Faith based services, spirituality, and aging. *Aging Internet information notes.* Washington DC: Author. [On-line]. Available: www.aoa.gov/naic/notes/faithandaging.html

RESOURCES

American Society on Aging (ASA)
Forum on Religion, Spirituality and Aging

833 Market Street, Suite 511
San Francisco, CA 94103-1824
415-974-9600
http://www.asaging.org/
The Forum on Religion, Spirituality and Aging explores the role of religion and spirituality in the lives of older adults. http://www.asaging.org/forsa.html

Association for Senior Adult Ministry
1714 Big Horn Basin
Wildwood, MO 63011-4819
636-273-6898
http://www.senioradultministry.com
An ecumenical organization of people working with older adults in churches and church-related organizations, the Association for Senior Adult Ministry (ASAM) publishes a monthly curriculum guide and offers a national certification in senior adult ministry.

Bureau of Primary Health Care (BPHC), Health Resources and Services Administration (HRSA)
The Faith Partnership Initiative
Center for Communities in Action
Bureau of Primary Health Care
4350 East West Highway, 3rd Floor
Bethesda, MD 20814
301-594-4494
http://bphc.hrsa.gov/faith/default.htm
The Bureau of Primary Health Care's Faith Partnership Initiative is a strategy designed to foster and build partnerships between its federally funded community health centers and faith-based organizations to increase access to quality primary and preventive health care, reduce health disparities and better coordinate health assets at the local level.

Center for Aging, Religion and Spirituality (CARS)
2481 Como Ave.
St. Paul, MN 55108-1496
651-641-3581
http://www.luthersem.edu/cars
The Center for Aging, Religion and Spirituality is an independent graduate level institution with an interfaith and multi-disciplinary ap-

proach to issues related to aging, religion and spirituality. The Center
for Aging, Religion and Spirituality provides education of religious
leaders about aging; research into religion, spirituality and aging issues;
and publication of quality research for scholarly and general reading.

The Center on Aging Studies Without Walls
University of Missouri-Kansas City
5215 Rockhill Road
Kansas City, MO 64110
816-235-1747
http://iml.umkc.edu/casww/
The Center on Aging Studies Without Walls is a joint venture between
the Center on Aging Studies at the University of Missouri-Kansas City
and University of Missouri Outreach and Extension, University of Missouri-Kansas City.

The Center for Gerontology, Spirituality and Faith
Sunny View Retirement Community
22445 Cupertino Road
Cupertino, CA 95014
408-253-4300 x67
http://www.spirituality4aging.org/
The Center for Gerontology, Spirituality and Faith is founded on the
belief that issues of spirituality and faith have central importance to
elders and people who work with them.

Faith in Action—The Robert Wood Johnson Foundation
Wake Forest University School of Medicine
Medical Center Boulevard
Winston-Salem, NC 27157-1204
336-716-0101 or 877-324-8411
http://www.fiavolunteers.org/
Faith in Action is a national volunteer movement that brings together
religious congregations from many faiths and other community organizations. Their common mission is to help people who are aging and
chronically ill maintain their independence by providing them assistance with everyday activities.

The Journal of Religious Gerontology
The Haworth Press Inc.

10 Alice St.
Binghamton, NY 13904
800-429-6784
http://bubl.ac.uk/journals/soc/jrelger/index.html
This journal offers research and information for practitioners working
with the spiritual and religious concerns of older adults.

National Council on the Aging
National Interfaith Coalition on Aging
409 Third St., SW, Suite 200
Washington, DC 20024
202-479-1200
http://www.ncoa.org/nica/nica.htm
National Interfaith Coalition on Aging is a diverse network of religious
and other related organizations and individual members which promotes the spiritual well-being of older adults and the preparation of
persons of all ages for the spiritual tasks of aging. The Coalition serves
as a catalyst for new and effective approaches to spiritual growth in aging
through research, networking opportunities, resource development,
service provision, and dissemination of information.

National Federation of Interfaith Volunteer Caregivers
One West Armour Blvd., Suite 202
Kansas City, MO 64111
816-931-5442
http://www.interfaithcaregivers.org/
That congregations of many faiths participate in a national network of
Interfaith Volunteer Caregivers programs that alleviate human suffer-
ing, enrich the human spirit, and build caring communities.

Shepherd's Centers of America
One W. Armour Blvd., Suite 201
Kansas City, MO 64111
816-960-2022 or 800-547-7073
http://www.shepherdcenters.org
Shepherd's Centers of America is an interfaith umbrella organization
that coordinates nearly 100 independent Shepherd's Centers throughout the United States. The various programs, activities and home services
of Shepherd's Centers all are built around four main emphases: life
maintenance, life enrichment, life reorganization, and celebration.

Union Theological Seminary and Presbyterian School of Christian Education
3401 Brook Road
Richmond, VA 23227
804-355-0671 or 800-229-2990
http://learn.union-psce.edu/aging/
The Union Theological Seminary and Presbyterian School of Christian Education Pastoral resources for older adults and their families. The Web site offers an annotated bibliography of over 1,500 books, articles and dissertations dealing with religion, spirituality and aging in both document and fully searchable formats.

PART SIX

Conclusion

CHAPTER TWENTY-TWO

Creating a Culture of Philanthropy

MARY

The first time I saw Mary was about 12 years ago. She was patiently sitting between her mother and brother waiting for the bell to ring for lunch. Mary had worked all her life, never married, and once retired became the caregiver for her mother and brother who had never recovered from the trauma of World War II. Their daily routine was always the same—they arrived at Vintage by bus around 9:30 a.m. and sat in the same chairs, and occasionally spoke to friends or staff until lunchtime.

Because Mary's mother, Vicky, was frail and elderly, they would enter the dining room ahead of the others and Mary would busy herself serving her mother and brother. Following lunch they would leave the center, returning home again by bus. Always the dutiful daughter, Mary had little time for herself. None of us can remember how or when we discovered that Mary had a real interest in billiards, but with the pool room a mere 50 feet from where they sat each day, it wasn't long before we convinced mother and brother that Mary would only be gone a short time and staff would always be there to help in any way. Reluctantly, Vicky agreed to this plan, and at last Mary had an opportunity for some fun.

As Vicky became even more frail, it was suggested that she be placed in Vintage's adult day care. Around the same time, Mary's brother was admitted to the local Veterans' Hospital. Suddenly, the dutiful daughter was free and she immediately began showing up in the pool room. Vintage was also in the midst of a capital campaign to purchase and renovate the property adjacent to the original building. One day Mary came to the director's office with a check for a large sum of money in appreciation for the care her mother received in adult day care. Her attorney had advised her to give some of her assets to charity and she chose Vintage. Mary was beaming with pride because she was able to help Vintage.

The old dining room where Mary had served her family daily became the new and enlarged pool room. This space was large enough to accommodate three pool tables plus a Ping-Pong table and lots of chairs for people to just hang out and relax. It didn't take long for Mary to go into full decorating mode with the help of her friend Charles. She purchased lights for both pool tables, racks for storing the cue sticks, and numerous other items to make the room comfortable. The first thing one notices upon entering the room are the hundreds of small stuffed animals hanging from the ceiling, another of Mary's contributions.

Mary arrives at Vintage every day around 10:00 in the morning and leaves around 3:30. She makes coffee first thing in the morning for everyone and is the volunteer responsible for getting all the players to sign in each day. The men have accepted Mary and the other women in the pool room, and she is clearly respected as a worthy opponent as well as a friend. Though Mary is always ready with a friendly hello if we meet her in the hallway and eager to show us a new outfit she has purchased for herself, she has little or no interest in other activities in the center.

Mary has continued to be a generous financial supporter of Vintage, providing funds for a garden in the adult day care, which is named in honor of her mother. In recognition of her generosity, the pool room has been appropriately named Mary's Pool Parlor. Vintage appreciates her generosity, at the same time realizing how important just one program can mean to ensuring and improving the quality of life for just one person.

How will senior centers fund their programs? Statistics from the New Nonprofit Almanac IN BRIEF: Facts and Figures on the Independent Sector 2001 reveal that the nonprofit sector has experienced dramatic growth in the last 10 years with 501(c)(3) organizations increasing by 74%. The total number of nonprofits grew to 1.6 million organizations in 1998 from 1.3 million in 1987. The increased competition among nonprofits for funds from government, corporations, and foundations will increase dependence on individual giving. Senior centers and other nonprofits will increasingly need to look inside for future sources of support. Fortunately, giving by individuals has grown steadily over the past 3 decades.

Gifts from individuals have consistently been the key source of contributions to nonprofit organizations. The Independent Sector report shows that individuals gave 76% of all contributions in 1997. Persons who are between the ages of 55 and 75 are more generous than any other age group. Significant gifts are usually from donors who are more than 60 years old. In addition to financial support, older persons are more likely to volunteer their time than their younger counterparts. The more directly involved in the senior center, organization, or event, the more likely they are to understand the need for charitable support.

In 1995, older people gave charitable gifts totaling $9.8 billion, primarily to churches, universities, hospitals, and medical research associations. Over the next 20 years, older people will leave between $200 billion and $400 billion to nonprofit organizations. Unfortunately, only a very small fraction of the gifts given by older individuals has gone to aging programs because the programs have not asked for these gifts.

Senior centers need funds for many different purposes and it needs individuals who will give annually. The annual fund lays the groundwork for all other fund-raising activities. The annual fund produces a large number of donors making relatively small gifts, generally through direct mail. Memorial giving programs allow people to make gifts in memory or in honor of deceased family members and friends or to recognize special occasions. Giving-clubs and other leadership giving programs help establish a healthy annual fund by providing recognition to donors at various levels. These programs develop a strong donor base from which future major donors can be identified.

A strong donor base provides more than financial support; it is a source of support from which goodwill and community interest in the center's efforts can grow. Building relationships is an essential part of effective fund-raising and senior center staff are experts at it. It is important to nurture the relationship with current donors, for they can serve as donors for years to come. Current donors can also help generate new referrals. A high priority must be placed on donor relations and creating a culture where philanthropy is perceived positively by center participants and supporters. This can be challenging in centers that receive government funding, because many seniors have adopted a philosophy of entitlement, developed years ago to get seniors to accept center services. Convincing participants that their gift is critical to the ongoing support of the center will take time and effort but it is time well spent. Not only does giving contribute to well-being, but it can also increase pride and sense of ownership of the senior center.

Planned gifts are another important resource that senior centers need to capitalize on. A planned gift is a deferred gift that is legally provided for during a donor's lifetime, but whose principal benefits do not accrue to the recipient until a later date, typically upon the death of the donor. Bequests are growing, increasing almost 1000% since

1967. Bequests are popular because of the tax benefits and because many wealthy people hold onto their wealth while they are living for the status, prestige, and security it provides. Likely prospects for planned gifts include current donors, board members, and senior center partici- pants. Recent studies suggest that more people are starting some form of gift planning and at younger ages than previously. Good cultivation processes can help identify donors who are willing to consider planned gifts, even when an outright cash or securities gift is not feasible.

DONOR CULTIVATION

Organizations needs to be committed to learning about donor interests and improving the donor experience. All employees and volunteers should be educated about their role in cultivating philanthropic sup- port. Giving a gift should be an enjoyable and rewarding experience. Donors must feel that making a gift, regardless of its size, is handled so well and so reliably that it is enjoyable. At every turn donors should know that they are important and held in high regard. Donor clubs can be used as mechanisms to provide special donor services to the most loyal and generous donors. Major donors who choose your organization should be told how deeply their partnership and support are appreci- ated. They should be thanked quickly, accurately, publicly, privately, frequently, creatively, appropriately, and gratefully.

The Independent Sector national survey of characteristics of those who gave and volunteered in the past year helps identify those who are more likely to give to charity. Those who attended religious services contributed a higher percentage of their average household income than those who did not attend (2.3% compared with 1.3%). Respon- dents 75 years and older gave nearly 5% of their household income; many had low incomes and were contributing from accumulated wealth. Retirees reported giving a higher than average proportion of their household income to charitable causes. College graduates reported the highest participation of all groups, giving an average of 2% of their household income. Eighty-one percent of households contributed when asked. As the level of household income increased, more households reported making a contribution. Most households make gifts from their income rather than from their wealth. Respondents were twice as likely to contribute when asked to give by someone they knew well.

People who volunteer are the most likely to donate and they are more likely to be generous than nonvolunteers. According to the Independent Sector, 84% of all charitable contributions were given by households that also volunteered. A senior center's most important asset is a volunteer base that will take the first step by giving themselves and then take the senior center's case to potential donors. Informed volunteer solicitors, who know the senior center's story and can tell it with their own story, are keys to successful fund-raising.

Each person gives for a different reason. People will give if they are motivated by a reason that is personally significant. A survey of more than 200 affluent persons who had given $50,000 or more to a single nonprofit was conducted by Russ Prince and Karen File. They describe seven major donor types and their motivations for giving in their book *The Seven Faces of Philanthropy*.

- The *communitarian* (more than 25%) is devoted to a place; helping the community reinforces businesses relationships; doing good makes sense. The communitarian expects individual attention from the charity as a condition of the gift.
- The *devout* (21%) gives primarily to religious institutions. Doing good is God's will.
- The *investor* (15%) bases decisions on financial motives, preferring charities that operate efficiently and effectively. Doing good is good business.
- The *socialites* (11%) must see that they have a direct impact through charitable giving. Doing good is fun.
- The *repayer* (10%) makes a charitable gift in gratitude for care received or because of a life-changing situation. Doing good in return.
- The *altruist* (9%) gives because doing good feels right. The altruist expects individual attention, consideration, and thoughtfulness, not special treatment.
- The *dynast* (8%) is very wealthy and gives to address community needs and societal problems. Doing good is a family tradition.

In a survey of families with net worths of more than $5 million, the most important motivating factor to give more is finding a cause they feel passionate about. Another survey of 1,000 donors conducted by Fidelity Investments Charitable Gift Fund in 1999 found that more than 90% agreed that giving makes them feel good and that their giving makes a difference to the causes they support.

WOMEN IN PHILANTHROPY

There are gender differences in giving, as well. Women give as a personal response to need, to make a difference, for personal satisfaction, and to organizations with which they are personally involved. Men give for recognition, for networking, for practical or business reasons, and because it is traditional.

Women represent a growing source of volunteer fund-raising leadership and major gifts. They have the passion and concern for the future that motivates philanthropists. Through philanthropy, women have begun to see their potential to help solve problems and create a better environment for future generations. Their clout is greater now because they are better educated, increasingly independent, and more affluent than ever before. They have risen in the ranks of the professional and business communities and gained control over their own wealth. Just 30 years ago, women owned less than 5% of American businesses. Today, more than 40% are owned by women, and it is estimated that women hold more than half the wealth in the United States.

Focus groups conducted by Martha Taylor and Sondra Shaw have found that women's motivations for giving can be summarized in six words: create, change, connect, collaborate, and celebrate. Women like to *create* new projects. They respond positively to programs they believe would effect societal *change*. Women want to *connect* to the programs they support. They will *commit* to serve as volunteer leaders. Women want to *collaborate* with others so that their contributions have a greater impact. Women noted that they liked to *celebrate* their accomplishments. They also found that women who are major donors expected accountability from the nonprofits they support. They want to be acknowledged personally for their gifts and receive information about how their gifts were used and how they helped. Women need details about a project before making a decision

BABY BOOMERS

The baby boom generation is entering its peak earning years and peak giving years. As they mature, boomers have demonstrated a commitment to philanthropy that outpaces other age groups. They are likely to become even more generous as they grow older and more affluent. Baby boomers are predicted to inherit $10 trillion in the next 30 years—

the largest transfer of wealth ever. They represent a potential source of gifts as future participants and caregivers of elderly parents.

Studies examining boomer interests show that they favor local over national organizations and they prefer to keep their funds in the community, often seeking out the hottest causes to support. Target baby boomers by cultivating relationships and gaining their trust. Provide boomers with practical information and the clear benefits of their philanthropy because they are information gatherers. Organizational reputation, integrity, cost-effectiveness, and efficiency are important to them, and they demand greater accountability from the charities they donate to. They also expect to be cultivated extensively.

DIVERSITY AND PHILANTHROPY

The National Society of Fundraising Executives' fund-raising dictionary defines diversity as the quality or state of being different; and the quality or state of encompassing people of a different race, ethnicity, gender, religion, physical ability, age, sexual orientation, and income. A key task for successful fund-raisers who are working in diverse environments is to understand these differences and use this knowledge to raise funds more effectively.

Today's typical donor is White, 55 to 64 years old, married or widowed, and generally predictable in response to fund-raising appeals. According to the Independent Sector, in 1999 more than 70% of households contributed to charity and the average contribution represented 2.2% of household income. Seventy-five percent of White households, 52% of Black households, and 63% of Hispanic households contribute to charities. The profile of tomorrow's donor will change, given that Whites are projected to be the largest segment of the U.S. population only through the first third of this century. It is important to understand the giving traditions of minority groups, especially Blacks, Hispanics, and Asian Americans, and create fund-raising strategies that recognize those traditions. Take the opportunity to ask relationship-building questions about traditions and observances. Increased giving among minority groups will reflect the extent to which effective new strategies have been created.

Diversify the funding base and the organization's leadership by looking deeper into the community for people who have never been approached about giving and to reach new constituencies. Look among business owners, professionals, executives, and others who are "on the rise" as resources that can lead to future major gifts.

FUND-RAISING MANAGEMENT

Donors who are engaged in an organization, committed to its cause, and loyal to its mission will continue to give and recruit new advocates for the organization as long as the organization provides good stewardship and accountability. Successful fund-raising organizations apply sound principles of fund-raising management and stewardship, including a compelling mission and a clearly stated case for support. Organizations that have a strong case for support are in position to attract the gifts needed. Fund-raising and development should be integrated into the organization's overall management process.

The organization must communicate and demonstrate that it provides critical services to at-risk populations. The case for support must document the needs that are to be addressed and construct a logical plan to meet those needs. The case for support should answers questions like the following:

- how the senior center or project helps older people and the community—how lives are changed
- what vital services are provided
- the track record of the organization
- future plans
- why the agency merits support

The Internet is another important medium to educate the public about the work of nonprofits and stimulate giving and volunteering. A Web site enables potential donors to use the Web to find out information about the senior center. It should include information on how to donate to the organization. As those seniors surfing the Web are more likely to be affluent and college educated, they make good donor prospects.

SUGGESTED ACTIVITIES

- recognition societies
- recognition gifts

- donor events
- educational programs for philanthropists
- financial-planning workshops featuring charitable giving options
- profiling major donors in newsletters and annual reports

BIBLIOGRAPHY

American Association of Fund-Raising Council Trust for Philanthropy. (1998). *Giving USA 1998. The annual report on philanthropy for the year 1997*. New York: Author.
American Association of Fund-Raising Council Trust for Philanthropy. (2001). *Giving USA Update*. Issue 2. New York: Author.
Hart, T. R. (1996, December). Putting the donor first. *Fund Raising Management*, 20–24.
Independent Sector. (1999). *Giving and volunteering in the United States. 1999 National Survey*. Washington, DC: Author.
Independent Sector. (2001). *The new nonprofit almanac in brief: Facts and figures on the independent sector 2001*.Washington, DC: Author. [On-line]. Available: www.indepsec.org
Jewish Healthcare Foundation. (1999, November). Raising the value of health philanthropy. *Branches*. Pittsburgh, PA: Author.
Kaminski, A., & Taylor, M. A. (1998, Spring). Barriers to giving/motivations for giving. *AHP Journal, 10*.
Kaminski, A., & Taylor, M. A. (1998, Spring). Women in philanthropy. *AHP Journal*, 5–12.
Kirkman, K. (1995, September). Thanks again and again. *Case Currents*, 38–40.
Marchetti, D. (1999, July 15). Most Americans made a gift to charity in past two years. *The Chronicle of Philanthropy*.
National Society of Fundraising Executives. (1996). *The NSFRE Fund-Raising Dictionary*. Alexandria, VA: Author.
Precourt, P. (1999, Spring). 'You're not from around here, are you?' Working across cultural boundaries. *Advancing Philanthropy*, 12–17.
Prince, R. A., & File, K. M. (1994). *The seven faces of philanthropy. A new approach to cultivating major donors*. San Francisco, CA: Jossey-Bass.
Resnik, R., Hudson, M., Carnell, P., Woodward, L., Quinn, J., & Krause, D. (1999, October 6). *Targeting baby boomers: Turning the next generation of wealth holders into philanthropists*. Presentation at the Association for Healthcare Philanthropy International Conference, San Diego, CA.
Scott, M. Building strong relationships. Advancing philanthropy. *Journal of the National Society of Fundraising Executives*, 47–48.
Singletary, P. (1999, Spring). Diversity. Challenge or opportunity? Advancing philanthropy. *Journal of the National Society of Fundraising Executives*, 8–9.
Snyder, A. A. (1993). *Senior center fund-raising: A technical assistance guide for providers of services to the aging*. Washington, DC: The National Council on the Aging.

Stelter, L. (2001, Spring). Silver surfers. Can you afford to ignore seniors on the Web? *AHP Journal*, 10–12.

Thompson-Haas, A. (1999, Fall). Using pyschographics to prepare for the 21st century. Understanding tomorrow's 'ideal' donor. *AHP Journal*, 19–22.

Von Schlegell, A., & Hickey, K. (1993, Winter). Women as donors: The hidden constituency. Advancing philanthropy. *Journal of the National Society of Fundraising Executives*. Reprint.

Whitley, F. V., & Staples, P. (1997, August). Womenpower: The growing factor in gifts fund raising in the decade ahead. *Fund Raising Management*, 14–18.

RESOURCES

American Association of Fund-Raising Council Trust for Philanthropy
25 West 43rd Street
New York, NY 10036
212-354-5799
http://www.aafrc.org
American Association of Fund-Raising Council Trust for Philanthropy advances research, education, and public understanding of philanthropy. Publishes *Giving USA*, the annual report on philanthropy.

Association for Healthcare Philanthropy (AHP)
313 Park Avenue, Suite 400
Falls Church, VA 22046
703-532-6243
www.go-ahp.org
The Association for Healthcare Philanthropy is dedicated exclusively to advancing and promoting the health care development profession.

Association for Fundraising Professionals (AFP)
1101 King Street Suite 700
Alexandria, VA 22314
703-684-0540
http://www.afpnet.org
The Association of Fundraising Professionals works to advance philanthropy through advocacy, research, education, and certification programs. (Formerly the National Society of Fund Raising Executives.)

Association of Professional Researchers for Advancement (APRA)
414 Plaza Drive, Suite 209

Westmont, IL 60559
630-655-0177
http://www.aprahome.org/
The Association of Professional Researchers for Advancement promotes standards that enhance the expertise of its members who conduct development research and prospect information management.

BBB Wise Giving Alliance
4200 Wilson Boulevard, Suite 800
Arlington, VA 22203
http://www.give.org
BBB Wise Giving Alliance is a merger of the National Charities Information Bureau and the Council of Better Business Bureaus' Foundation and its Philanthropic Advisory Service, CBBB Standards for Charitable Solicitations.

Canadian Centre for Philanthropy
425 University Avenue, Suite 700
Toronto, ON M5G 1T6
416-597-2293
http://www.ccp.ca/
The Canadian Centre for Philanthropy is a national charitable organization dedicated to advancing the role and interests of the charitable sector for the benefit of Canadian communities.

Chronicle of Philanthropy
1255 23rd Street, NW, Suite 700
Washington, DC 20037
202-466-1200
http://philanthropy.com/
A newspaper for the nonprofit world, its web site includes news summaries, job listings, and announcement of upcoming conferences and workshops.

The Evergreen State Society
Post Office Box 20682
Seattle, WA 98102-0682
206-329-5640
http://nonprofits.org/
The Internet Nonprofit Center, the Nonprofit Locator, the Library, and the Form 990 Project are projects of The Evergreen State Society.

The Evergreen State Society is a Seattle-based nonprofit organization addressing policy issues and management questions in order to strengthen the nonprofit sector in Washington state and beyond.

Foundation Center
79 Fifth Avenue/16th Street
New York, NY 10003-3076
212-620-4230 or 800-424-9836
http://fdncenter.org/
The Foundation Center provides print, CD-ROM, and online resources to help grantseekers identify appropriate funders and develop targeted proposals.

Independent Sector
1200 Eighteenth Street, NW, Suite 200
Washington, DC 20036
http://www.indepsec.org/
The Independent Sector is a national leadership forum fostering private initiative for the public good. Publishes books, pamphlets, and videos for nonprofits.

Indiana University Center on Philanthropy
The Center on Philanthropy at Indiana University
317-274-4200
The Fund Raising School
317-684-8933 or 800-962-6692
550 W. North St., #301
Indianapolis, IN 46202-3272
http://www.philanthropy.iupui.edu/
The Center on Philanthropy at Indiana University offers a masters of arts in philanthropic studies. Its mission is to increase the understanding of philanthropy through research, teaching and public service.

National Center for Charitable Statistics
2100 M St. NW
Washington, DC 20037
202-261-5801
http://nccs.urban.org/
The National Center for Charitable Statistics is the national repository of data on the nonprofit sector in the United States. Its mission is to

develop and disseminate high quality data on nonprofit organizations and their activities for use in research on the relationships between the nonprofit sector, the government, the commercial sector, and the broader civil society.

National Center for Nonprofit Boards
1828 L Street NW, Suite 900
Washington, DC 20036-5114
http://www.ncnb.org/main.htm
202-452-6262 or 800-883-6262
Provides board development services, satellite workshops, an annual leadership conference and books, videos, audio tapes, and periodicals concerning nonprofit governance.

National Committee on Planned Giving®
233 McCrea Street, Suite 400
Indianapolis, IN 46225
317-269-6274
http://www.ncpg.org
The National Committee on Planned Giving® is a professional association for people whose work includes developing, marketing, and administering charitable planned gifts.

Nonprofit Resource Center
http://not-for-profit.org/
Provides a comprehensive list of links to Web sites of interest to nonprofits.

The Prospect Research Page
David Lamb
1710 Stagecoach Road
Grand Island, NE 68801
308-398-1856
http://www.lambresearch.com/
A list of helpful prospect research resources compiled by consultant, David Lamb.

CHAPTER TWENTY-THREE

Looking Ahead

Senior centers are a source of vital, community-based social, nutrition, and health-promotion programs that help millions of older adults and their families bridge the gap between full independence and limited support. Funding for the Older Americans Act's supportive services and senior center programs has failed to keep pace with inflation or with the rapidly growing older population, especially the 85-plus population for whom home- and community-based assistance are essential. Strong government programs are absolutely essential if seniors with modest incomes are to get the help they need to age successfully. Senior centers must work to preserve and strengthen the government programs upon which so many older adults rely.

The senior center network also needs to be strengthened at the national, state, and local levels. Only the National Institute of Senior Centers (NISC) of the National Council on the Aging is dedicated to senior centers. Some states do have senior center associations or senior-center-directors associations. These have been successful in providing educational and networking opportunities for senior center staff; advocacy at the state and local level for funding, recognition, and support; linkages with aging and other state and local departments such as mental health; and galvanizing older adults to advocate on their own behalf. Pennsylvania Senior Centers has its own Web site, an initiative of the state Senior Center Joint Committee of the Pennsylvania Association of Senior Centers and the Pennsylvania Association of Area Agencies on Aging. The Web site was developed with funding from the Pennsylvania Department of Aging. The primary purpose of the site is to provide Pennsylvania's senior centers with opportunities to exchange information and ideas on topics of vital interest. Through the Web site, Pennsylvania senior centers have a way of sharing their wealth of ideas and successes with other centers throughout the state.

Part of the solution to meeting the diverse and unmet needs of older persons is to make better use of untapped resources, especially senior centers. Senior centers are not adequately recognized nor are they developed and utilized to their full potential. Many senior centers provide a limited range of services because they lack the staffing, funding, and resources to be the best they can be.

If senior centers focus on the failure of traditional funding sources to keep up with the needs of older adults, they will become an increasingly marginal part of the inevitable boom in aging services. Those centers that embrace the opportunities to tap into new revenue sources and greatly expand services and programs will be successful in the future. NCOA's 2001 a National Survey of Health and Supportive Services in the Aging Network found that high-quality programs in the study made extensive use of partnerships and cost-sharing to leverage funding and meet client needs. The study also identified training and technical assistance as barriers to expansion and targeted several areas for development:

- Accessibility—motivating hard-to-reach older adults to participate; marketing through the mass media
- Self-care—improving clients skills in self-care
- Funding—engaging the broader community to meet funding needs
- Outcomes—measuring change in health status and health behaviors

James Firman, president and chief executive officer of the National Council on the Aging, believes the aging network and the organizations that comprise it are paralyzed by a pervasive and powerful belief that there are not enough resources and they are frustrated by the constant struggle to raise funds to meet needs. Firman believes that "struggling to stay afloat" will continue to be the dominant reality for organizations that do not shift the perceptions that impede their ability to succeed.

Senior centers must diversify their revenue sources. James Firman identified at least ten potential revenue sources aging programs could tap into:

1. *Expand private pay programs*, such as fees for computer classes and services for caregivers. Don't ignore the needs of seniors who have resources to spend. Organizations that focus exclusively or pri-

marily on low-income seniors will find their options for growth severely limited. Private-pay clients can strengthen an organization financially and enhance its ability to serve low-income seniors. People who pay for things themselves often demand improvements in services and programs that eventually benefit all participants of all income levels. A survey of members of the National Institute of Senior Centers about fee practices found that most currently charge fees for some of their services. Several of those who do not charge fees said they are not permitted to do so because they are government agencies. Yet even those senior centers that are only partially government-funded have struggled to implement fees for services because of government restrictions or rigid interpretations at the local level. The most commonly mentioned services that fees are collected for are home-delivered and congregate meals, adult day services, exercise classes, and transportation. Fees can help boost attendance because the participant makes a commitment by paying a fee. Requiring prepayment for some programs allows program managers to better plan and deliver existing services or add new ones. Charging fees also helps subsidize or provide scholarships for those who can't afford to pay for activities. NISC members believe that fees are part of the future because of financial pressures and the need for independence from shrinking funding sources. They also said fees help ensure quality programs and guarantee that key services are available to all seniors, regardless of income. Charging a fee can increase the perceived value of a service or program, making it more desirable to certain segments of the older population.

2. *Help older adults identify strategies to increase their income.* Ensure that seniors, especially those with low incomes, take advantage of all of the federal, state, and local benefits to which they are entitled.

3. *Request bequests and donations.* Institute a charitable planned-giving program.

4. *Tap into Medicare, Medicaid, and managed care.* Community support services can help improve chronic care outcomes, keep older people out of hospitals and nursing homes, and save a great deal of money for managed care companies and for the government. By enhancing current services, such as home safety checks, medication compliance services, blood pressure monitoring, and health-promotion and disease-prevention services, aging programs could tap into these revenue sources. The challenge is to learn how to target these services in ways that will produce cost-effective results and generate the evaluation data that prove the value of these services.

5. *Apply for foundation and government grants.* Government grants for behavioral and social research are an excellent yet largely untapped source of revenue. There is a mistaken belief that the philanthropic activities of foundations are decreasing but foundation-giving is actually growing. Learn to use grants to transform organizations and tap into other more sustainable sources of support.

6. *Identify corporate partners.* Be aware of all the opportunities that aging programs have to affiliate and work with the private sector. Companies spend billions of dollars developing and marketing services and products to older people. Besides charitable contributions, there are many other sources of corporate support potentially available through other departments of companies, including their marketing, human resources, and R&D departments. Staff expertise and knowledge can be used to help companies do a better job of reaching and serving older people. Corporate marketing departments can support education efforts on issues related to the services and products the company offers. Human resource departments need help in meeting the eldercare needs of their employees and retirees. The R&D departments need help in developing better services and products.

7. *Identify new volunteers.* The volunteer labor of millions of Americans, including those of older adults, is another largely untapped potential resource. Volunteers not only help defray labor costs, but they are also more likely to give donations to the organizations they volunteer with.

8. *Implement creative fund raisers.* Fund-raising events can be a major source of revenue and can also increase the organization's visibility in the community, lead to new partners, and produce new clients.

9. *Develop strategic alliances* with other nonprofit organizations, both inside and outside the aging field. Strategic alliances can result in better services to clients and improved bottom lines and enable both organizations to focus more on the activities they do best and eliminate duplication of effort. They can make it possible to tap into revenue streams that would otherwise be unavailable to them. Community-based organizations serving older persons need to organize themselves into effective networks if they are to thrive.

10. *Utilize the Internet* as a strategy to increase program resources. For example, funding sources can be researched and applied for online. Web sites can attract a new generation of participants and donors.

Senior centers are in the successful-aging business, helping older people to maintain maximum health, independence, and fulfillment. If senior centers can prove that they can achieve these outcomes, they will be well positioned to sit at the table with public and private partners and negotiate significant new revenue streams. Anecdotal stories, like those featured in this book, abound, of how senior centers have benefited older adults. Longitudinal studies that follow senior center participants have been lacking. Though the evidence mounts that the services provided by senior centers (socialization, education, health promotion, I&R, meals, etc.) contribute to successful aging, there is a lack of data proving the effectiveness of senior centers on the lives of participants. Such "proof" could help senior centers with their funding needs.

BIBLIOGRAPHY

Firman, J. (2001). Scarcity or abundance? An update. Practical strategies for achieving organizational prosperity. *Innovations, 1.* National Council on the Aging. [On-line]. Available: www.ncoa.org/publications/inno1_01/firman01.html

Joyce, E. (2001). *Scarcity or abundance. Stronger programs through fees for services.* Washington, DC: National Council on the Aging. [On-line]. Available: www.ncoa.org/publications/innovations/abundance/fees_for_services.htm

The National Council on the Aging, Inc. (2001). *A national survey of health and supportive services in the aging network.* Washington, DC: Author. [On-line]. Available: www.ncoa.org/research/cbo.html

National Council on the Aging. (2001, June). Older Americans act appropriations. Supportive services. *NCOA Issue Brief.* Washington, DC: Author.

RESOURCES

Alliance for Aging Research
2021 K Street, NW, Suite 305
Washington, DC 20006
202-293-2856
http://www.agingresearch.org/
The Alliance for Aging Research is dedicated to improving he health and independence of Americans as they age through public and private funding of medical research and geriatric education.

American Federation for Aging Research (AFAR)
1414 Avenue of the Americas, 18th floor

New York, NY 10019
212-752-2327
http://www.afar.org/
http://www.infoaging.org/
The American Federation for Aging Research supports both basic and clinical biomedical research into aging and age-related diseases to promote healthier aging.

Grantmakers in Aging
5335 Far Hills Avenue, Suite 220
Dayton, OH 45429
937-435-3156
http://www.giaging.org/
Grantmakers in Aging is an educational nonprofit membership organization for staff and trustees of foundations and corporations, is the only national professional organization of grantmakers active in the field of aging.

Pennsylvania Association of Senior Centers
c/o Info to Go
5912 Ricky Ridge Trail
Orefield, PA 18069
http://www.paseniorcenters.org/

Pioneer Network
1900 South Clinton Avenue
PO Box 18648
Rochester, NY 14618
716-244-8400 ext. 115
http://www.pioneernetwork.net/
The Pioneer Network is a national resource center for changing the culture of aging in America. The Pioneer Network seeks to identify and promote innovative transformations in practice, services, public policy and research being developed around the country.

Retirement Research Foundation
8765 W. Higgins Road, Suite 430
Chicago, IL 60631-4170
773-714-8080

http://www.rrf.org/
The Retirement Research Foundation is the nation's largest private
foundation devoted solely to serving the needs of older Americans and
supporting efforts in aging-related research and improve the care of
the elderly.

Afterword

On September 11, 2001, as we worked to complete this book and send it to the publisher, America's heart was torn apart. Using American planes filled with innocent passengers as missiles, terrorists flew into the World Trade Center and the Pentagon. A fourth plane, diverted by heroic passengers, crashed in Somerset County, 80 miles southeast of Pittsburgh.

The following Friday a service was held at Vintage as part of the National Day of Remembrance and Prayer. Well over 150 people were in attendance. I want to share this with you because so many of the people whose stories appear in this book were an integral part of the program, and they were cast on that day in roles similar to the roles they play each day at Vintage.

- Annette marshaled her troops, calling more than 40 people on Thursday, not inviting them to come, but telling them they must attend, and of course they did!
- Michael agreed to play the piano, as his hands were feeling somewhat better. He, along with two choral groups, led us in singing songs from "God Bless America" to "Amazing Grace."
- Sidney led us in a responsive reading, parts of which were written by Thomas Jefferson and Abraham Lincoln.
- Jay, as president of house council, lighted three memorial candles for all the people who had died as a result of the terrorist attack and he lit the unity candle for our country.
- Helen, in a green polyester dress and white blouse, joined Albert in one of the two choral groups.
- George provided several large American flags that he had painted in the art studio, which were proudly hung on the walls in the auditorium.
- Cheryl read scripture and Paula led us all in singing the "Star-Spangled Banner."

- "Smokey" Joe's son, our state representative, spoke and thanked Vintage for being such a special place for his dad. He encouraged us to remain steadfast in the days ahead.
- Jayne and Ruth handed out programs and red-white-and-blue ribbons.

Vintage, as well as other senior centers across the country, would be nothing but brick and mortar if it were not for the hundreds of thousands of older adults who come for the services, the programs, and as has been the case these past few days, for the support.

In writing their stories for this book there was a common thread that was woven among their tales, and it is that we are indeed a family. Never was that more true than on September 14, 2001.

Index

Academic/technical level, in creativity, 97
Access-Able Travel Source, LLC, 223
Accreditation, 7
Acculturation, 30
Acting classes, 122–123
Activities:
  arts, 103–138
  computers, 139–152
  health promotion, 153–174
  horticulture, 175–188
  humanities, 189–197
  intergenerational programs, 198–218
  physical fitness, 153–174
  travel, 219–223
Activities of daily living (ADLs), 26, 314–315, 317–319
Activity specialists, 177
Administration for Children and Families, 268
Adult day services, 6
Adult learners, see Lifelong learning programs
  interests of, 70–72
  language learners, 70–72
  learning styles, 75–79
  multiple intelligences, 75–79
Adventure-travel services, 37
Advocacy assistance, 6, 232
Aerobic exercise, 161
AgeLight LLC, 150

Age Power: How the 21st Century Will Be Ruled by the New Old (Dychtwald), 36
Age segregation, 199–200
Aggressive behavior, 178
Aging population, growth in, 293. See also Aging population profile; Older adult needs
Aging population profile:
  cultural diversity, 30–32
  disability, 25–26
  education, 24–25
  ethnic population, 21–22
  generational differences, 28–30
  health status, 25–26
  income, 23
  life expectancy, 26–27
  living arrangements, 22–23
  marital status, 22
  poverty, 23
  racial population, 21–22
  sexual orientation, 27–28
  socioeconomic status, 23–24
Aging process, generally:
  negative perceptions of, 93
  sedentary lifestyle and, 154, 159
  success factors, 8–11
  vision loss and, 272
Aging with Dignity, 332
AIDS, 28, 301, 317
Ailing outgoers, defined, 40
AIRS/INFO Line Taxonomy of Human Services, 233

Albert, Marilyn, 11
Alcohol abuse, 27. *See also* Substance abuse
Alcoholism, 303–304
Allegheny East Mental Health/Mental Retardation, 306
Alliance for Aging Research, 368
Alliance for Information and Referral System (AIRS), 229, 237–238
Alliance for Technology Access, 142
Alliance for Technology Success, 151
Alliance of Information and Referral Systems, 234
Altruist, defined, 355
Alzheimer Center of University Hospitals of Cleveland/Case Western Reserve University, Minority Recruitment Satellite (MRS), 341
Alzheimer's Association, 107, 307–308
Alzheimer's disease, 296–297, 300, 306, 317
Alzheimer's Disease Education and Referral Center (ADEAR), 308
American Antiquarian Society, 194
American Art Therapy Association (AATA), 124–125
American Association for Geriatric Psychiatry, The, 308
American Association of Fund-Raising Council Trust for Philanthropy, 360
American Association of Museums, 191
American Association of Retired Persons (AARP):
    Andrus Foundation, 209
    caregiving, 315
    functions of, 23, 71, 87, 107, 143, 150–151, 162, 332
    Grandparent Information Center, 251
    grandparenting survey, 243–244
    Widowed Persons Service program, 331
American Association on Mental Retardation (AAMR), 255

American Community Gardening Association, 185–186
American Federation for Aging Research (AFAR), 368–369
American Folklife Center, 1235
American Foundation for the Blind (AFB), 287
American Geriatrics Society, 45
American history, *see* Humanities
American Horticultural Society, The, 186
American Horticultural Therapy Association, 186
American Library Association, 211
American Life Project, 144
American Music Therapy Association, Inc. (AMTA), 125
American Psychological Association, Division of Adult Development and Aging, 308
American Self-Help Clearinghouse, 238
Americans for the Arts, 125
American Society on Aging (ASA), 45, 332, 343–344
American Speech-Language-Hearing Association (ASHA), 287
Amigos del Valle, 125–126
Andragogy, 72–75
Anticipatory caregiver, 326
Anxiety, 159
Anxiety disorders, 298
Apathy, 300
Aphasia, 285–286
Appalshop, 119, 126
Appetite changes, implications of, 298
Apprenticeships, 37
Arboreta, 183
Arc of the United States, The, 268
Art & Humanities Resource Center for Older Adults (AHRC), 126
ArtAge Publications, 126
Art therapy, 116
Arthritis, 26, 155
Arthritis Foundation, The, 171
Arts:

and aging programs, 118–121
art therapy, 116
audience attendance statistics,
    109–110
benefits of, 107
creative writing, 117
folk art, 113–114, 121–122
information resources, 124–138
involving older adults, 121
music therapy, 114–115
participation in, 108–112
performing arts, 112–113
public policy on, 107–108
quilting, 114–116
significance of, case illustrations,
    103–106
suggested activities, 117–118,
    121–123
Arts and crafts programs, 121–122, 181
Arts Council of Oklahoma City, The,
    119, 126
Arts for the Aging, Inc. (AFTA),
    126–127
Arts Midwest, 127
Artswatch, 120, 127
Assisted Living Federation of America,
    332
Assistive devices, 328
Associated Writing Programs, 127
Association for Fundraising Profession-
    als (AFP), 360
Association for Healthcare Philan-
    thropy (AHP), 360
Association for Research on Nonprofit
    Organizations and Voluntary Ac-
    tion (ARNOVA), 58
Association for Senior Adult Ministry,
    344
Association for the Study of African
    American Life and History, 194
Association for Volunteer Administra-
    tion (AVA), 58
Association of Professional Researchers
    for Advancement (APRA),
    360–361
Asthma, 157

Auditory training, 275
Autobiographies, 94–95, 342
Autonomy issues, 261

Baby-boom generation:
    aging of, 21
    arts participation, 108–112
    characteristics of, generally, 7, 23,
        29–30
    philanthropy and, 356–357
    recreational activities, 65
    substance abuse, 303–304
    travel, 220–221
Baby busters, 109
Ballet, 110
Baseball, 167
Batesville Area Arts Council, 127–128
BBB Wise Giving Alliance, 361
BenefitsCheck*Up*, 238
Bequests, 353–354, 366
Bereavement:
    dealing with, 301–302
    programs, 325
*Best Practices: Health Promotion and
    Aging,* 165
Bible-study classes, 342
Bilingual staff, 31–32
Bipolar disorder, 292, 298
Birdwatching, 37
Bisexual persons, 27
Blindness, *see* Visual impairments
Bodily-kinesthetic intelligence, 77
Body language, 285
Boom, Bust and Echo 2000 (Foot),
    36–37
Botanical gardens, 183
Bown, Denise, 325
Brain cells:
    creativity process and, 93
    growth of, 10
Bridging, 86
Brookdale Center of Aging, intergener-
    ational programs:
    as information resource, 211–212
    model of, 206

Brookdale Foundation Group, The, 251
Bureau of Primary Health Care (BPHC), Health Resources and Services Administration (HRSA), The Faith Partnership Initiative, 344
Byrock, Ira, 325

Camping, 65
Canadian Association for Music Therapy, 128
Canadian Centre for Philanthropy, 361
Canadian Horticultural Therapy Association (CHTA), 186–187
Cancer, 158, 301
Cardiovascular disease, 300
Caregiver:
  in loss, 327
Caregiver(s), *see* Caregiving
  at-risk, 323–324
  counseling services, 323, 327, 330
  defined, 315
  family as, 315–316
  grandparent-grandchild relationship, 245–246, 248–249
  help for, 317
  in loss, 327
  of mentally impaired, 294
  needs, 325–327
  resource center/library, 329
  secondary, 319
  stress, 316–317
  support groups, 323, 327, 330
Caregiving:
  case illustration, 312–314
  cognitive impairments, 317–318
  educational programs, 328–329
  effects of, 42–43, 320–324
  end-of-life care, 324–325
  family as caregivers, 315–319
  formal, 320, 324
  incidence of, 314–315
  informal care, 318–320, 324
  information and referral services, 329

information resources, 331–334
  long-distance care, 315–316
  opportunities for senior centers, 327–330
  outreach programs, 329
  preventive health care, 328
  rewards of, 321–322
Caregiving Boom, 327
Careguide, Inc., 332
Carpeting, safety guidelines, 283
Carstensen, Laura, PhD, 9
Cataracts, 26, 272
Center Care Program, 262–263
Center for Aging, Religion and Spirituality (CARS), 344–345
Center for Gerontology, Spirituality and Faith, The, 345
Center in the Park, 119, 128
Center on Aging, Health & Humanities, The, 194–195
Center on Aging Studies Without Walls, The, 345
Centers for Disease Control and Prevention (CDC), 158, 164, 171
Ceramics, 123
Cerebrovascular disease, 155
Charles Schwab & Co., 144
Chicago Botanic Garden, 187
CHIPS (Computers for Homebound and Isolated Persons), 146, 151
Cholesterol levels, 160, 256
Choral groups, 122
Chronic disease, 155, 158
Chronicle for Philanthropy, 361
Cigarette smoking, 27, 160
Cincinnati Opera Outreach Program, 126
CineSol Latino Film Festival, 119
City Farmer, Canada's Office of Urban Agriculture, 187
City Lore: The New York Center for Urban Folk Culture, 128
Closing the Digital Divide, 151–152
Cognitive impairment, 10, 317–318
Cohen, Gene, 94
College for Seniors programs, 134

Colon cancer, 158
Communication skills, 178
Communication strategies:
  aphasia and, 285–286
  hearing impaired, 284–285
  importance of, 31–32
  visually impaired, 283–284
Communication techniques, cognitive
  impairment and, 317
Communitarians, defined, 355
Community activism, 95
Community awareness, 202
Community-based services, 5
Community gardens, 183–185
Community integration, developmental disabilities, 258
Complementary and alternative medicine (CAM), 166–167, 172–173
Compulsive behavior, 179
Computers:
  case illustration, 139–140
  cost factors, 142–143
  digital inclusion statistics, 141–142,
    145–146
  e-mail, 144–146
  implementation suggestions,
    146–148
  information resources, 142, 150–152
  internet use, 143–144
  participation and use of, 140–141,
    144–145
  suggested activities, 148–148
Congregate meals, 366
Conservatories, 222
Consortium for Pacific Arts & Cultures, 128
Consumer behavior, 35
Container gardening, 176
Continuing education programs, 37
Coping mechanisms, 96
Coping skills, 178, 299, 322, 337
Cornea, scars on, 272
Cornell University Applied Gerontology Research Institute, model in-
  tergenerational programs,
  206–207

Coronary artery disease, 155, 160
Coronary heart disease, 158
Corporate partnerships, 367
Council for Adult and Experiential
  learning, 89
Council of Senior Centers, 107
Counseling services, for caregivers,
  323, 327, 330
Crazy Quilt Society, 135
Creating for Life workshop, 132
Creative writing, 106, 117
Creativity:
  benefits of, 92, 94–96
  case illustration, 91–92
  defined, 92
  developmental phases, 95
  horticultural therapy and, 179
  importance of, 9
  information resources, 99
  levels of, 97
  potential, enhancement of, 97–98
  research studies, 93, 96
  significance of, 92–93
Creativity Discovery Corps, The, 99
Creutzfeldt-Jakob disease, 297
CTCNet, 148, 151
Cultural competency, 30, 32
Cultural diversity, 30, 32, 75
Cultural enrichment, 191–192
Cultural outings/events, 122
Custodial grandparents, 245–246
Cyber-volunteers, 51–52
CYFERnet, 212

Dance, 106, 122
Dead Quilt Society, 135
Delirium, 297
Dementia, 155, 293, 296–298, 301,
  317, 319, 324
Demographics, aging population:
  profile, 17–33
  wants, needs and interests, 34–45
Denver Botanic Garden, 187
Depression:
  access to care, 299
  in caregivers, 321

Depression *(continued)*
    causes of, 301–302
    impact of, 96, 108, 157, 159, 177,
        295, 297–298
    incidence of, 300–301
    prognosis, 300–301
    risk factors, 300, 305
    symptoms of, 298–300
    treatment of, 299–301
Depressive disorders, 303
Developmental disabilities:
    adaptive behaviors, 254–255
    case illustration, 253–254
    daily living skills, 254
    defined, 254
    demand for services, 255–258
    evaluation of integration program,
        266
    incidence of, 177
    inclusion, 258–262
    information resources, 255, 268–269
    integration models, success factors,
        262–265
    leisure experiences/skills, 255,
        261–262
    site evaluation criteria, 265–266
    support groups/service, 257, 261
Devout, defined, 355
Diabetes, 26, 155, 158–159, 300
Diabetic retinopathy, 272
Digital technology, impact of, 192–193
Digital television, 192–193
Dining out, 38
Disability:
    developmental, *see* Developmental
        disabilities
    disuse, 154
    primary prevention of, 161
Disabled elderly, 25–26
Disch, Robert, Dr., 202
Discretionary income, 35
Divorce, 22, 24, 29
Donor cultivation, 354–355
Do not resuscitate (DNR) orders, 325
DOROT, 207, 212
Drawing classes, 123

Dumont, Matthew, 184–185
Dunn, Marian E., PhD, 162
Dychtwald, Ken, 36
Dynast, defined, 355

Early boomers, defined, 108, 110
Eastern Michigan University, Institute
    for the Study of Children, Fami-
    lies and Communities, 252
Ecotourism, 37, 220
Educational attainment, 24–25, 29, 51
Educational programs, *see* Lifelong
    learning programs
    in arts, 123
    caregiving, 328–329
Educational Resources Information
    Center (ERIC), 89
Elder abuse, 234–235, 240
Eldercare, 330, 334
Elderhostel, 212
Elders Share the Arts (ESTA):
    Center for Creative Aging/Elders
        Share the Arts, 208–209, 212–213
    functions of, 119, 128–129
eMarketer, 143
Emotional state, successful aging and,
    9
Emotional support, importance of, 9
Employment opportunities, 221
Empowerment, in creativity, 94–96
Empty-nesting, 42
Encore phase, in creativity, 95
End-of-life care, 324–325
Endocrine disorders, 300
Energy healing, 166
Entrenched caregiver, 326–327
Environmental Alliance for Senior
    Involvement (EASI), 65, 67
Environmental factors, creativity, 97
Environmental modifications, sensory
    impaired:
    color contrast, 281
    environmental issues, generally, 281
    furniture, 280–281
    lighting, 280
    printing, 282

programmatic, 281–282
signs, 282
telephones, 283
Erikson, Erik, 8, 94
Ethnic music and dance, 122
Ethnic population, 21–22. *See also* Racial differences
Evergreen State Society, The, 361–362
Exercise:
  benefits of, 9–10, 37, 161
  disability prevention, 159
  importance of, 154–155
Existential ability, 78
Extended family households, 245

Faith in Actionhe Robert Wood Johnson Foundation, 345
Falls, 159
Family Caregiver Alliance, 332
Family caregivers:
  coresidents, 318
  developmental disabilities, 255, 257
  end-of-life care, 324–325
  incidence of, 316
  informal care, 318–319
  grandparents as parents, 242–246
Family crises, grandparent role in, 245
Family history kits, 191
Family volunteering, 52
Fatigue, implications of, 300
Federal Communications Commission, 234
Fee practices, 366
Fifty-Plus Fitness Association, 172
File, Karen, 355
Firman, James, 365
FirstGov, 238
Flexibility training, 161
Floor covering, safety guidelines, 283
Florida Alliance of Information and Referral Services, 234
Flower-arranging, 179
Focus groups, 43
Folk art, 113–114, 121–122
Folk Art Society of America, 129
Folk dancing, 122

Folk remedies, 166
Foot, David, 36–37
Foreign language, adult learners, 84–86
Formal volunteering, 52
Foundation Center, 362
Foundation grants, 367
Fractures, 158
Frail elderly:
  mental health needs, 295
  physical fitness and, 159, 161
Frail recluses, defined, 40
Freshman caregiver, 326
From Age-ing to Sage-ing: A Profound New Vision of Growing Older (Schacter-Shalomi/Miller), 339
Functional ability, 25, 154–155
Funding resources, 5, 365–366
Fund-raising management, 358
Furniture arrangements, safety guidelines, 283
Future trends:
  accessibility, 365
  funding resources, 365–366
  information resources, 364–365, 368–370
  outcome, 365
  self-care, 365

Gardening, *see* Horticulture
  benefits of, 37–38
  physical difficulties of, 183
  popularity of, 176
Gardner, Howard, Dr., 76
Gay population, 27, 295
Generational differences:
  baby boom generation, 29–30
  GI generation, 28–29
  impact of, 28
  silent generation, 29
Generation Connection Society (GCS), The, 213
Generations on Line, 146, 152
Generations Together, 213
Generations United, 107, 213, 252
Generation X, 109

Genius level, in creativity, 97
Gerontographics, 39–40
Gerontological Society of America, 45
Gesturing, communication strategies, 285
Get Fit-Stay Fit Challenge, 165
Giambra, Leonard, PhD, 9
GI generation, 28–29
"Giving back" phase, 94
Giving-clubs, 353
Glaucoma, 272
Goal-oriented adults, 73
Golfing, 37–38, 167
Government grants, 367
GRACE (Grass Roots Art and Community Efforts), 129
Grandchildren:
    raising, 244
    relationship with, 38, 42, 243–244
Grandparenting issues, *see* Grandparents as caregivers
Grandparents as caregivers:
    caregiving functions, 245–246, 248–249
    case illustrations, 242–243
    day care, 246
    extended family households, 245
    family crises, 245
    financial assistance, 249
    grandmother-only households, 246
    grandparenting styles, 244–245
    health concerns, 247
    information resources, 251–252
    isolation, 247–248
    legal, 248
    mental health issues, 249
    parenting demands, 247
    relationship with grandchildren, 243–244
    split-generation households, 245
    suggested activities for, 250
    support for, 249–250
Grandparents as Parents, 206
Grant funding, 367
Grantmakers in Aging, 369
Graphic design, 123

Greenhouse, 176
Grief, dealing with, 178, 301, 306, 340
Grooming routines, 39
Group work, 80

Hamilton Stores, 221
Hard of Hearing Advocates (HOHA), 287
Harvard Project Zero, 89–90
Head injury, 317
Health education programs, 259–260
Health insurance counseling services, 230
Health promotion programs:
    case illustrations, 153
    chronic disease, 155
    developmental disabilities and, 259
    importance of, 154–156, 163–166
    information resources, 171–174
    medication misuse, 156–158
    physical activity, 154–155
Health status, aging population statistics, 25–26, 75
Healthy hermits, defined, 39
Healthy indulgers, defined, 39
Healthy People 2010, 163–164
Hearing aids, 275
Hearing impairments:
    communication strategies, 284–285
    defined, 275
    hearing aids, 275
    incidence of, 26, 274–275
    isolation and, 276–277
    problems associated with, 276–77
    rehabilitation devices, 275–276
    staff training, 279, 281
    telephone modifications, 283
    treatment for, 275
Heart disease, 26, 155, 297, 301
Helping.org, 58
Herbal medicine, 166
Highmark Blue Cross Blue Shield, 165
Hiking, 64
Hip fracture, 155, 159
Hipskind, Donna Grove, 325
HIV, 28

H-Net, 195
Hobbies, 37, 183
Hockey, 165
Holiday blues, 302
Home-delivered meals, 6, 230, 366
Homeopathy, 166
Hormone disorders, 297
Horticultural Intergenerational Learning as Therapy (HILT), 206
Horticultural therapy:
characteristics of, 177–178
emotional growth, 179
intellectual benefits, 178
physical benefits, 179–180
social benefits, 179
Horticulture:
adaptations, 182–183
case illustration, 175–176
community gardens, 183–185
defined, 176
implementation suggestions, 180
information resources, 186–188
suggested activities, 180–182
therapy, *see* Horticultural therapy
Hospital admissions, 157
Humanities:
case illustration, 189–190
cultural sites, 191
digital technology, impact of,
192–193
historical sites, 191
information resources, 194–197
overview, 190–192
suggested activities, 193
Humor, in adult learning programs,
81
Huntington's disease, 297
Hypertension, 26, 155, 158, 160
Hypothermia, 159

I&R specialists, role of, 230–231. *See
also* Information and referral (I&
R) programs
Incarceration, 245
Income levels, 23
Incontinence, 317

Independent Sector, 59, 352, 354–355,
362
Indiana University Center on Philanthropy, 362
Infection, long-term, 297
Info Line, 238–239
Information and referral (I&R)
programs:
assistance requests, 231
caregiving, 329
case illustration, 227–229
eligibility for, 230
enhanced, 232
functions of, 229–231
information resources, 237–241, 236
on-line support groups, 235
outcomes, 231–232
publicizing strategies, 232–233
regular, 232
resource accessibility, 231
Sentinel Project, 234–235
structure of, 233–234
suggested activities, 236
Innovation level, in creativity, 97
Intellectual disabilities, 258–261
Interfaith Caregivers Alliance, 332–333
Intergeneration Day, 214
Intergenerational Entrepreneurship
Demonstration Project: Howe-to
Industries, 209
Intergenerational Innovations, 214
Intergenerational programs:
benefits of, 200–202
case illustration, 198–199
evaluation of, 204
implementation of, 202–204
information resources, 211–218
mentors, 205
model programs, 205–210
need for, 199–200
success factors, generally, 203–204
Intergenerational Shared Site (IGSS)
programs, 204
International Association for the Scientific Study of Intellectual Disabilities, 258

International Association for Volunteer Effort (IAVE), 59
International Association of Physical Activity, Aging and Sports (IAPAAS), 172
International Quilt Study Center, The, 129–130
International Society for the Performing Arts Foundation (ISPA), 129
Internet:
  funding resources, 367
  on-line support groups, 235
  philanthropy information resource, 358
  travel information, 221
Interpersonal intelligence, 77
Intrapersonal intelligence, 76–77
Inventive level, in creativity, 97
Investor, defined, 355
Iowa State University Extension, 213–214

Jazz performances, 110, 112
John Carter Brown Library, The, 194
John D. and Catherine T. MacArthur Foundation, 8–9
Join Hands Day, 57
Journal of Music Therapy, 125
Journal of Religious Gerontology, The, 345–346

Kaiser Permanente's Educational Theater Programs, 130
Keepers of the Treasures—Cultural Council of American Indians, Alaska Natives and Native Hawaiians, 120, 130
Kinship training, 252
Koop, Surgeon General C. Everett, 166
Korrnet, 146
Kotulak, Ronald, 10

Landscaping, 179
Language learning, intergenerational, 206

Large-print type, 282
Last Acts, 333
Late boomers, defined, 109
Late-life creativity, 93. *See also* Creativity
Late-life depression, symptoms of, 299
Leadership giving programs, 353
Leisure activities, survey of, 38
Leisure market, 37
Lesbian population, 27
Lewy body disease, 297
Liberation phase, in creativity, 95
Life expectancy, implications of, 26–27, 243, 256
Lifelong learning programs:
  attrition, 78–79
  barriers to learning, 75, 78
  benefits of, 37, 86–87
  case illustration, 69–70
  computer opportunities, 146–147
  digital technology, 192–193
  information resources, 89–90
  learning styles, 75–79
  literacy and, 82–84
  motivation, 79
  multiple intelligences, 75–79
  older adult learners, interests of, 70–72
  older language learner, 84–86
  principles of adult learning and education, 72–75
  reinforcement, 79–80, 82
  retention, 80
  suggested activities, 87–88
  support system, 74, 80–82
  transference, 80
  women in, 82
  workshops, 71
Lifelong working, 86–87
Lifestyle, generally:
  needs, 42
  sedentary, 154, 159
  trends, 65
Lighthouse International, 288
Lighthouse National Survey on Vision Loss, 272

Lighting, safety guidelines, 280
Lindeman, Eduard, 72
Linguistic competence, 31
Linguistic intelligence, 76, 78
LinkAge 2000, 214
Lipreading, 275
Literacy skills, 82–84
Living arrangements:
  aging population statistics, 22–23
  caregivers, 319–320
Liz Lerman Dance Exchange, 130–131
Logical-mathematical intelligence, 76, 78
Loneliness, 295–296
Long-distance care, 315–316
Long-term care, 318, 322

Macular degeneration, 272
Major depression, 292
Major depressive disorder, 298. *See also* Depression
Make a Difference Day, 57
Managed care, 366
Mannsman's Gallery, 98
Marital status, 22
Marketing strategies, 41–43
Martin Luther King Day, 57
Massage, 166
Masters Race, 153–154, 167
Matter of the Heart and Mind grief workshop, 341
Mature America in the 1990s, 70
Meaning of Adult Education, The (Lindeman), 72
Media arts, 123
Media Metrix, 144
Medicaid, 366
Medicare, 157, 366
Medication, generally:
  misuse, 156–158
  workshops, 158, 169
Megavitamins, 166
Memoirs, 342
Memory function, aging process, 10
Memory loss, 300–301, 306
Mental disorders:

caregivers, 294
case illustration, 290–292
dementia, 293, 296–298
depression, 298–302
development/etiology, 294–296
diagnosis, 292, 297
incidence of, 292–293
information resources, 307–311
psychological intervention, 292
senior support services, 305–306
substance abuse, 302–304
suicide, 305
treatment of, 292
types of, 292
Mental health, *see* Mental disorders
aging process and, 292–293
loneliness, impact of, 295–296
public education programs, 296
senior support services, 305–306
service delivery, 293
suggested activities, 306
support, importance of, 295
Mental illness, 177, 245
Mental retardation, *see* Developmental disabilities
Mental training, 10
Mentoring, 56, 117, 201, 205, 263
Mid Atlantic Arts Foundation, 132
Mid-America Arts Alliance, 131
Middle age, 96
Midlife crisis, 96
Mill Street Loft, 131
Miller, Ronald S., 339
Mineta, Norman, 145
Mission statements, 31
Mobility impairment, 259
Mobility instructors, 280
Modeling, 263
Modern adult learning theory, 72
Modern Maturity, 38, 70, 162, 220
Moody, Rick, Dr., 202
Motor skills, 177
Mourning process, 341. *See also* Bereavement; Grief
Muscle-strengthening exercise, 159, 161

Museum(s):
attendance statistics, 191
cooperative programs, 222
Museum One, Inc., 119–120, 131–132
Music, enjoyment of, 106. *See also* Musi-
cal activities; Musical intelligence;
Musical theater
Music therapy, 114–115
Musical activities, 122
Musical intelligence, 77
Musical theater, 109–110
Myocardial infarction, 160
Myths and Realities of Aging 2000, 154

National Adult Literacy Survey, 83
National Aging I&R Support Center
(NIRSC), 229, 239–240
National Aging Information Center
(NAIC), 239
National Alliance for Caregiving, 315,
332–333
National Alliance for the Mentally Ill,
308–309
National Assembly of State Arts Agen-
cies (NASAA), 132
National Association for Music Ther-
apy, 125
National Association of Area Agencies
on Aging (N4A), 13, 239, 333
National Association of Professional
Geriatric Care Managers, 332–334
National Association of State Units on
Aging (NASUA), 229, 239
National Center for Charitable Statis-
tics, 52, 362–363
National Center for Complementary
and Alternative Medicine,
172–173
National Center for Nonprofit Boards
(NCNB), 59, 363
National Center on Elder Abuse, 240
National Committee on Planned Giv-
ing, 363
National Council for the Traditional
Arts, 132–133
National Council on Aging (NCOA):

/AARP (NAC/AARP), caregiving re-
search, 316, 318
on the arts, 107–108
Health Promotion Institute, 165
as information resource, generally,
12, 165, 172, 195, 365
Myths and Realities of Aging 2000, 154
National Interfaith Coalition on
Aging (NICA), 339, 346
National Institute of Senior Centers
(NISC), 5, 364
National Survey of Health and Sup-
portive Services, 7, 365
National Depressive and Manic De-
pressive Association, 309
National Endowment for the Arts
(NEA), 107, 118, 121, 133
National Endowment for the Humanit-
ies (NEH), 107, 190–193,
195–196
National Eye Institute Information
Center, 288
National Family Caregiver Support Pro-
gram (NFCSP), 315
National Federation of Interfaith Vol-
unteer Caregivers, 346
National Federation of the Blind, 288
National Foundation for Depressive Ill-
ness, Inc., 309
National Gardening Association,
187–188
National Health Interview Survey, 25
National Hospice and Palliative Care
Organization, The, 334
National Humanities Institute, 196
National Institute for Literacy, 90
National Institute of Mental Health
(NIMH), 309–310
National Institute of Senior Centers,
12
National Institute on Aging (NIA), 240
National Institute on Alcohol Abuse
and Alcoholism (NIAAA), 309
National Institute on Deafness and
other Communication Disorders,
288

National Institute on Disability and Rehabilitation Research, 268
National Institute on Senior Centers, 43
National Institutes of Health, 173–174
National Library Service for the Blind and Physically Handicapped, 288–289
National Mental Health Association (NMHA), 310
National Quilting Association, Inc., 133
National Recreation and Parks Association, 68
National Rehabilitation Information Center (NARIC), 268
National Resource Center for Rural Elderly, 310
National Senior Games Association, 167, 173
National Senior Softball League, 167
National Society of Fundraising Executives, 357
National Survey on Drug Abuse, 304
National Therapeutic Recreation Society, 261, 269
Naturalistic intelligence, defined, 77–78
Networking, recreational activities and, 66
Newberry Library, 196
New England Foundation for the Arts (NEFA), 133
New York Public Library, 197
New York State Intergenerational Network (NYSIgN), 214–215
Nonprofit Resource Center, 363
Normal aging, 155
Normal physical activity, 154
North Carolina Arts Council, 119, 133–134
North Carolina Center for Creative Retirement (NCCCR), 134
Nurses, functions of, 177
Nursing home admissions, 296
Nutrition:
    importance of, 10
    physical fitness and, 160

Oasis Institute, 40
Obesity, 155, 256, 259
Obsessive-compulsive behavior, 292
Occupational therapists, functions of, 177, 280
Older adult needs:
    identification of, 35, 40–41
    market strategies, 41–43
Older Americans 2000: Key Indicators of Well-Being, 63
Older Americans Act, 5–6
Omohundro Institute of Early American History and Culture, 197
Oral hygiene, 259
Oriental medicine, 166
Orientation instructors, 280
Orthopedic impairments, 26
Osteoarthritis, 155
Osteoporosis, 155, 157, 159
Outreach programs, caregiving, 329
Over-the-counter medications, 156–157

PACE (People with Arthritis Can Exercise), 156
Pain management, 179
Painting, 106, 123
Palliative care, 325
Parental abuse/neglect, 243, 248
Parkinson's disease, 300–301, 317
Partner gap, 162
Partners Project, 264
Partnerships:
    as funding resource, 367
    recreational activities, 66
Patient education, 305–306
Peer support programs, 56
Penn Hills Senior Center, 167, 173
Penn State Cooperative Extension and Outreach: Generation Celebration, 209
Pennsylvania Association of Senior Centers, 369
Pennsylvania Senior Centers, 364

Pennsylvania Senior Environment
Corps, 65–66
Pennsylvania Spelling Championship
for Older Adults, 91
Pennsylvania State University, 215
Pension plans, 23
People Plant Council, 188
Performing arts, 112–113
Personal health issues, 37–39
Pew Internet, 144
Pharmacokinetics, 302
Philadelphia Senior Learning Center,
145–146
Philanthropy:
baby boomers, 356–357
bequests, 353–354, 366
case illustration, 351–352
diversity and, 357–358
donor base, 353
donor characteristics, generally, 52,
94–95
donor cultivation, 354–355, 366
fund-raising management, 358
gifts, types of, 352–354
information resources, 360–363
planned gifts, 353–354
suggested activities, 358–359
women in, 356
Photography, 123
Physical activity:
categories of, 154
decline in, 154
importance of, 9–10
suggested activities, 169
Physical fitness:
health benefits, 162–163
importance of, 158–162
information resources, 171–174
sexuality and, 162–163
sports and, 167–168
Physical therapists, functions of, 177
Pick's disease, 297
Pictograms, 285–286
Pioneer Network, 369
Planned gift programs, 353–354
Poetry Society of America, 134

Poets & Writers, 134
Points of Light Foundation, The, 57,
59
Population statistics, *see* Demographics,
aging population
Positive Adults Taking Health Seri-
ously (PATHS), 165
Positive aging experiences:
creativity, 91–99
lifelong learning, 69–90
recreation, 60–68
volunteerism, 49–59
Positive mental attitude, 9
Pottery, 123
Poverty, 23–24, 246
Prescription drug abuse, 304
*Presence of the Past: Popular Uses of His-
tory in American Life, The,* 191
Preventive health care, 328
Prevocational training, 178
Primitive/intuitive expression, 97
Prince, Russ, 355
Problem-solving ability, 10
Productivity, in aging population, 8
Progressives, defined, 108
Project EASE (Exploring Aging
through Shared Experiences),
206
Project GUIDE (Growth and Under-
standing of Intergenerational Pro-
gramming through Distance
Education), 206–207
Prospect Research Page, The, 363
Pseudodementia, 301
Psychotherapy, 299
Public libraries, 191
Public offenders, 177
Public policy:
on arts, 107–108
faith-based organizations, 339
health promotion programs, 165
Public television, 192

Quality of life, 107, 162, 261, 277, 303,
325
Quicksilver, 127

Quilt Heritage Foundation, 134–135
Quilting, 114–116, 129–130, 133–135
Quilt Rescue Squad, 135
Quilt Restoration Conference, 135

Racial differences:
  aging population, 6
  caregiving, 319
  educational attainment, 25
  health status, 26
  life expectancy, 26
  mental retardation in, 255–256
  philanthropy, 357–358
  population statistics, 21–23
  socioeconomic status, 24
  spirituality, 340–341
  substance abuse, 303
Radio programs, 192
Ready or Not, 113
Recreational activities:
  benefits of, 63
  case illustration, 60–62
  importance of, 62–64
  information resources, 67–68
  outdoor recreation, 64–66
  physical fitness and, 160
  suggested activities, 66–67
  types of, 37–38
Recreation therapists, functions of, 177
Reevaluation phase, in creativity, 95
Rehabilitation, impact of, 160
Rehabilitation counselors, 280
Rehabilitation Research and Training
  Center on Aging with Mental Re-
  tardation, 269
Rehabilitation specialists, functions of,
  177
Relevancy-oriented adults, 73
Religion, importance of, 336–337,
  339–340. *See also* Spirituality
"Remembering Old New York" Project,
  intergenerational, 206
Reminiscence, 342
Repayer, defined, 355
Research network, 9
Resistance exercises, 164

Resource Directory for Older People,
  2340–241
Response time, 74
Retirement income, 23
Retirement Research Foundation,
  369–370
Retirement years, changes in, 7, 42, 96
Risk-taking activities, 96
Roaring '20s, defined, 108
Rock climbing, 65

Sabbaticals, 37
Sage-ing Center movement, 339
Sarcopenia, 159
SASE: The Write Place, 135
Schacter-Shalomi, Zalman, 339
Schizophrenia, 292–294
Schomburg Center for Research in
  Black Culture, 197
Scuba diving, 65
Sculpture, 123
Seattle Longitudinal Study, 10–11
Secondary caregivers, 319
Sedentary lifestyle, 154, 159
Self-awareness, 338
Self-care, 166, 342, 365
Self-control, 178
Self-directed learning, 56, 73
Self-discovery learning techniques, 80
Self-esteem, 177, 201, 205
Self-expression, 106, 179
Self-Help Clearinghouse, 173, 235
Self-help groups, 166, 306
Self-worth, 106
Senior Adult Theater Program, 135
Senior Arts, 120, 135–136
*Senior Center Self-Assessment and National
  Accreditation Manual,* 7
Senior centers, generally:
  accreditation, 7
  defined, 5
  focal points of, 6–7
  funding, 5, 353, 365
  population statistics, 5–6
  social activities, 3–5
Senior.com, 152

SeniorNet, 143, 145
Seniornet.com, 152
Senior Softball World Series, 167
Senior Support Services, 306
Sensory impairments:
  case illustration, 270–271
  communication strategies, 283–286
  developmental disability and, 259
  environmental modifications,
    280–283
  hearing impairments, 274–277
  information resources, 287–289
  participation in senior centers, im-
    portance of, 277–280
  suggested activities, 286
  visual impairments, 271–274
Sensory perceptions, 178
Seven Faces of Philanthropy, The (Prince/
    File), 355
Sexual orientation, 27–28
Sexuality:
  developmental disabilities and, 259
  influences on, 162–163
  mental disorders and, 295
Shepherd's Centers of America, 346
Silent generation, 29
Simonton, Dean Keith, PhD, 94
Sinusitis, 26
Sleep disturbance, implications of,
    298, 300
Social activities, sample of, 3–5, 17–20
Socialites, defined, 355
Socially disadvantaged, 177
Social relationships, 79
Social Security, 23, 257
Social services programs, 229. *See also*
    Information and referral
    programs
Social support network, 299
Social support programs, development
    of, 9
Social support system, importance of,
    8–9
Social welfare, 79
Society for Accessible Travel & Hospi-
    tality (SATH), 223

Socioeconomic status, 23–24, 35–36,
    111
Softball, 167
Somatic disorders, 301
Southeast Florida Center on Aging,
    136
Southern Arts Federation, 136
Spatial intelligence, 76
Special needs population:
  caregiving, 312–334
  developmental disabilities, 253–269
  grandparenting issues, 242–252
  information and referral programs,
    227–241
  mental health, 290–311
  sensory impairments, 270–289
  spirituality and aging, 335–347
Speech-reading, 275
Spellbinders, 209, 215
Spiritual Eldering Institute, 338–339
Spirituality:
  case illustration, 335–336
  cultural traditions, 340–341
  information resources, 343–347
  life-changing events, 338
  significance of, 336–337, 339–340
  spiritual development, 337–338,
    341–342
  spiritual-wellness skills, 337
  strength of, 338
  spiritual well-being, 339
Split-generation households, 245
Sports-related injuries, 155, 167
Staff training/development programs,
    31
Stagebridge Theater, The, 136–137
Stairways, safety guidelines, 283
Stanford Geriatric Education Center,
    33
Storytelling, 94–95, 123
Strategic alliances, 367
Strength training, 159, 161
Stress management, 178
Stroke, 26, 155, 272, 301, 317
Strom Thurmond Institute of Govern-
    ment and Public Affairs, Retire-

ment and Intergenerational
  Studies Laboratory, 215–216
Substance abuse:
  alcoholism, 303–304
  causes of, generally, 302–303
  impact of, 96, 177, 245, 248, 298
  incidence of, 302–304
  prescription drug abuse, 304
  self-medication, 303
  treatment of, 304
Substance Abuse and Mental Health
  Services Administration (SAM-
  HSA), 310–311
Substance abuse disorders, 301
Successful aging, 8–11, 259
Successful Aging (Rowe/Kahn), 8
Suicide, 305
"Summing-up" phase, in creativity,
  94–95
Supply and demand economics, 36–37
Support groups:
  for caregivers, 323, 330
  developmental disabilities, 257
  horticultural therapy, 182
  on-line, 235–236
  self-help, 286
Support networks, importance of, 201,
  306. *See also* Social support
Survey of Family Caregivers in New
  York City, 322–323

TDD (Telecommunication Device for
  the Deaf), 283
Telephone(s):
  for hearing impaired, 283
  reassurance programs, 6
Temple University, Center for Inter-
  generational Learning, 216
Terrariums, 176
Texas Agricultural Extension Service:
  Youth Exchanging with Seniors
  (YES), 210
Texas I&R Network, 234
Texas Tech University, College of
  Home Economics, 216
Theater, 106, 122–123

Theatrical groups, 112–113
Theatrical plays, 110
Thought process, 93–94
Time management, 178
Traditions, preservation of, 202
Transgender persons, 27
Travel:
  arboreta, 183
  benefits of, generally, 37–38
  botanical gardens, 183
  case illustration, 219–220
  cultural sites, 191
  field trips, 183, 222
  frequency of, 220–221
  historical sites, 191
  information resources, 223
  internet, as information resource,
    221
  popularity of, 220
  suggested activities, 222
  types of, 220–221
Tribal Preservation Program, 137
211 designation, information and referral program, 234
2-1-1.org, 241

Unconditional love, 201
UN International Plan of Action on
  Aging, 260
Union Theological Seminary and Pres-
  byterian School of Christian Edu-
  cation, 347
United Hospital Fund, 323
U.S. Administration on Aging:
  functions of, 12, 107, 240, 264, 334
  Region VIII, 216
U.S. Census Bureau, 33
U.S. Department of Health and Hu-
  man Services, 172–174
U.S. Preventive Services Task Force,
  161
United Statewide Community Arts As-
  sociation (USCAA), 137
United Way of America, 234
United Way of Atlanta, Georgia, 234
United Way of Connecticut, 234

University of Maryland, Adult Health and Development Program (AHDP), 216–217
University of Massachusetts, Division of Continuing Education, 137
University of Minnesota Extension Service: Elder's Wisdom, Children's Song: Community Celebration of Place, 210, 217
University of Southern California, Intergenerational Health Research Team, 217
University of Wisconsin-Extension, 252

Vascular dementia, 297
Veterans' benefits, 230
Vintage, programs provided by, *see specific case illustrations*
Violence, 179
Vision rehabilitation, 273–274
Visiting Nurse Service, 323
Visual arts, 123
Visual impairments:
    adaptation to, 274
    assessment of, 272–273
    communication strategies, 283–284
    defined, 271
    degree of, 272
    fear of, 274
    impact of, generally, 155
    incidence of, 271
    medical care for, 273
    rehabilitation services, 273–274
    risk for, 271–272
    staff training, 279–281
Vitamin/mineral imbalance, 300
Vocational training, 178
Volunteer Center National Network, Seasons of Service Opportunities, 57
Volunteerism, *see* Volunteers
    benefits of, 53–54, 94
    case illustration, 49–50
    information resources, 58–59
    encouragement of, 50
    statistics, 50–53

suggested activities, 57
summing-up phase, 95
volunteer management, 54–57
Volunteers:
    benefits of, 367
    horticulture therapy, 177
VSA Arts, 137

Walking, benefits of, 37, 64, 155, 159
Washington Business Group on Health (WBGH), 334
Weatherization programs, 230
Web sites, interactive, 192. *See also* Internet
Weight loss, implications of, 300
Weight training, 161, 164
Well-being, influential factors, 25, 63, 92, 159, 258, 337, 339
Wellness Works, 165
Wellsource, Inc., 174
Western Folklife Center, 138
Western Pennsylvania Hospital, 164–165
Western States Art Federation, 138
West Penn-Vintage Community Care for Seniors, 164, 174
White House Conference on Aging, 29, 107–108, 339
White-water rafting trips, 65
Widowhood, 22, 42, 301
Wisdom, 106, 201
Withdrawal, social, 96
Women:
    as caregivers, 316, 318–319, 323
    grandmother-only homes, 246
    with intellectual disabilities, 261
    in learning programs, 82
    with mental retardation, 256–257
    in philanthropy, 356
    postmenopausal athletes, 160–161
    spirituality in, 340
Worchester State College, Intergeneration Urban Institute, 217–218
Word processing training, 147
Work-choice patterns, 87
Work ethic, 28–29

Workforce Investment Act (1998), 83
Work-leave programs, 37
Workshops:
  arts, 117, 122
  grief, 341
  health promotion, 158, 169
  lifelong learning programs, 71
  spirituality development, 342
World Health Organization, 163, 258
World War II, 108, 111
World War II Veterans Project, intergenerational, 206

Worry, dealing with, 178
Writer-to-writer mentorships, 117

YMCA, 165
Young at Heart, 164–165
Younger older adults, 43–44
Young-old population, 35–36

Zoos, trips to, 222